Physiology of Spinal Anesthesia

FOURTH EDITION

Physiology of Spinal Anesthesia

FOURTH EDITION

NICHOLAS M. GREENE, M.D., M.A.,
F.R.C.Anaesth.

Professor of Anesthesiology, Emeritus
Yale University School of Medicine
New Haven, Connecticut

SORIN J. BRULL, M.D.

Assistant Professor of Anesthesiology
Yale University School of Medicine
New Haven, Connecticut

With a Foreword by the late
JOHN GILLIES, C.V.O., M.C., F.R.C.P.E., F.R.C.S.E.,
F.F.A.R.C.S.
James Y. Simpson Reader in Anaesthetics
University of Edinburgh
Edinburgh, Scotland

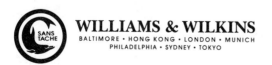

WILLIAMS & WILKINS
BALTIMORE · HONG KONG · LONDON · MUNICH
PHILADELPHIA · SYDNEY · TOKYO

Editor: Timothy H. Grayson
Project Manager: Marjorie Kidd Keating
Copy Editor: Joseph Pomerance
Designer: Norman W. Och
Illustration Planner: Lorraine Wrzosek
Cover Designer: Norman W. Och

Printed in the United States of America

First Edition, 1958
Second Edition, 1969
Third Edition, 1981

Library of Congress Cataloging in Publication Data

Greene, Nicholas M., 1922–
    Physiology of spinal anesthesia / Nicholas M. Greene, Sorin J.
Brull ; with a foreword by the late John Gillies. — 4th ed.
        p.   cm.
    Includes bibliographical references and index.
    ISBN 0-683-3555-X
    1. Spinal anesthesia—Physiological effect.   2. Anesthetics—
Pathophysiology.   I. Brull, Sorin J.   II. Title.
    [DNLM: 1. Anesthesia, Spinal.   WO 305 G811p]
RD85.S7G7   1993
617.9′64—dc20
DNLM/DLC
for Library of Congress   92-5578
                                                                    CIP

                                              92 93 94 95 96
                            1   2   3   4   5   6   7   8   9 10

FOREWORD
To The First Edition

It is gratifying to observe in the present generation of specialists in anaesthesia an increasing urge to found their practice on rational study and pertinent knowledge of the basic sciences, particularly physiology and pharmacology. In consequence of this somewhat overdue trend clinical empiricism and impressionism must surely cease to determine fashions in anaesthetic procedure although emancipation from such thralldom is still around the corner and may remain there awhile.

A new outlook is now imperative since the complexity of modern methods and management of the pharmacologically stricken patient involve the anaesthetist in an acute responsibility which is not exceeded in any other field of medicine.

Appreciating the urgent need for a full review and assessment of the extensive physiological trespass that frequently may be associated with spinal anaesthesia Dr. Greene has successfully contrived to present not merely a narrative but a comprehensive and definitive appraisal of the considerable volume of research that has so far been done in this recurrently controversial subject.

A foreword is not an essential part of any book but in appropriate circumstances it provides an acceptable opportunity to commend the scholarship and industry of the author. In the present instance, having been privileged to see Dr. Greene's book in the making I can proffer such commendation unreservedly and with the assurance that he has made a notable contribution to the literature of his specialty.

John Gillies
Edinburgh, 1958

v

PREFACE
To The Fourth Edition

Spinal anesthesia remains one of the basic techniques in the arsenal of the modern anesthesiologist despite the waxing and waning of its popularity over the 90 years since its introduction into clinical practice. We have now had more clinical experience with spinal anesthesia than we have had with any other anesthetic technique in use today. The primary reason for the continuation of spinal anesthesia as an integral part of anesthetic practice, and, in fact, a reason for its renaissance in recent years, is the realization that spinal anesthesia has a unique potential to provide anesthesia with a combination of, on the one hand, a low degree of what Dr. John Gillies referred to as physiologic trespass, with, on the other hand, profound degrees of sensory denervation and muscle relaxation.

The combination of anesthesia, muscle relaxation, and minimal physiologic trespass means that spinal anesthesia has the potential for being a uniquely safe anesthetic technique. Safety of spinal anesthesia is of a dual nature: pharmacologic and physiologic. The availability today of local anesthetics demonstrably free of neurologic side effects means that the neurologic safety of spinal anesthesia is no longer an issue. Not so with physiological and, thus, with clinical safety of spinal anesthesia, neither of which have been quantified.

Our inability to quantify the safety of spinal anesthesia is due in large part to the unfortunate but real fact that clinical experience alone is unreliable as a basis for judging clinical safety when dealing with a field as filled with uncontrollable variables as is clinical anesthesia. The hazards and the Byzantine complexities of demonstrating safety on the basis of epidemiologic studies of outcome are so great that we are left with but little choice except to fall back on understanding, as best we can, the physiologic changes wrought by spinal anesthesia as a gauge, however flawed, of the safety of spinal anesthesia. A clear differentiation must be made in this regard between physiologic changes and "physiologic trespass." Changes in physiologic function do not necessarily represent

vii

physiologic trespass. Changes in function represent real or potential trespass only when of such magnitude that they become dangerous. Changes associated with exercise, for example, represent normal physiologic responses to increased metabolic demand. They represent physiologic trespass only if they become so extreme as to endanger otherwise healthy individuals or when, with lesser levels of exercise, the changes occur in individuals with preexisting physiologic limitations due to disease. Similarly, decreases in blood pressure during spinal anesthesia do not necessarily represent physiologic trespass. They become trespass only when severe in normal individuals or when, with lesser decreases, they occur in patients with preexisting physiologic limitations.

The safety of spinal anesthesia rests upon understanding both the causes of physiologic responses, and the technique and effects of these responses on organ function in health and disease. The purpose of *Physiology of Spinal Anesthesia* is to examine, in detail, causes and effects of physiologic changes produced by the subarachnoid injection of local anesthetics. Techniques of spinal anesthesia, that is, how and where to inject the local anesthetic and the clinical indications and contraindications to do so, are not considered. Pharmacologic aspects of spinal anesthesia are considered only insofar as they relate to physiologic responses. Mode of action of local anesthetics, a pharmacologic, not physiologic topic, is not reviewed in depth. Factors that govern distribution of local anesthetics within cerebrospinal fluid, and thus sensory levels of anesthesia, involve complexities beyond the scope of this monograph. Similarly, the pharmacokinetics of uptake of local anesthetics into tissues within the subarachnoid space are considered only to define which neuronal structures are affected thereby defining the basis of physiologic responses. The pharmacokinetics of elimination of local anesthetics from cerebrospinal fluid, though clinically important because they dictate duration of anesthesia, are also not considered.

Readers will observe the curious but lamentable fact that our knowledge of the physiologic changes associated with spinal anesthesia is in many instances surprisingly and substantially below our level of understanding of physiologic changes associated with general anesthesia. This is most apparent in the paucity of information one would expect on the cardiovascular effects of spinal anesthesia in view of the extensive data so widely reported in such exquisite detail on the effects of general anesthesia on minute cardiovascular functions. It is to be hoped that eventually those who have available such techniques and know how to use them will apply them to patients having regional, including spinal, anesthesia. We know just about everything we need to know about all the parameters of subendocardial blood flow, myocardial biomechanics, and myocardial oxygenation in patients with coronary arterial insufficiency having opioid-nitrous oxide anesthesia for coronary arterial bypass surgery. We know little about the same patient having spinal anesthesia for urethral prostatic resection. We must rely, therefore, on articles, even those from the paleoanesthetic literature, to fill in gaps in our knowledge as best we can. This is one reason that readers will find this monograph to be so rich in citations of literature often decades old. No apologies need be offered for doing so. The older literature is cited because those are the only references available, and not just in cardiovascular areas. Exposure to some of this older literature also has the fringe benefit of broadening one's perspective of the historic foundations of our specialty.

Physiologic responses to epidural and other forms of regional anesthesia are intentionally not reviewed in depth in this monograph. Epidural and spinal anesthesia are indeed related to each other, but only to the same extent as cousins or, at best, siblings; monozygotic twins they are not. However, because of the well-deserved popularity of epidural anesthesia, and because there are indeed several noteworthy similarities to spinal anesthesia, a chapter on epidural anesthesia is included that briefly compares physiologic responses to spinal anesthesia and physiologic responses to epidural anesthesia. The chapter on epidural anesthesia is not designed to provide a complete review of the physiology of epidural anesthesia, a mission ably accomplished by others elsewhere.

Finally, the subject of this monograph is spinal *anesthesia*, emphasis on *anesthesia*. Local anesthetics produce local anesthesia. Anesthesia is loss of sensation, all types of sensation, which is why lidocaine, bupivacaine, et al., are called local *anesthetics*. They are not called local analgesics; they produce anesthesia, not analgesia. Analgesia is a state characterized by alteration in perception of an otherwise painful stimulus, not loss of all tactile sense. Spinal anesthesia, not spinal analgesia, is our topic. We will not deal with physiologic responses, or any other responses, to the intrathecal injection of opioids or other analgesics, which do indeed produce spinal analgesia, but with physiologic consequences so different from physiologic consequences of spinal anesthesia as to constitute a totally different subject. If omission of consideration of responses to intrathecal injection of opioids in a treatise on the physiology of spinal anesthesia is a sin, it is a sin of commission, not omission.

Nicholas M. Greene
Sorin J. Brull

CONTENTS

CHAPTER 1

The Central Nervous System

Spinal anesthesia may be defined as the temporary interruption of transmission of nerve impulses produced by the injection of a local anesthetic into the subarachnoid space. The physiologic effects of spinal anesthesia are entirely dependent on the action of the local anesthetic on nerve tissue within the subarachnoid space. Local anesthetics injected into the lumbar subarachnoid space do not result in concentrations of local anesthetic in cisternal and much less in ventricular cerebrospinal fluid (CSF) adequate to have intracranial effects (p. 61). Similarly, unlike the case with epidural anesthesia (Chapter 10), the amounts of local anesthetics used for spinal anesthesia are so low and rate of their vascular absorption from the spinal subarachnoid space is so slow that peripheral plasma concentrations of local anesthetics (Howarth, 1949; Giasi, *et al.*, 1979) and their metabolites (Helrich, *et al.*, 1950) are too low to have any pharmacologic and, therefore, any physiologic effects. The peak levels of lidocaine in venous plasma after subarachnoid injection of 75 mg average only $0.32 \pm 0.07 \ \mu g \cdot ml^{-1}$ (Giasi, *et al.*, 1979) while following IM injection of the same amount (75 mg), peak plasma lidocaine concentration was nearly double ($0.80 \ \mu g \cdot ml^{-1}$) (Orr, *et al.*, 1986). Subarachnoid injection of 15 mg of bupivacaine is associated with no detectable plasma levels (Meyer and Nolte, 1978).

All physiologic responses to spinal anesthesia being brought about by actions of local anesthetics within the subarachnoid space, it is appropriate to consider in detail the nature and sites at which spinal anesthesia produces its effects on both nerve fibers crossing the subarachnoid space and the spinal cord itself.

Effects of local anesthetics on the central nervous system are brought about by their uptake into subarachnoid neural structures. The where, why, and how of this uptake are a necessary prelude to consideration of the effects on neuronal function produced by such uptake. Other pharmacokinetic aspects of local anesthetics injected into the subarachnoid space, including distribution within, and elimination from, CSF, clinically important though they are, are too complex for consideration in a book devoted to physiologic, not pharmacologic or pharmacokinetic aspects of spinal anesthesia.

Uptake

One of the more important factors contributing to where local anesthetics are taken up into nerve tissue from cerebrospinal fluid (Table 1.1) is accessibility of nerve tissue to the anesthetic.

1. *Accessibility* involves the proximity of a potential neuronal site of local anesthetic uptake to CSF. Uptake of local anesthetics into nerve roots as they traverse the subarachnoid space, bathed on all surfaces by spinal fluid containing local anesthetics, is greater than uptake into neural elements located within the substance of the cord simply because of greater accessibility. Uptake of local anesthetics into the cord itself does, however, occur. It occurs on the pia-covered surface of the cord. It occurs at sites beneath the surface of the cord through invaginations of the subarachnoid space accompanying vascular structures penetrating into the cord, the spaces of Virchow-Robin (Fig. 1.1)..

2. *Concentration* of local anesthetics in cerebrospinal fluid also determines the site of their uptake, especially into neuronal tissues within the substance of the cord. High concentrations of local anesthetic in spinal fluid compensate in part for the decreased accessibility of intracordal structures by increasing the concentration gradient down which local anesthetics move by simple diffusion.

Concentration of local anesthetics in CSF is determined by uptake into tissues within the subarachnoid space, by movement away from the site of injection, by volume of the subarachnoid space, and by elimination of local anesthetic from the subarachnoid space. The concentration of local

---

Table 1.1.
Determinants of Site of Subarachnoid Uptake of Local Anesthetics Injected into Cerebrospinal Fluid

---

Accessibility of potential sites of uptake

Concentration of local anesthetic in CSF
- Tissue uptake
- Movement from injection site
- Volume of CSF
- Elimination from CSF

Diffusion of local anesthetic
- Concentration gradient
- Time from injection into CSF
- Molecular weight
- Molecular configuration
- Tissue barriers

Lipid content of tissues

Lipid solubility of local anesthetic

pKa of local anesthetic

Blood flow to sites of uptake

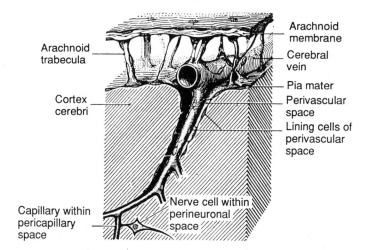

Arachnoid membrane

Arachnoid trabecula

Cerebral vein

Pia mater

Cortex cerebri

Perivascular space

Lining cells of perivascular space

Capillary within pericapillary space

Nerve cell within perineuronal space

Figure 1.1. Spaces of Virchow-Robin. (Reproduced with permission from Strong, O.S., and Elwyn A., *Human Neuroanatomy*. First Edition. Baltimore: Williams & Wilkins Co., 1943).

anesthetic in (CSF at the site of injection decreases sharply immediately following injection (Fig. 1.2) as shown for procaine by Koster, *et al.*, (1936). Similar curves have also been described for procaine by Küstner and Eissner (1930), for lidocaine by Mörch, *et al.*, (1957), and for bupivacaine by Meyer and Nolte (1978). The rapid decrease in concentration at the site of injection within the first few minutes after intrathecal injection is due to a combination of spread of the local anesthetic away from the site of injection and absorption of the anesthetic into tissues within the subarachnoid space (Lipschitz, *et al.*, 1953). A later, more gradual decrease in concentration is mainly a reflection of removal of the anesthetic from the subarachnoid space by vascular absorption from the subarachnoid space and, pharmacokinetically probably more important, by vascular absorption from the epidural space following diffusion of the local anesthetic across the dura.

Movement of local anesthetic in spinal fluid away from the site of injection results in a decrease in concentration as a function of distance from the site of injection (Fig. 1.3). The site at which concentration of local anesthetic is greatest is defined as the epicenter of local anesthetic concentration. A decrease in concentration of local anesthetic at the site of injection can also be due to movement of the epicenter of anesthetic concentration away from the site of injection. In either case, the concentration of local anesthetic falls off as a function of distance from the site of maximum concentration (Koster, *et al.*, 1938; Helrich, *et al.*, 1950; Kitahara, *et al.*, 1956).

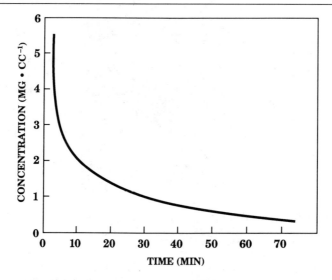

Figure 1.2. Effect of time on concentration of procaine in spinal fluid at the site of injection. (Adapted with permission from Koster, *et al.*, Am. J. Surg. *33*: 245, 1936.)

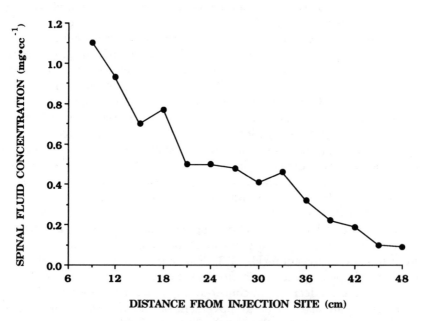

Figure 1.3. Procaine concentrations in spinal fluid at various distances cephalad to the site of injection. (Reproduced with permission from Helrich, *et al.*, J. Pharmacol. Exp. Ther. *100*: 78, 1950.)

The level at which the epicenter lies determines both the dermatomal level of sensory anesthesia and, in part, the duration of anesthesia at that level. The location of the epicenter immediately following injection into the subarachnoid space depends not only on the site at which the injection was made, but also even more on the baricity of the local anesthetic solution injected and the position of the patient at the time of injection and over the next 5–15 min. The baricity of a local anesthetic solution is the ratio between the weight in grams of 1 ml of the anesthetic solution to be injected into CSF and the weight in grams of 1 ml of CSF at the same temperature. Baricity is a more accurate reflection of the direction in which a local anesthetic solution will move in the subarachnoid space as a function of position than is its specific gravity. Specific gravity of a solution is the ratio between the weight in grams of 1 ml of solution and the weight of 1 ml of water at the same temperature. Using specific gravity as an index of movement of local anesthetic within CSF therefore relies on the ratio between two ratios, each of which has water as a common denominator.

If an isobaric local anesthetic solution (i.e., one of the same density as CSF at 37°C) is injected, the epicenter of local anesthetic concentration in spinal fluid remains at the site of injection regardless of the position of the patient during and after injection. If a hyperbaric anesthetic solution (one with a density greater than that of spinal fluid) is injected, gravity causes the epicenter of concentration to lie above, craniad to, the site of injection when injection is made while the patient is in the head-down position. Alternatively, gravity causes caudad movement of the epicenter if injection is made while the patient is in the head-up position. The epicenter of a hypobaric solution (one with density less than that of spinal fluid) moves cephalad from the site of injection if injected in the head-up position or caudad if injected in the head-down position.

Regardless of where the epicenter of local anesthetic concentration lies, the concentration of local anesthetic in spinal fluid decreases as a function of distance both above (craniad to) and below (caudad to) the point of maximum concentration in spinal fluid as shown diagrammatically in Figure 1.4. These concentration curves are clinically and physiologically important because the level at which nerves are blocked is determined in part by the concentration of local anesthetic in spinal fluid. As shown in Figure 1.4, the concentration curves of local anesthetic in spinal fluid below a site of injection may be truncated when hyperbaric solutions are injected while the patient is in the head-up position, or when hypobaric solutions are injected in the head-down position. Similarities in local anesthetic concentrations at the epicenters when hyper- and hypobaric solutions are injected are infrequently present in the clinical situation because the amount (in milligrams) of local anesthetics injected is usually less with hypobaric solutions.

Similarity of the shape of the concentration curves at a given time in

Figure 1.4 regardless of baricity emphasizes that baricity alone does not determine concentration as a function of distance from the epicenter. That the areas under the curves in Figure 1.4 are less at 10 min than at 5 min (and equally less) with different baricities emphasizes that baricity alone does not affect rate of loss of local anesthetic from spinal fluid.

The concentration curves illustrated in Figure 1.4 also suggest that zones of differential blockade during spinal anesthesia associated with differences in spinal fluid concentrations of local anesthetics (pp. 15–18) are similar with hypo-, iso-, and hyperbaric solutions. The concentration curves furthermore indicate the important fact that concentration-related zones of differential blockade during spinal anesthesia can exist both caudad and cephalad to the epicenter of concentration. Equality of zones of differential blockade above and below the epicenter of concentration is not seen, of course, if the epicenter is so low in the subarachnoid space

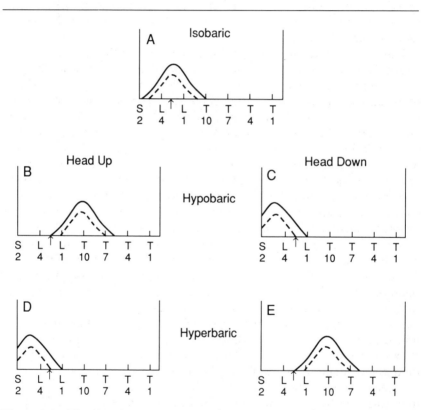

Figure 1.4. Diagramatic representation of concentrations of local anesthetics in spinal fluid (vertical scale) at different levels within the subarachnoid space (horizontal scale) 5 (solid line) and 10 (dashed line) min after injection into the same lumbar interspace of the same amount and volume of local anesthetic either isobaric with patient in any position (A), hypobaric with patient in the head up (B) or head down (C) position, or hyperbaric with patient in the head up (D) or head down (E) position.

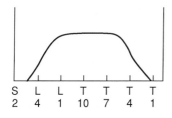

S	L	L	T	T	T	T
2	4	1	10	7	4	1

Figure 1.5. Diagramatic representation of plateau of highest concentration of local anesthetic as a function of distance from site of injection when the amount and volume of anesthetic solution injected is that which produces the curves seen in Figure 1.4.

that the concentration curve caudad to the epicenter is truncated (Fig. 1.4).

Finally, the idealized concentration curves may not be seen in clinical practice when the amount and volume of local anesthetic solution injected are so great that bulk displacement of cerebrospinal fluid from the site of injection causes the bell-shaped concentration curve of Figure 1.4 to be replaced by a concentration curve that contains a plateau (Fig. 1.5). The distance over which the plateau part of the concentration curve extends (Fig. 1.5) depends on the dose (amount) of anesthetic administered and the volume in which it is given. The cephalad decrease in concentration curve in Figure 1.5 is, however, similar to that seen in Figure 1.4.

The significance of the difference in the concentration curves portrayed in Figures 1.4 and 1.5 lies in the extent of total neural blockade within the subarachnoid space. In Figure 1.4, peak concentrations may be adequate to block all fibers traversing the subarachnoid space only over a relatively small area of two to three spinal segments, resulting in a narrow band of segmental anesthesia. In Figure 1.5, the band of segmental anesthesia will be wider or even eliminated if the caudad distribution of local anesthetic is so great that there is no trailing off of concentration in that direction (i.e., caudad truncation).

Volume of the spinal subarachnoid space and, thus, volume of CSF fluid also affect concentration of local anesthetic in cerebrospinal fluid (Table 1.1). A decrease in volume of the subarachnoid space means, of course, a proportional decrease in volume of CSF. When the volume of spinal fluid decreases, there is less dilution by CSF fluid of the highly concentrated anesthetic solution injected into the subarachnoid space, and the concentration of anesthetic in spinal fluid therefore increases. The resulting effects of increased concentration on drug uptake have been described above. Spread of local anesthetic within the subarachnoid space is also increased by decreased volume of CSF.

Acute decreases in volume of the subarachnoid space are rarely encountered. Sustained decreases in volume of the subarachnoid space with associated decreases in spinal fluid volume are more frequent. A frequent cause of decreased volume of the spinal fluid is chronic engorgement of veins in the epidural spaces brought about by compression of venous effluent channels as occurs with large intra-abdominal tumors and the gravid uterus at term. Acute elevations of intra-abdominal pressure associated with coughing, the Valsalva maneuver, or acute engorgement of epidural veins increase spinal fluid pressure transiently but have no effect on volume of fluid in the spinal subarachnoid space.

The importance of concentration of local anesthetics in spinal fluid in determining uptake of local anesthetics within the subarachnoid space is illustrated by the reversibility of spinal anesthesia when the concentration of local anesthetic in the subarachnoid space is reduced to near zero by flushing of the subarachnoid space with anesthetic-free solution. Koster, et al. (1939), for example, found in 13 patients that the duration of action of procaine injected into the subarachnoid space could be decreased by flushing the subarachnoid space with three to five 10-ml injections of saline, if flushing were performed within about 22 min of injection of procaine. In the absence of flushing, the time to return of motor function averaged 45 min from the time of injection. When flushing was done within 22 min of injection, the average time from flushing to recovery of motor function was 7 min. Flushing more than 22 min after injection had no effect on the time of recovery of motor function. Thus it is perhaps not unexpected that Converse, et al., (1954) were unable to decrease the duration of tetracaine spinal anesthesia significantly in three patients when the subarachnoid space was irrigated with 40 ml saline 30 min after injection of the tetracaine. Sargent, et al. (1971) found that effective decrease in the duration of spinal anesthesia required flushing of the subarachnoid space even sooner after injection than Koster, et al. reported. They found that in dogs, to decrease the duration of procaine spinal anesthesia significantly, irrigation of the subarachnoid space had to be accomplished during onset of anesthesia (i.e., when the concentration of local anesthetic in spinal fluid was still high). Duration of anesthesia was decreased by 80% if irrigation was started within 1 minute, but was decreased by only 30% if irrigation was performed 15 min after injection. Once the local anesthetic is adsorbed onto nerve tissue, irrigation of the subarachnoid space has relatively little effect.

3. *Diffusion* is another determinant of anatomic sites within the subarachnoid space into which local anesthetics may be taken up during spinal anesthesia (Table 1.1). *Diffusion* can, for present purposes, be defined as the passive movement of molecules of local anesthetics in the absence of physical or thermal agitation down a concentration gradient from areas of high concentration to areas with lesser or no levels of local anesthetics (potential uptake sites within the subarachnoid space). Ideally, diffusion can be quantitated in terms of mass (μmol), of local anesthetic moving a given distance (100 nm, say) per unit of gradient (say, 100 μmol/100 nm) per unit time (10 sec). Such precise quantitation of diffusion of local anesthetics in vivo has not been reported, but concepts regarding diffusion are helpful in understanding uptake of local anesthetics during spinal anesthesia.

One of the fundamental concepts in considering rates of diffusion of local anesthetics in spinal fluid and, thus, the sites at which they may be absorbed, centers about the obvious fact that the rate of diffusion is related to initial concentration of local anesthetic in spinal fluid. The greater the initial concentration, the greater the mass of anesthetic moving down the concentration gradient. Rate of diffusion decreases as a function of time, however, because of the progressive decrease in the concentration gradient. Molecular weight also determines the rate of diffusion. The greater the molecular weight, the slower the rate of diffusion, as seen, for example, in the well-recognized difference between rates of diffusion of carbon dioxide and oxygen in hypoventilated alveoli. During spinal anesthesia, the less the molecular weight of a local anesthetic, the more rapid its diffusion down a concentration gradient from CSF into the spinal cord.

Molecular structure may also influence the rate of diffusion of molecules across nonlipid barriers such as the dura. In a study of a variety of nonanesthetic pharmacologic and physiologic compounds, Moore, *et al.* (1982) found that, in the presence of equal concentration gradients, spherical molecules diffuse more readily across the dura than do molecules of similar molecular weight but with a straight-line molecular configuration. Ester-linked local anesthetics have, in general, straight-line molecular configurations. Amide-linked local anesthetics have more spherically shaped molecules. Amide-linked local anesthetics would be expected, therefore, to diffuse more rapidly across the dura than ester-linked local anesthetics. Perhaps the two types of local anesthetics diffuse at different rates not only across the dura but also within biologic liquids.

4. *Tissue lipids* (Table 1.1), whether macro- or microscopic, increase the rates of diffusion of local anesthetic molecules down a concentration gradient. They do so in proportion to the level of lipid solubility of the molecules.

5. *Lipid solubility of local anesthetics* (Table 1.1) influences the rate at which they diffuse into lipid-containing tissues across lipid-containing membranes. Uptake of highly lipid-soluble anesthetics into a highly lipid site increases the steepness of the concentration gradient to that site, and so, increases the rate of diffusion to the site. "Soaking up" of lipid soluble molecules into lipid-rich tissues may, however, delay diffusion across the tissue despite the increase in rate of diffusion to the tissue.

6. *pKa* (Table 1.1). The degree to which local anesthetics are ionized at normal levels of pH, a function of their negative log of dissociation constant (pKa), is another determinant of the site of uptake because anesthetics are taken up into the lipid of cell membranes (and other lipid sites) in their undissociated form. The greater the percent of a local anesthetic existing in the un-ionized state at a physiologic pH of 7.4, the greater their uptake into lipids and, therefore, the steeper the slope of the concentration curve and, as mentioned above, the more rapid the

Table 1.2.
Effect of pH on Dissociation of Local Anesthetics

	pK$_a$	Total Drug in Cationic Form (%)		
		pH 7.0	pH 7.4	pH 7.8
Procaine	8.9	99	97	93
Tetracaine	8.2	94	86	72
Bupivacaine	8.1	93	83	67
Lidocaine	7.9	89	76	56
Mepivacaine	7.6	80	61	39

Table 1.3.
Changes in pH of Cerebrospinal Fluid of Humans at the Site of Injection of 3 ml (15 mg) of Bupivacaine 0.5% With (N = 15) and Without (N = 7) 1:200,000 Epinephrine (mean ± SE)[a]

	Time (min)							
	0	5	10	15	25	60	120	180
Without epinephrine	7.38 ± 0.008	7.31 ± 0.004	7.30 ± 0.004	7.30 ± 0.003	7.31 ± 0.025	7.32 ± 0.003	7.33 ± 0.003	7.34 ± 0.003
With epinephrine	7.39 ± 0.006	7.24 ± 0.01	7.26 ± 0.01	7.28 ± 0.01	7.28 ± 0.01	7.28 ± 0.01	7.30 ± 0.01	7.31 ± 0.01

[a] Adapted with permission from Stark, et al., Anaesthesist 26: 395, 1977.

rate of diffusion to the site of uptake. The pKa values of several local anesthetics are presented in Table 1.2, together with the effect of changes in pH on the degree of ionization and, in Table 1.3, the changes in pH of spinal fluid that occur at the site of injection of a local anesthetic solution.

7. *Tissue blood flow* (Table 1.1) to sites of neuronal uptake of local anesthetics during spinal anesthesia, though not a determinant of uptake *per se*, is another determinant of the amount and concentration of local anesthetic within the various sites of uptake. The greater the blood flow to tissue, the greater the rate of removal of local anesthetic from its site of uptake and the lower the concentration of local anesthetic in the tissue. Conversely, the lower the blood flow, the lower the rate of removal from a site of tissue uptake.

The above theoretical considerations emphasize some of the complexities involved in determining site and rate of uptake of local anesthetics by and into neural elements during spinal anesthesia. The realities of these considerations have been quanitated in measurements of uptake of local anesthetics during experimental spinal anesthesia by Cohen

(1968) and, earlier, by Howarth (1949) and Grodinsky, *et al.* (1933). Cohen injected 1 ml of anesthetic solution containing 25 mg radioactive labeled procaine or lidocaine in 10% dextrose into the subarachnoid space at L_2 in six dogs. Thirty minutes later the animals were killed and tissues from the lumbar spinal cord were obtained. Cohen found local anesthetic present in all tissues, non-neural as well as neural (Table 1.4). Notable is the fact that the highest concentrations were in the lateral and posterior columns. The lowest concentrations were in dorsal root ganglia, in anterior horn grey matter, and in extradural fat. Intermediate tissue levels were in the dura, dorsal roots, anterior columns, posterior horn grey matter, and ventral roots. The effect of time on the concentrations of local anesthetics in various tissues following induction of spinal anesthesia injection into the subarachnoid space is seen in the results reported by Howarth (Table 1.5). He injected 3.3 mg radioactive dibromoprocaine into the subarachnoid spaces of cats and obtained tissue for analysis of drug concentrations 10, 20, and 30 min later. The concentration of dibromoprocaine in neural tissue decreased quite rapidly. Like Cohen, Howarth found significant concentrations of local anesthetic within the cord, more so in superficial portions of the cord than in deeper, more central areas. On the other hand, the concentration of anesthetic was higher in nerve roots than in superficial portions of the cord. In Cohen's animals the concentration of anesthetic was somewhat less in dorsal roots than in certain relatively superficial tracts. The difference is proba-

Table 1.4.
Concentrations of Lidocaine or Procaine in Lumbar Spinal Cords of Dogs Killed 30 min Following Subarachnoid Injection of 25 mg of Anesthetic at L_2[a]

Source	Concentration of Local Anesthetic (μg/mg of tissue)[b]
Lateral column	1.38 ± 0.12
Posterior column	1.36 ± 0.18
Dura	0.98 ± 0.30
Dorsal root	0.87 ± 0.20
Anterior column	0.73 ± 0.24
Grey matter (posterior horn)	0.53 ± 0.09
Whole grey matter	0.34 ± 0.13
Ventral root	0.32 ± 0.10
Whole cord	0.27 ± 0.10
Extradural fat	0.25 ± 0.10
Grey matter (anterior horn)	0.21 ± 0.08
Dorsal root ganglion[c]	0.16
Cerebrospinal fluid	0.83 ± 0.15

[a] Reproduced with permission from Cohen, Anesthesiology *29:* 1002, 1968.
[b] Mean ± SEM
[c] Mean of two specimens.

Table 1.5.
Concentrations of Dibromoprocaine in Spinal Cords of Cats 10, 20, and 30 min
Following Subarachnoid Injection of 3.3 mg of Anesthetic[a]

	Average Concentration ($\mu g \cdot gm^{-1}$ or $\mu g \cdot ml^{-1}$)		
	10 min	20 min	30 min
Roots	320	246	63.7
Periphery of lumbar cord	138	66	30.9
Central lumbar cord	5.3	2.6	18
Periphery of cervical cord	0.5	0.42	6.5

[a] Adapted with permission from Howarth, Br. J. Pharmacol. 4: 333, 1949.

bly related to the fact that Cohen determined concentrations in specific areas whereas Howarth measured average concentrations in all superficial areas of the cord, thereby obscuring the differential concentrations observed by Cohen. In addition, Cohen measured the concentration only in dorsal roots; root concentrations reported by Horwath may have included anterior nerve roots.

Local anesthetics get into the substance of the spinal cord during spinal anesthesia by diffusion down a concentration gradient from spinal fluid to tissues. Diffusion would be both through the pia mater as well as diffusion into the substance of the cord from spinal fluid in spaces of Virchow-Robin within the substance of the cord (p. 2–3). These spaces ultimately connect with perineuronal clefts that surround the bodies of nerve cells in several portions of the spinal cord. This arrangement suggests that this route may be more important for delivery of local anesthetics into the substance of the cord itself than diffusion inward from the pial surface, which is a slow process.

The reason why local anesthetics are more concentrated in certain areas and in certain structures within the subarachnoid space than they are in others is not related to any one of the above factors, but instead, to a combination of accessibility, lipid solubility, diffusion, and tissue blood flow. How accessible to anesthetics neural elements within the cord are is, to a considerable degree, a function of the number of spaces of Virchow-Robin per unit of surface area of the cord. These spaces accompany blood vessels, and the blood supply of the spinal cord in humans is primarily derived from the anterior spinal artery, branches of which pass through the anterior median fissure into the substance of the cord. Therefore, it might be expected that the concentrations of local anesthetics within the cord would be greater and more deeply located anteriorly than they are posteriorly. That this is not the case is probably due to the role played by lipid solubility. Local anesthetics are more soluble in lipids than they are in water. Myelin contains lipids. Posterior and lateral spinal cord tracts are more heavily myelinated than are anterior tracts (with the exception of the anterior corticospinal tract). Posterior nerve roots are also more heavily myelinated than are anterior nerve roots. Heavy myelination tends to concentrate local anesthetics, provided accessibility through the spaces of Virchow-Robin is the same, and providing the third factor involved in determining tissue concentration, tissue blood flow, is also the same. The rate at which local anesthetics are removed from the spinal cord is governed to a substantial degree by blood flow. The greater the blood flow per volume of spinal cord tissue, the more rapidly anesthetics are borne away. The greater the blood flow, therefore, the lower the tissue concentration of local anesthetics. This may partially explain the fact that the concentrations of local anesthetics are lower in the anterior portions of the cord than they are posteriorly, despite greater accessibility anteriorly through the spaces of Virchow-Robin. It is unlikely, however, that tissue blood flow is the sole or even the most important determinant of cord concentrations of local anesthetics during spinal anesthesia. Higher concentrations are probably achieved in posterolateral portions of the cord because of their higher myelin content. In considering the balance between accessibility, lipid solubility, and circulatory removal, we should note that the posterior spinal column is also supplied by an artery that penetrates the cord directly and which also supplies the posterior roots. Furthermore, grey mater of the spinal cord has a substantially greater blood supply than does white mater. Higher concentrations of local anesthetics are found in some areas of the cord despite their higher blood flows because they contain material (i.e., lipids) in which local anesthetics are so soluble.

The presence of local anesthetics within the cord during spinal anesthesia does not necessarily mean they are there in concentrations adequate to have pharmacologic effects on neuronal function. The pharmacologic and functional significance of accumulations of local anesthetics in the cord during spinal anesthesia is addressed on pp. 48–55.

It should be noted that uptake of local anesthetics within the subarachnoid space is, in contrast to what is observed peripherally, not influenced by binding of local anesthetics to proteins or other substances in cerebrospinal fluid. The amount of local anesthetic bound by human spinal fluid is negligible (Tucker, et al., 1970).

The effect of epinephrine on neuronal uptake of local anesthetics has not been studied directly. It can be assumed, however, that, since epinephrine decreases vascular absorption of local anesthetics through its vasoconstrictive effect, concentrations of local anesthetic increase in subarachnoid neural structures when epinephrine is used to prolong the duration of anesthesia.

Anesthetic Action

The term "anesthetic action" would be a misnomer if we implied that the pharmacologic basis of action of local anesthetics is to be addressed in this section. How local anesthetics produce their effects will not be addressed. Instead, anesthetic action applies to a consideration of where local anesthetics act during spinal anesthesia as foundation for understanding the neurologic basis for the physiologic responses produced by injection of local anesthetics into CSF.

One of the questions to be considered is: exactly where in the subarachnoid space do local anesthetics act to produce sensory denervation so profound as to produce complete blockade of all sensory afferent impulses? What neuronal tissues are involved? Are they nerves crossing the subarachnoid space? Are they dorsal root ganglia? Nociceptive neurons in spinal cord dorsal horn tissue? Or are they axons in nerve tracts within the substance of the spinal cord?

With regard to dorsal root ganglia as a site of action of local anesthetics used to produce spinal anesthesia: though technically root ganglia are not deep to the arachnoid and, thus they are not in the subarachnoid space, local anesthetics injected into the subarachnoid space can affect dorsal root ganglia by diffusing from spinal fluid through the arachnoid and dura to the ganglia. Local anesthetics are taken up by dorsal root ganglia (Table 1.4). Indeed, in 1954 Frumin, *et al.* suggested that dorsal root ganglia represent *the* primary sites of action of local anesthetics injected into the subarachnoid space on sensory afferent fibers. This concept was subsequently supported by the observations of Galindo and Witcher in 1982. In studies by both Frumin, *et al.*, and by Galindo and Witcher, root ganglia were found to be more susceptible to the blocking action of local anesthetics than were sensory afferent nerve axons. This effect was most evident during high-frequency transmission of nerve impulses. Together, these papers provide compelling evidence that dorsal root ganglia can indeed be included as a site of action (i.e., blockade) of local anesthetics injected into the subarachnoid space. It is an overstatement, however, for this site of action to be considered the only, or even the major, anesthetic site of action of local anesthetics when injected into the subarachnoid space in amounts, volumes, and concentrations adequate to provide operative anesthesia. More likely, local anesthetics injected into the CSF in concentrations adequate to produce sensory blockade also act directly on somatic sensory afferent nerves as they cross the subarachnoid space. Whether nociceptive neurons in Rexed laminae within the spinal cord dorsal horns also constitute sites of anesthetic action of local anesthetics that have diffused into the cord from the subarachnoid space during spinal anesthesia also is a possibility. This possibility has been evaluated in review of the effects of spinal anesthesia on the spinal cord itself, including (pp. 48–51) the possibility that local anesthetics within the cord can also affect axonal transmission of impulses along nerve tracts within the cord.

More difficult, more studied, more contentious, and more important is the question as to whether or not spinal anesthesia is associated with dermatomal zones of differential nerve blockade. This involves yet another question: are different types of nerves blocked by different concentrations of local anesthetics? If so, then zones of differential blockade of nerve fibers in the subarachnoid space result in zones of differential blockade of sensory and motor nerves as measured peripherally in spinal dermatomes. If there is no differential sensitivity of nerves to the blocking action of local anesthetics, then a dermatomal level in which, for example, pinprick sensation is blocked must represent the spinal segmental level at which all nerves, sympathetic, sensory and motor, are blocked. That controversy even exists about this subject in the face of overwhelming clinical evidence that zones of differential blockade do indeed exist during spinal anesthesia and is due in part to the difficulty in proving beyond all pharmacologic doubt that, under rigidly controlled conditions, such a thing as differential sensitivity of nerve fibers does exist and, if so, why and how?

Since this is a book on the physiology of spinal anesthesia, not a monograph on the pharmacology and mode of action of local anesthetics, there is no need to review the monumental numbers of articles published that address the issue of differential sensitivities of different types of nerve fibers to different concentrations of local anesthetics. The reader interested in undertaking even a superficial review of the subject should read, at the very least, the papers of Courtney (1975); Courtney, *et al.* (1978); Covino and Vassalo (1976); Douglas and Malcolm (1955); de Jong (1980); Fink (1989); Fink and Cairns (1983, 1984 b, 1985, 1987); Ford, *et al.* (1984); Franz and Perry (1974); Galindo and Witcher (1982); Gasser and Erlanger (1929); Gissen, *et al.* (1980, 1982); Heavener and de Jong (1974); Lorente de Nó and Condouris (1959); Nathan and Sears (1961); Paintal (1967); Raymond, *et al.* (1989); Rosenberg and Heinonen (1983); Rosenberg, *et al.* (1980); Scurlock, *et al.* (1978); Staiman and Seeman (1977); Truent and Lanzoni (1952); and Wildsmith, *et al.* (1985, 1987, 1989).

The reader who has undertaken the task of reviewing the articles cited above would be justified in drawing two conclusions. First, it is possible to demonstrate under nonclinical experimental conditions the existence of differential sensitivity of different types of nerves to the blocking actions of local anesthetics. Second, the etiology of differential blocking effects of local anesthetics is multifactorial. For example:

1. Frequency-dependence of local anesthetic action means that even under "basal" conditions different types of nerves with different frequencies of nerve impulse transmission have different sensitivities to local anesthetics. Physiologic or experimentally induced increases in frequency of nerve impulse transmission increase anesthetic sensitivity depending on both the type of nerve fiber and the degree of increase in stimulation frequency.

2. Duration of exposure of nerves (or axons) to local anesthetic solutions alters perceived sensitivity to local anesthetic action. Rate of penetrance of local anesthetic into nerves depends on pKa, lipid solubility, and the pH at which the experiments are carried out. Rates of penetrance, and so, rates of onset of anesthetic action, are to be differentiated from measurements of anesthetic action made under steady state conditions when concentrations of local anesthetic within and outside nervous tissue are fully equilibrated.

3. Most, though perhaps not all investigators believe that axonal diameter is, by itself, not a determinant of nerve sensitivity to the blocking action of local anesthetics. There may be a general association between fiber size and sensitivity, but close scrutiny indicates that such a general association is unreliable. Deviation from the general rule that fiber size and minimum anesthetic concentration are directly related is evident, for example, in the fact that though different in size, A delta-fibers and C-fibers are almost equally sensitive to the effects of local anesthetics. Furthermore, though preganglionic myelinated B-fibers are larger than unmyelinated C-fibers, they are three times more sensitive to the effects of a local anesthetic such as lidocaine. Therefore, although axonal diameter and nerve function are related (Table 1.6), it does not necessarily follow that nerve function and nerve sensitivity to local anesthetics are necessarily related to each other.

Table 1.6.
Classification of Nerve Fibers

Fiber Class	Myelin	Diameter (μm)	Conduction Velocity (m·sec^{-1})	Function
A-α	Heavy	12–20	70–120	Motor
A-β	Moderate	5–12	30–70	Deep pressure, touch, vibration
A-γ	Moderate	5–10	30–70	Proprioception, muscle tone
A-δ	Moderate	2–5	12–30	Pain (sharp), temperature
B	Light	1–4	3–15	Preganglionic sympathetics
C-sC	None	0.3–1.3	0.7–1.3	Postganglionic sympathetics
C-dγC	None	0.4–1.2	0.1–2.0	Crude touch, pain (dull), temperature

4. Results of in vitro studies of sensitivity to local anesthetics depend in part on whether nerves normally sheathed remain intact, or whether they have been desheathed.

5. The ability to demonstrate differential sensitivity of nerves to local anesthetics varies with the type of local anesthetic (amide- or ester-linked) as well as within the same type of anesthetic (e.g., amide vs. amide).

6. Local anesthetics block myelinated nerves at the nodes of Ranvier. Axonal conduction block is produced only when several, not just one, nodes are exposed to pharmacologically active concentrations of local anesthetics. Length of nerve exposed to local anesthetic also, therefore, influences sensitivity to local anesthetics.

Despite all the complexities and difficulties involved in demonstrating and, when demonstrating, explaining differential sensitivities of different concentrations of local anesthetics, it is a pragmatic and ineluctable if inexplicable fact that, in clinical practice, regional anesthesia is routinely associated with differential blockade of different types of nerves. Differential blockade can be seen when local anesthetics are injected in the vicinity of large mixed peripheral nerves or nerve trunks. This type of differential blockade can be explained largely on neuroanatomic grounds and on the basis of the pharmacokinetics of uptake of local anesthetics into large, mixed peripheral nerves: nerve fibers in the outer, more peripherally located parts of such nerves are more readily blocked than are more centrally located nerve fibers in the core of the mixed nerve. This is so because the perineurally injected anesthetic diffuses into the mixed nerve (i.e., toward the core) from the outside.

The role of possible differential sensitivity of different types of nerves to the effects of local anesthetics during peripheral nerve blocks is difficult to identify because of the anatomic arrangement of nerve fibers. This is not the case during spinal anesthesia. During spinal anesthesia, the clearly evident zones of differential blockade are but peripherally related to anatomic factors. They are, instead, directly associated with aforementioned differences in concentrations of local anesthetic within spinal fluid as a function of distance from the site of injection or the site of the epicenter of anesthetic concentration (pp. 2–7). The term "associated with" is used advisedly. Absolute proof that the association is due entirely to different concentrations of local anesthetic in CSF, intuitively logical though it may be, is lacking. But the clinical evidence is compelling that there exist zones of differential nerve block during spinal anesthesia, zones of differential blockade most often evident cephalad to the site of injection.

Though zones of differential blockade can be identified cephalad to the site of injection by testing function of various sensory and motor nerves during onset and maintenance of spinal anesthesia, the same cannot always be done with equal reliability during regression of spinal anesthesia. Misinformation about zones of differential block may result when measurements are made during regression of spinal anesthesia because of the anatomy of nerves originating in the spinal cord at and below the level of the second lumbar segment. The most distal preganglionic sympathetic fibers exit from the subarachnoid space at the level of L_2. Somatic sensory fibers arise from spinal segments below L_2 and exit from the subarachnoid space at levels often well below L_2. Therefore, when spinal anesthesia wears off and the level of anesthesia descends (as local anesthetic is absorbed from the subarachnoid space), a spinal fluid level of local anesthetic is reached that is no longer adequate to block sympathetic outflow at L_2. Complete sympathetic activity will return. There can, however, still be concentrations of local anesthetic in spinal fluid below L_2 adequate to produce sensory anesthesia at lower lumbar and sacral levels. Testing sympathetic and sensory function in the lower extremity at this time shows sympathetic innervation to be normal at a time when sensory anesthesia is still present. This does not mean, as has been suggested (Roe and Cohen, 1973), that sensory nerves are more sensitive to the effects of local anesthetics than are preganglionic sympathetic fibers. Such a pharmacologically paradoxical finding is readily explicable on a neuroanatomic basis.

Mention should be made of clinical situations in which pharmacologic action of local anesthetics used in spinal anesthesia is not as great as anticipated. One is development of *tachyphylaxis*, which is defined as the progressive decrease, often acute in onset, in responses to a drug following its repeated administration. Tachyphylaxis is seen most frequently during spinal anesthesia in association with repeated injections of a local anesthetic intrathecally through a spinal catheter, and resulting in a decrease in anesthetic effectiveness (Cohen, *et al.*, 1968; Bromage, *et al.*, 1969; Smith and Rees, 1970; Kroin, *et al.*, 1986; Baker, *et al.*, 1991). Anesthesia lasts for a shorter period of time after the third injection of local anesthetic than it did after the first injection; more anesthetic needs to be injected on the third injection than on the first to achieve the same degree of anesthesia. Local anesthetic tachyphylaxis develops acutely and it disappears rapidly. Tachyphylaxis is not evident when spinal anesthetics are administered on successive days, only, as with continuous spinal anesthesia, when subsequent injections are made before or immediately after recovery of function following the preceding injection.

Tachyphylaxis during spinal anesthesia has been attributed to changes in CSF pH produced by the injection of local anesthetic solutions which often have pH substantially lower than 7.0 (Table 1.3). In humans the pH of CSF decreases from a normal value of 7.39 to 7.24 within 5 min of the injection of 3 ml (15 mg) of bupivacaine 0.5 percent (Stark, *et al.*, 1977). It returns only slowly toward normal, still being in the range of 7.31–7.34 3 hr later (Table 1.3). Decreases in spinal fluid pH resulting from injection of highly acidic solutions into CSF with its limited buffering capacity have been hypothesized to induce such a decrease in the amount of lipid-soluble free-base form of local anesthetics, that pharmacologic activity decreases (Cohen, et al., 1968). This effect of pH subsequently has been shown by Baker, et al. (1991) to be unlikely as a cause of local anesthetic tachyphylaxis during spinal anesthesia. Baker, et al. found that injections of 0.25% bupivacaine at pH 4.2 or 6.8 into a surgically implanted irrigating system adjacent to the sciatic nerve in rats resulted in development of tachyphylaxis. The degree of tachyphylaxis and the rapidity with which it developed were similar, however, with solutions of both pH values, 4.2 and 6.8, despite the 400-fold difference in hydrogen ion concentration. This observation effectively renders untenable the theory that local anesthetic tachyphylaxis during spinal anesthesia is caused by changes in CSF pH.

It has also been shown that local anesthetic tachyphylaxis is not associated with a decrease in anesthetic activity or potency at the level of the nerve itself. Lippert, et al. (1989) exposed rabbit aortic nerves isolated from surrounding tissues to increasing concentrations of bupivacaine until nerve transmission was completely blocked. The bupivacaine concentration was then decreased to a point where the block was only partial, and then maintained there for 4 hr. Lippert, et al. found that, during the period of exposure to a constant concentration associated with partial block, nerve activity did not increase, as would be expected in the presence of tachyphylaxis, but instead decreased. In addition, nerve activity during partial block was consistently less during exposure to a constant concentration of bupivacaine than it was during the initial nerve block. Both observations indicate than an increase, not a decrease, in bupivacaine anesthetic activity occurred over time during exposure to the local anesthetic that would be expected during tachyphylaxis. This makes it unlikely that changes in axonal conduction (induced by changes in concentration) are involved in the development of tachyphylaxis. The results of this study and those reported by Baker, et al. (1991) suggest the possibility that local anesthetic tachyphylaxis might be related to a pharmacokinetically mediated reduction of local anesthetic at the axon, or to a hypothetical increase in input to the central nervous system during long-term block of axonal conduction. As Lippert, et al., also note, their observations support the suggestion that tachyphylaxis occurs only in intact animals or humans.

A different type of tolerance to local anesthetics is that reported with chronic ethanol consumption. Fassoulaki, et al. (1990), for example, found, in intragroup comparisons of rats given lidocaine spinal anesthetics before and 9 days after being on a high alcohol diet, that the dose of lidocaine needed to produce sensory blockade was statistically significantly less after 9 days of ethanol ingestion than it had been earlier. Curiously, when intergroup comparisons between rats given alcohol and rats having two spinal anesthetics 9 days apart but with a regular diet and no alcohol in the intervening days, the intergroup difference in the amount of lidocaine needed to provide sensory denervation was not statistically significant. Aside from providing a striking example of the difference between baseline data for making intragroup comparisons and true control data for making intergroup comparisons, the biologic, pharmacologic, or statistical significance of these data remains obscure. The data obtained were totally different when yet another spinal anesthetic was administered in both groups of rats 14 hr after the second spinal anesthetic. Here the amounts of lidocaine needed to produce sensory denervation were significantly *greater* after the rats given alcohol had sobered than they were in the same rats when drunk 14 hr before. The amounts of lidocaine needed were also significantly greater in the now-sober rats than in rats that were never drunk over the period of 9 days and 14 hr. It would seem likely that sensitivity to local anesthetics, not kinetic changes, explains the latter results since the duration of sensory blockade did change significantly. Also, somatic motor blockade by intrathecal lidocaine remained unaltered during and after the high alcohol diet. The clinical significance of these findings remains to be defined. It may be that they are clinically relevant only when using a spinal catheter for injections of dilute concentrations of local anesthetics in the production of diagnostic or therapeutic differential spinal anesthesia in alcoholic patients.

Clinically more devastating to patient and anesthesiologist than either of the two above situations is failure of any anesthesia to develop following the apparently successful injection of local anesthetic solution into the subarachnoid space despite free aspiration of CSF into the syringe before and after injection. The majority of instances in which there is total failure of spinal anesthesia to develop are the result of technical failures (Sechzer, 1963; Cohen and Kallos, 1972; Levy, et al., 1985; Manchikanti, et al., 1987; Munhall, et al., 1988). Specifically, the most frequent explanation is that the injection has been made into the subdural, not the subarachnoid space. This is testified to by the frequency with which flawed myelograms are seen radiologically because of subdural, not subarachnoid, injection of contrast media. Subdural injection occurs when the tip of the spinal needle has tented and even partially penetrated the arachnoid thereby opening the otherwise only potential subdural space and allowing spinal fluid to be aspirated, even though the whole bevel of the needle has not entered the free subarachnoid space (Sechzer, 1963; Cohen and Kallos, 1972).

Failure of anesthesia to develop following injection into what was believed to be the free subarachnoid space, has been ascribed to use of spinal anesthetic solutions that are no longer pharmacologically active (Sinclair, 1973). This is an unlikely explanation. Rarely if ever in 1992 do pharmaceutical companies market pharmacologically inactive substances. That the local anesthetic injected is pharmacologically active can be readily proven by taking advantage of the fact that there always remains a bit of local anesthetic solution in the ampule following aspiration of most of its contents for injection into the subarachnoid space. Saving this residual local anesthetic until spinal anesthesia developed became a personal policy of N.M.G. over 40 yr ago. When, as indeed did happen on occasion, no anesthesia developed, the residual solution was tested for pharmacologic activity by placing a drop of it on the tip of the tongue. Pharmacologic inactivity was never encountered. The anesthetic had almost surely been injected subdurally.

There are, however, a few very rare instances in which there is no apparent explanation for failure of anesthesia to develop. Weiskopf (1970), for example, reported a patient who was given two catheter spinal anesthetics 2 wk apart. Repeated injections of local anesthetic on both occasions failed to produce anesthesia. Spinal fluid could be readily aspirated through the catheters at both times. Injection of contrast material through the catheter confirmed its placement in the subarachnoid space. Intradermal injection of the same anesthetic (tetracaine) produced anesthesia. Dripps (1950) also reported comparable instances of failure of spinal anesthesia to develop in 7 of 486 patients with catheters in the subarachnoid space. The etiology of these failures remains obscure, but the description (Miller, 1981) of a familial insensitivity to local anesthetics or incredible brevity of action, or both, in twins in one instance and in two sisters and in their mother in another instance, raises the possibility of a genetically based abnormality of the membrane site(s) at which local anesthetics act.

Effects of Spinal Anesthesia on the Sympathetic Nervous System

Block of afferent sensory and efferent somatic motor fibers is the clinical *raison d'être* for spinal anesthesia. Spinal anesthesia is also, however, associated with significant physiologic effects that cannot be ascribed to afferent sensory or efferent somatic blockade. Nor can they be ascribed to systemic blood levels of local anesthetics injected into the subarachnoid space and reaching plasma concentrations great enough to have direct peripheral pharmacologic effects. Blood levels of local anesthetics used in spinal anesthesia are too low to have any direct, peripheral effects (Giasi, *et al.*, 1979; Greene, 1979). Nor, finally, can physiologic responses to spinal anesthesia be ascribed to any hypothetical diffusion of local anesthetic injected in the lumbar subarachnoid space upward into the cisterna magna and from thence out of the cisterna, through the foramina of Magendie and Luschka against the flow of CSF in amounts adequate to produce local anesthetic concentrations sufficient to induce direct depression of physiologically important brainstem centers.

The vast majority of the physiologic effects of spinal anesthesia, and essentially all of the cardiovascular effects of spinal anesthesia, are mediated simply and solely by the preganglionic sympathetic blockade produced by the local anesthetic injected into the subarachnoid space. It is this sympathetic denervation that is the *sine qua non* of the physiology of spinal anesthesia. For this reason it is appropriate to consider in some detail exactly how to measure the existence of sympathetic denervation during clinical spinal anesthesia and, if present, its extent. Measurement of the existence and extent of sympathetic denervation might seem to be simple indeed: just measure the extent to which local anesthetic has spread in the subarachnoid space by measuring the extent of sensory anesthesia and assume that preganglionic sympathetic fibers are blocked to the same level. Or, alternatively, simply measure magnitude of physiologic, especially cardiovascular responses and assume there is a direct relation between the two. In general, the more extensive the sensory anesthesia, the more extensive the extent of sympathetic denervation and the greater the physiologic trespass. This is not accurate enough, though. It is not accurate enough because there are no reliable, straightforward, and direct relationships between the level of sympathetic denervation and magnitude of physiologic trespass, cardiovascular or otherwise. There are no relationships for physiologic, pharmacologic, and anatomic reasons. The physiologic reasons are considered in Chapter 2. The pharmacologic factors, including differential sensitivities of different types of nerve fibers to the blocking effects of local anesthetics, are considered on pp. 15–18. The anatomic factors contributing to the lack of clinically reliable relationships between the above factors center about the anatomy of the spinal part of the sympathetic nervous system. Given the importance of the sympathetic nervous system in the genesis of physiologic responses to spinal anesthesia, it is worthwhile to review the anatomy of this important component of the nervous system.

Sympathetic preganglionic axons arise from cells in the intermediolateral column of the spinal cord. These cells are present in the cord only from the first thoracic to the second lumbar spinal segments, inclusive; their axons leave the spinal cord as the anterior spiral roots, traverse the subarachnoid space and pass through the dura and epidural space. At this stage they are thinly myelinated. Because of the difference between the level of the cord segment at which an efferent nerve has its origin and the level of the intervertebral foramen by which it leaves the theca, the sympathetic fibers pass obliquely downward across the subarachnoid space. The obliquity of this angle becomes more marked distally, so that the sympathetic fibers arising in the second lumbar segment (opposite the twelfth thoracic vertebra) travel in the subarachnoid space for a distance of two vertebral bodies before emerging through the dura at the level of the second lumbar vertebra. After passing through the dura, the preganglionic fibers course in the white (myelinated) *rami communicantes* to the paravertebral sympathetic ganglia. Within the ganglia each vasoconstrictor, pilomotor and sudomotor axon comes into synaptic relationship with a number of postganglionic fibers which rejoin, by way of the gray (unmyelinated) *rami communicantes*, the spinal nerves and then are distributed to the trunk and limbs. Other preganglionic fibers destined to innervate the muscles of the abdominal viscera pass through the paravertebral ganglia and synapse with postganglionic fibers in the prevertebral celiac, preaortic, and hypogastric ganglia. Although some preganglionic fibers end in the paravertebral ganglia nearest the point at which they leave the vertebral column, the majority either ascend or descend in the sympathetic chain for up to as many as six spinal segments before forming synapses with postganglionic fibers. Furthermore, each preganglionic fiber may form synapses with as many as 22 postganglionic fibers (White, *et al.*, 1952). Thus, sympathetic motor pathways are not distributed in a segmental manner as are somatic sensory fibers, and stimulation or paralysis of a single preganglionic sympathetic fiber produces a diffuse response. Stimulation of the anterior root of the fourth thoracic nerve produces, for example, pilomotor activity in the sensory areas innervated by the fifth cervical through the sixth thoracic anterior roots (White, *et al.*, 1952). Paralysis of a preganglionic sympathetic fiber, as during spinal or extradural block, will also produce effects that are manifest in sensory dermatones at some distance from the spinal level at which the sympathetic block occurred.

Viscerosensory afferent sympathetic fibers travel with the sympathetic trunks, pass uninterrupted through the sympathetic ganglia, and then proceed in the white *rami communicantes* to the spinal nerves. These fibers, like those of the somatic sensory nerves, have ganglionic cells in the posterior root ganglia. Central fibers from the ganglion cells pass through the subarachnoid space and enter the gray matter of the lateral horns of the spinal cord.

The autonomic motor distribution to various parts of the body is summarized in Table 1.7, while the sympathetic afferent innervation is in Table 1.8.

Essential to understanding the effects of spinal anesthesia on function of the sympathetic nervous system is the realization that there is no direct relationship between sensory levels of spinal anesthesia and extent of sympathetic denervation. Anatomic reasons for this include the fact

Table 1.7.
Segmental Motor Innervation of the Viscera[a]

Organ	Higher Cranial Segments	Vagus Nerve	Second to Fourth Sacral Nerves	T1	T2	T3	T4	T5	T6	T7	T8	T9	T10	T11	T12	L1	L2
				Thoracic												Lumbar	
Eyes	+			+	+	+	+										
Salivary glands	+			+	+	?											
Blood vessels of meninges and brain	+			+	+	?											
Blood vessels of head and neck				?	+	+	+										
Sweat glands of head	+			?	+	+	+										
Blood vessels, sweat glands, and erector pili muscles of arms				?	+	+	+	+	+	+	+	+					
Heart		+		+	+	+	+	?									
Lungs		+			+	+	+	?									
Esophagus, stomach, liver, pancreas, and small intestine		+						+	+	+	+	+	+	+			
Adrenal		?									+	+	?	+	+	+	
Kidney													?	?		?	?
Bladder			+											+	+	+	+
Genitalia			+												+	+	+
Colon and rectum			+													+	+
Blood vessels, sweat glands, and erector pili muscles of legs													+	+	+	+	+

Column group headers: *Segments That Give Off Parasympathetic Neurons* (Higher Cranial Segments, Vagus Nerve, Second to Fourth Sacral Nerves); *Segments that Give Off Sympathetic Neurons* (Thoracic, Lumbar).

[a] Reproduced with permission from White, Smithwick, and Simeone, *The Autonomic Nervous System*, The Macmillan Company, New York, 1952

Table 1.8.
Segmental Sensory Innervation of the Viscera[a]

Organ	Superficial Areas to Which Pain is Referred	Thoracic 1	2	3	4	5	6	7	8	9	10	11	12	Lumbar 1	2	Sacral 2	3	4	Peripheral Visceral Pathway
Heart	Precordium and inner arm	+	+	+	?														Middle and inferior cervical and thoracic cardiac nerves
Lung	No referred pain																		
Liver and gallbladder	Right upper quadrant and right scapula						?	+	+	?									Major splanchnic nerve
Stomach	Epigastrium						?	+	+	?									Major splanchnic nerve
Small intestine	Umbilicus									+	+	?							Major splanchnic nerve
Colon Ascending, sigmoid and rectum	Suprapubic Deep pelvis and anus											?	+	+		+	+	+	Lumbar chains and preaortic plexus
Kidney	Loin and groin											?	+	+					Renal plexus via least splanchnic nerve and upper lumbar rami
Ureter	Loin and groin													+	+				Renal plexus and upper lumbar rami
Bladder Fundus	Suprapubic											+	+	+					Lower intercostal nerves
Bladder neck	Perineum and penis															+	+	+	Pelvic nerves
Uterus Fundus	Suprapubic region and lower back											+	+	+					Superior hypogastric plexus
Cervix	Perineum															+	+	+	Pelvic nerves

Segments at Which Visceral Afferent Axons Enter Spinal Cord

[a] Reproduced with permission from White, Smithwick, and Simeone, *The Autonomic Nervous System*, The Macmillan Company, New York, 1952.

that the highest, most cephalad preganglionic sympathetic fibers arise from first thoracic spinal segment. Spinal anesthesia blocks sympathetic fibers only preganglionically. A sympathetic preganglionic block at the first thoracic level results, therefore, in total sympathetic blockade following lumbar injection of local anesthetic solution, a site of injection that also assures blockade of the lowest, most caudad preganglionic sympathetic fibers that arise at the second lumbar spinal segmental level. Also, for reasons stated below (pp. 33–37), the level of sympathetic blockade usually lies about two spinal segments above the level made anesthetic to pinprick. This means that sensory levels of anesthesia to pinprick at the third thoracic segmental level are associated with total preganglionic sympathetic block. Because the extent of sympathetic denervation during spinal anesthesia determines cardiovascular responses to spinal anesthesia, changes in cardiovascular function during cervical levels of spinal anesthesia are no greater than they are in the presence of T_3 levels of sensory anesthesia. Emphasis of this point is redundant in view of the preceding discussion, but it is often clinically implied that the physiologic changes of spinal anesthesia with a sensory block at the fifth cervical level are more profound than they are with a sensory block at T_3. The sympathetic paralysis is the same, that is, complete, in each case.

A second anatomic reason for absence of a direct relationship between sensory levels of anesthesia and the extent of sympathetic denervation lies in the fact that a single preganglionic fiber ascends and descends in the paravertebral sympathetic chain before synapsing with as many as 18 postganglionic sympathetic fibers. These fibers are then distributed peripherally to structures whose sensory segmental innervation does not correspond with the level from which the preganglionic sympathetic fiber arose. Stimulation (or paralysis) of a single preganglionic sympathetic fiber produces diffuse peripheral responses in sensory dermatomes above and below the spinal segmental level at which there is stimulation of the preganglionic fiber.

Finally, a third anatomic reason for differences between extent of sensory and sympathetic denervation, already alluded to on p. 18, is illustrated by the fact that while sympathetic denervation persists longer than does sensory blockade on the trunk (Daos and Virtue, 1963; Pflug, et al., 1978), sympathetic tone in the toes may start to return (as evidenced by return of skin temperature to preanesthetic levels) during regression of spinal anesthesia even though pinprick anesthesia persists in the lower extremity (Roe and Cohn, 1973; Kim, et al., 1977). The concentration of local anesthetic at L_2 may decrease during regression of spinal anesthesia to the point where sympathetic fibers are no longer blocked at L_2 but the concentration of local anesthetic caudal to L_2 may still block sensory fibers innervating part or all of the lower extremity. Afferent input from the feet is thus present in the absence of sympathetic block purely on a neuroanatomic basis, not because sensory fibers are more sensitive than sympathetic fibers to the effects of local anesthetics.

Essential to the study of the effects of spinal anesthesia on the sympathetic nervous system are the sensitivity and accuracy of techniques used to determine in humans whether sympathetic activity is or is not blocked under clinical conditions, and, if blocked, the anatomic extent of the block. Review of the advantages and limitations inherent in methods for *in vivo* clinical measurement of sympathetic denervation is in order before comparing them with similar data on measurements of sensory levels of anesthesia, also in this chapter (p. 41). Such reviews are necessary for establishing a basis for answering questions such as: Do zones of differential blockade of sensory and sympathetic fibers exist during clinical spinal anesthesia? If so, how wide, how extensive are they? Do they change during onset, maintenance, and offset of spinal anesthesia? Are they different with different local anesthetics? Answers to these questions depend on the validity of measurements of sympathetic and sensory blockade. Here, the former is important; the latter is important below (p. 42).

The following review of techniques for evaluation of sympathetic activity during spinal anesthesia is and must be based solely on *in vivo* studies carried out in humans if the results are to be clinically relevant. Furthermore, the review must be limited to data derived only from studies of spinal anesthesia. Data on sympathetic denervation in humans during epidural anesthesia, paravertebral (including stellate ganglion) block, peripheral nerve block, and surgical sympathectomy are not necessarily applicable to spinal anesthesia. Valuable though such data may be in other contexts, they are associated with physical, pharmacologic, or other potentially confounding effects that differentiate them from the pure sympathetic block seen during spinal anesthesia (Greene, 1981). Problems inherent in transfer of data obtained in animal studies to the clinical situation also render studies not carried out in humans irrelevant.

Techniques for measurement of preganglionic sympathetic blockade in humans can be direct or indirect. Only direct studies of axonal conduction in sympathetic fibers in humans can prove beyond all doubt whether or not sympathetic blockade is present. Since data and conclusions from all other techniques are indirect, they are necessarily inferential.

One direct method for measurement of sympathetic denervation, the only one reported in humans, is intraneural measurement of postganglionic sympathetic activity in peripheral tissues. As described by Lundin, *et al.* (1989), this technique provides unequivocal evidence of sympathetic blockade at least during epidural anesthesia. The technique of intraneuronal measurement is so specific that it is also valid during spinal anesthesia. Though both sensitive and specific, this technique nevertheless has major limitations. It is invasive, and provides data on sympathetic conductivity in only one (postganglionic) fiber. Because of its invasiveness, this technique cannot be used for determining how many other sympathetic fibers are also blocked.

Indirect techniques are, thus, necessary for measurement of sympathetic activity during spinal anesthesia in humans. They fall into three categories. One of the three categories centers about measurement of physiologic functions expected to be altered by sympathetic denervation. The second is based on the assumption that there exists a consistent relation between unmeasurable preganglionic activity and more readily measured function of somatic sensory nerves. The third indirect technique involves simple visual examination for evidence of sympathetic denervation that is not dependent on physiologic changes measured in the first category above.

Indirect measurements of sympathetic activity based on altered physiologic responses to sympathetic activity include measurement of changes in cutaneous conductance as reflected by changes in sympathogalvanic reflex activity. The afferent arc of the sympathogalvanic reflex goes from a peripheral sensory site being stimulated to the central autonomic center in the brainstem. The efferent arc from the central autonomic center includes the entirety of sympathetic outflow with, among other responses, an increase in sudomotor activity. This increases the concentration of electrolytes on the cutaneous surface which, in turn, increases the conductivity on the surface of the skin. The change in conductivity can be measured by applying a small electrical current between two electrodes placed on the surface of the skin. The absence of a normal increase in skin conductance following application of an otherwise effective peripheral stimulus is considered to indicate that sympathetic innervation of the site at which the electrodes are placed has been interrupted.

The stimulus used to elicit the sympathogalvanic reflex may consist of immersion of a hand or a foot into ice water (i.e., cold pressor test). The reflex can also be elicited by cutaneous electrical stimulation at a point distant from the site at which galvanic activity is being measured, as well as by nonspecific benign stimuli such as breath-holding during inhalation, taking a short, deep breath, or exposure to a sudden, sharp sound. All the above, except for immersion in ice water, have been used in studies of the effect of spinal anesthesia on skin conductance in humans by a group of Swedish investigators (Löfström, et al., 1984; Bengtsson, et al., 1985). In their 1984 paper these investigators found that skin conductance measured in the hand, the foot and at dermatomal levels of T_5, T_9, and T_{12}–L_1 responded to all the above stimuli, thereby demonstrating that the same stimuli and the same sites of cutaneous conductance measurements could be used for measuring cutaneous conductance during spinal anesthesia. Preliminary clinical data in their 1984 paper indicated that changes in skin conductance normally produced by the stimuli were blocked during spinal anesthesia. Detailed discussion of the usefulness of cutaneous galvanometric changes as an index of the extent of preganglionic sympathetic denervation during clinical spinal anesthesia is delayed until results of studies using it are compared with results using other techniques (below). At this point, however, it should be noted that Kirnö, *et al.* (1991) have raised serious questions above the validity of the assumptions on which the use of galvanic skin response as a measure of sympathetic activity depends. Kirnö, *et al.* confirm that galvanic skin response does indeed measure sweat production. They also found, however, that sweat production itself is a complex function that is not linearly related to sympathetic activity.

Other methods used for measurement of sudomotor activity have included application to the skin of indicators as simple as starch and iodine, whose color changes as a function of the amount of sweat present. Perhaps of some limited use in determination of sympathetic activity in the distal extremities, these methods are impractical during spinal anesthesia since ambient temperature must be increased enough to induce sweating by the patient. They are, furthermore, unreliable if applied to truncal skin in an attempt to define dermatomal levels in which sudomotor activity has been blocked.

A variety of measurements of alterations in peripheral vascular tone have been used as indices of sympathetic denervation. These include measurements of surface skin temperature, cutaneous blood flow, and peripheral arterial pulse wave contours.

Measurements of skin temperature reflect integrity of sympathetic innervation because vasodilation of cutaneous vessels normally associated with sympathetic denervation redistributes blood to the surface of the skin with an increase in its temperature. That skin temperature increases following sympathetic blockade during spinal anesthesia has been well known for many years (Brill and Lawrence, 1930; Foregger, 1943; Felder, *et al.*, 1951). It should be remembered, however, that increases in skin temperature following sympathetic denervation do not necessarily indicate increases in blood flow ($ml \cdot 100g^{-1} \cdot min^{-1}$). They reflect primarily redistribution of cutaneous blood, with an increase in tissue blood flow that may even be associated with vascular stagnation.

The value of changes in skin temperature in determining the extent of sympathetic denervation during spinal anesthesia is limited. Increases in skin temperatures are most easily measured and most pronounced in the feet and hands. If sympathetic innervation of the lower extremities (T_{11}–L_2; Table 1.7) is blocked during spinal anesthesia, skin temperature in the toes increases (Bengtsson, *et al.*, 1983). This provides no information, however, about the extent of sympathetic denervation above T_{11}, levels of considerable importance in mediation of the more profound systemic cardiovascular changes that may be associated with spinal anesthesia. Similarly, because the preganglionic innervation of the upper extremity is so extensive (Table 1.7), it is difficult to define exactly where the most cephalad level of sympathetic denervation lies during spinal anesthesia by measuring skin temperature of the fingers. Skin temperatures of the fingers may also, of course, decrease during spinal anesthesia. This happens when sympathetic function at the T_4–T_1 level remains intact during mid-thoracic levels of sensory anesthesia and participates in a reflex compensatory increase in sympathetic tone (Bengtsson, et al., 1983).

Changes in skin temperature on the trunk are more difficult to measure but physiologically of greater interest than changes in skin temperature of toes and fingers. They might indicate the integrity or lack therefore of mid-thoracic preganglionic sympathetic fibers more precisely than temperatures in digits. Cutaneous temperature probes on skin surfaces of the abdomen are, however, of limited value in measuring changes in skin temperature during spinal anesthesia even in the laboratory, much less in the operating room. More sophisticated, though not easy to use under clinical conditions, are thermographic techniques. Bengtsson (1984), for example, measured skin temperature using infrared thermography in a study that included both sham (everything except lumbar puncture) and operative spinal anesthetics. Sham spinal anesthesia was associated with an average decrease in skin temperature of 0.05 ± 0.6 °C (SD) in all thoracic dermatomes. During operative spinal anesthesia with sensory levels above T_{10}, marked increases in skin temperature were seen only in the feet. On the abdomen there was only a tendency for development of a transition zone between slight increases, slight decreases, or no changes in skin temperature. The level at which this tendency for development of a temperature transition zone lay below, i.e., caudad to, the level of analgesia. Thermographically measured changes in skin temperature on the abdomen were, in this study, modest, too modest to be of material value in measuring the level of preganglionic sympathetic block.

While changes in skin temperature on the trunk measured thermographically by Bengtsson were modest, those reported by Chamberlain and Chamberlain (1986) using infrared thermography were marked and extensive. In fact, 100% of 10 patients having tetracaine spinal anesthesia and 80% of 10 patients having lidocaine spinal anesthesia developed increases in skin temperature to the T_1 level within 26–30 min of injection of the local anesthetic. The authors felt this indicated that sympathetic block also extended to T_1. There was no relation between sensory segmental level of anesthesia and spinal segmental level of increased skin temperature. In this study, patients with T_{10} and even T_{11} levels of sensory anesthesia had total preganglionic sympathetic block as determined by thermographically measured increases in skin temperature. This result is difficult to explain (Greene, 1986). While the thermographic imagery techniques used in the study of Chamberlain and Chamberlain are of proven value in measurements of skin temperature, one wonders if the extensive increases in skin temperature that they recorded might have been related to, or even entirely due to, factors other than spinal anesthesia. Similar studies using double-blind techniques and including sham lumbar punctures appear to be in order.

It appears that while measurements of changes in skin temperature in toes and fingers are accurate indications of the presence or absence of sympathetic denervation of the extremities during spinal anesthesia in the absence of occlusive arterial disease, changes in skin temperature on the trunk, even using thermography, have yet to be proven reliable and accurate reflections of the level of preganglionic sympathetic denervation during spinal anesthesia. Skin temperature measurements give yes or no answers about sympathetic innervation of the toes and fingers but only in toes and fingers. Techniques are needed that provide data on the extent of sympathetic denervation at mid-cordal levels as reflected by changes in skin temperature of the abdomen during spinal anesthesia.

Incidentally, the sensation of warmth in the feet that occurs within 30 sec of injection of a local anesthetic into the lumbar subarachnoid space is not the result of elevation of skin temperature caused by cutaneous hyperemia in the feet. Saddle spinal anesthesia produces a sensation of warmth in the feet in the absence of sympathetic denervation of the feet. Furthermore, the feeling of warmth in the feet precedes by 1½–2½ min any increase in skin temperature in the feet during onset of levels of spinal anesthesia high enough to produce sympathetic denervation (Gordh, 1977). This suggests that the sensation of warmth in the feet soon after induction of spinal anesthesia may be due either to transient stimulation before block of afferent fibers transmitting the sensation of warmth, or to blockade of afferent fibers subserving cold discrimination before blockade of heat discriminatory fibers. To differentiate between these two possibilities under the rapidly changing conditions that take place during induction of clinical spinal anesthesia is difficult. Under more controllable conditions afforded by differential spinal anesthesia, vasodilation of skin vessels of the lower extremities has been observed before a change in temperature discrimination (Nathan, 1979). Indeed, under these circumstances when warmth discrimination was blocked, cold discrimination was often either normal or only diminished, but not eliminated. The early onset of pedal warmth during spinal anesthesia prior to elevation of skin temperature due to sympathetic block may, therefore, represent brief stimulation of fibers involved in transmitting the sensation of warmth. It is not a reflection of increased skin temperature in the feet.

Measurements of cutaneous blood flow instead of cutaneous temperature during spinal anesthesia is another technique that has been used to study the extent and frequency of sympathetic denervation associated with spinal anesthesia. While details of the effect of spinal anesthesia on cutaneous circulation are considered in Chapter 2, it can be said here that, not surprisingly, changes in skin blood flow in general parallel changes in skin temperature during spinal anesthesia when cutaneous flow is measured by Doppler flowmetry (Bengtsson, et al., 1983). However, when Bengtsson, et al., plotted individual relative changes in skin temperature against individual relative changes in skin blood flow, no consistent correlation was found. This suggests that in an individual case measurements of cutaneous blood flow or cutaneous temperature may be of finite value as an indication of sympathetic denervation even in fingers and toes. Even if they do give information about sympathetic innervation in fingers and toes, they, too, give no information about sympathetic activity in mid-thoracic dermatomes. These same limitations apply when digital blood volumes (ml·100 g^{-1}) are measured plethysmographically, or, when combined with occlusive techniques, are used to measure blood flow (ml·100 g^{-1}·min^{-1}). Changes in capillary oxygen tension as a result of changes in tissue blood flow consequent to sympathetic denervation have been reported (Bridenbaugh, et al., 1971), but the information derived is of limited physiologic usefulness in quantitation of the spinal segmental level of sympathetic denervation during spinal anesthesia.

Measurement of pulse wave contours is another method that has been used to evaluate sympathetic blockade on the basis that the vasodilation consequent to sympathetic denervation changes the volume and velocity of arterial pulses (Meijer, et al., 1988). These measurements, along with measurements of skin temperature, skin blood flow, and skin blood volume, are all of use principally in extremities. Pulse wave contours in arteries supplying the central nervous system or abdominal viscera during spinal anesthesia would be of interest but have not yet been reported.

Neither changes in heart rate nor changes in blood pressure are reliable indicators of the extent of preganglionic sympathetic blockade during spinal anesthesia. Too many other factors are involved in responses of heart rate and blood pressure to sympathetic blockade produced by spinal anesthesia, including age, position of the patient, blood volume, other autonomically active drugs given pre- or intraoperatively, the amount of intravenous fluids administered, sensory adequacy of the anesthesia, and intraoperative surgical manipulations.

The second category of methods available for measuring the extent of preganglionic sympathetic denervation during spinal anesthesia, techniques not based on studies of physiologic variables, assumes the existence of a relatively constant relationship between the levels of sensory somatic and preganglionic sympathetic denervation. The assumption that such a relationship exists may be reasonable, but that it actually exists and, especially, if it does exist, the specifics of the relationship are matters of controversy. Three possibilities exist: levels of denervation are the same with both sensory and sympathetic fibers; somatic sensory fibers are more sensitive to local anesthetic action than are sympathetic fibers and, thus more extensively blocked than preganglionic fibers; or, finally, sympathetic fibers are more sensitive to local anesthetic and thus they are more extensively blocked than somatic sensory fibers. The simplicity of measurement of dermatomal levels of sensory anesthesia under clinical conditions is so considerable that, if the existence of a constant relationship between levels of somatic sensory and preganglionic block could be established, the clinician could readily evaluate both the adequacy of the level of surgical anesthesia and the potential for physiologic trespass based on the level of sympathetic denervation.

Three cutaneous stimuli have been most frequently used to assess, both experimentally and clinically, the sensory levels of spinal anesthesia: temperature discrimination, pinprick, and light touch. Consistency of results is best achieved if these stimuli are always applied to the skin of the abdomen in the same plane, usually the midclavicular or the anterior axillary line. The latter is preferable when measuring high thoracic sensory levels of anesthesia, especially in females with large or pendulous breasts that make difficult definition of the T_4 dermatome anteriorly. When these three modalities are tested, each is found to be blocked at different dermatomal levels (Brull and Greene, 1989). During hyperbaric spinal anesthesia temperature discrimination is lost in dermatomes that lie at statistically significantly higher (more cephalad) segmental levels than do the dermatomes in which the sensation of pinprick is lost, which in turn lie at statistically significantly higher segmental levels than the dermatomes in which the sensation of light touch is lost (Fig. 1.6; Brull and Greene, 1989). The consistency of the width of the differential blockade between dermatomal levels of loss of temperature discrimination is remarkable. So is the loss of pinprick sensation when these two modalities were first used in 1958 to establish the presence of zones of differential blockade (Greene, 1958) and when they were used again under similarly controlled conditions for the same purposes more than 30 years later (Brull and Greene, 1989). In the 1989 study, it was also found that the zones of differential sensory blockade remained essentially unchanged during onset, maintenance, and offset of spinal anesthesia, and that the zones were similar with tetracaine and with bupivacaine spinal anesthetics.

Rocco, *et al.* (1985) used the same stimuli as used by Greene (1958) and by Brull and Greene (1989) to evaluate zones of differential sensory blockade during clinical spinal anesthesia. They, too, found that with both lidocaine and tetracaine dermatomal levels of anesthesia to touch

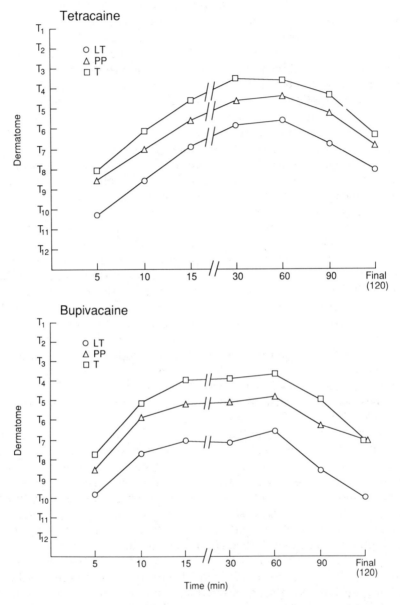

Figure 1.6. Levels of thoracic dermatomal blockade of light touch (LT), pinprick (PP), and temperature (T) discrimination as a function of time (min) during tetracaine (top) and bupivacaine (bottom) spinal anesthesia. (Reproduced with permission from Brull and Greene, Anesth. Analg. 69: 342, 1989.)

lay consistently and statistically significantly caudad to the levels of anesthesia to pinprick and cold sensation. Unlike the findings reported by Brull and Greene (1989), Rocco, *et al.* found that the extent (i.e., dermatomal levels) of the sensory denervations did not increase and decrease in a parallel manner during onset and offset of anesthesia. Segmental levels of blockade of different types of nerve fibers would be expected to change together, in parallel, during spinal anesthesia if there was a differential sensitivity to anesthetic blocking action of local anesthetics. Because of the absence of parallelism, Rocco, *et al.* concluded that differential anesthetic sensitivity of the nerves involved the type of stimuli used to detect it. In their study there were also no consistent, statistically significant differences in dermatomal levels of anesthesia to pinprick and to temperature discrimination. The reasons for failure to observe pinprick-to-temperature zones of differential blockade in this study are not clear, but the fact that levels of both pinprick and temperature anesthesia were consistently above levels or anesthesia to touch confirms the existence of differential zones of sensory blockade.

There is currently no doubt that, when studies under appropriately controlled conditions in statistically valid numbers of patients without hearing or cognitive disability, zones of differential sensory anesthesia can be identified during hyperbaric spinal anesthesia. Although there are no reported studies of zones of differential sensory blockade during iso- and hypobaric spinal anesthesia, it seems likely that they, too, would exist, since these spinal anesthetic techniques are also likely to be associated with gradients of concentration of local anesthetic in CSF on either side of the epicenter of highest concentration (Figs. 1.4 and 1.5).

The fact that zones of differential sensory blockade are present during hyperbaric spinal anesthesia supports the contention that it is likely that zones of differential sympathetic blockade also exist during spinal anesthesia. The first systematic attempt to define the extent of sympathetic blockade during clinical spinal anesthesia with a view toward determining the possible existence of a zone of differential sensory and sympathetic blockade was reported in 1958 (Greene, 1958). As mentioned above it is difficult to the point of impossibility to obtain reliable measurements under clinical conditions of the extent of sympathetic denervation on the trunk. This early attempt to measure sympathetic blockade in patients given hyperbaric spinal anesthesia was based on the hypothesis that loss of the ability to discriminate temperature might be at least an approximation of the level of the loss of sympathetic activity based on the closeness of degrees of myelination, axonal diameters, and conduction velocities (Table 1.6). The assumption was that spinal segmental sympathetic activity was blocked at least to the spinal segmental level at which temperature discrimination was lost. Appreciation of the sense of cold was measured by applying a sponge soaked in ether to the skin of the abdomen in the mid-clavicular line. Spraying a highly volatile liquid on the skin is equally useful. The technique has the disadvantage of being based on the assumption that temperature discrimination is an accurate index of sympathetic function. This limitation is offset, however, by the possibility that the extent of loss of temperature discrimination may underestimate rather than overestimate the extent of sympathetic denervation, probably by a relatively small amount. The advantage of this technique for estimation of sympathetic activity based on loss of temperature discrimination lies in a simplicity so great that it can be used under the difficult conditions of an operating room during anesthesia and surgery. This technique has been widely and frequently used by other investigators with similar results.

The observations of Meijer, *et al.* (1988) are confirmatory of loss of temperature discrimination as a reflection of preganglionic sympathetic denervation during spinal anesthesia. These investigators found that the onset of increased amplitude of pulse waves in the toes occurring following induction of spinal anesthesia, an indication of sympathetic denervation, is associated with equally prompt loss of the ability to sense cold when ice was applied to the dermatome corresponding to the level at which lumbar puncture was performed. The loss of temperature discrimination that occurred simultaneously with increase in pulse wave amplitude preceded the onset of complete sensory anesthesia in the same dermatome.

The third and last of the categories of indirect measurements of sympathetic denervation under clinical conditions is visual evidence of sympathetic denervation based not on vascular responses but on sympathetic neuroanatomy. This category of indirect measurement compellingly supports the existence of zones of differential sensory blockade during spinal anesthesia that presage the existence of zones of differential sympathetic blockade. The neuroanatomic factors providing visual evidence of sympathetic denervation are operative only during high sensory levels of spinal anesthesia. Specifically, repeated personal (N.M.G.) observations have shown that sensory (pinprick) levels of spinal anesthesia at the level of T_3 are associated with an extraordinarily high frequency of development of bilateral Horner's syndromes. Because they occur bilaterally, the Horner's syndromes are not conspicuous and may be missed. Ptosis, miosis, conjunctival injection, and anophthalmia may be seen, however, when the patient is carefully examined, though facial anhidrosis is difficult to detect. These changes are seen only, of course, if drugs altering sympathetic or parasympathetic activity have not been administered before or during the course of anesthesia. Horner's syndromes are never seen with pinprick levels of spinal anesthesia caudad to T_4, and only rarely with pinprick levels at T_4, but they are almost invariably present with pinprick levels of spinal anesthesia at T_3 when they are specifically sought, though if not sought, not seen.

The only way Horner's syndromes can develop in the presence of T_3 sensory levels of spinal anesthesia is by blockade of preganglionic sympathetic fibers at the level of T_1, T_2, T_3, and T_4. With most hyperbaric spinal anesthetics, sensory blockade to T_3 is therefore associated with complete sympathetic denervation. The existence of Horner's syndromes with sensory pinprick levels at T_3 means there must exist a zone of differential sensory blockade (at T_3) and preganglionic sympathetic blockade (at T_1). Measurements of the dermatomal level of loss of temperature discrimination at the T_1 level in the presence of Horner's syndrome associated with T_3 levels of pinprick anesthesia have not been carried out. Such measurements would test whether loss of temperature discrimination is an accurate measure of sympathetic blockade, but this would be unlikely, since temperature discrimination on the skin of the face is mediated by the trigeminal nerves, not spinal nerves.

The preponderance of evidence in the preceding review of methods used to evaluate the extent of sympathetic blockade leads to three conclusions. First, sympathetic denervation occurs during spinal anesthesia. Second, anatomically the denervation occurs preganglionically within the subarachnoid space. And, third, the dermatomal level at which the ability to discriminate cold is lost is a reasonable, reproducible, and consistent method for estimation of the extent of sympathetic denervation during spinal anesthesia under clinical conditions. The level of preganglionic blockade might lie a bit above or even a bit below the dermatomal level at which temperature discrimination is lost, but measurement of temperature discrimination as an indication of sympathetic denervation is simple to do and, above all, it is free of findings that cannot be explained on an anatomic basis or on the basis of technical limitations associated with other methods used for measuring sympathetic denervation. Loss of temperature discrimination never leads to the anomalous finding that preganglionic sympathetic denervation is essentially complete during all spinal anesthetics, regardless of sensory levels of anesthesia, as suggested by thermographic techniques for measurement of sympathetic denervation. Nor does the dermatomal level of loss of temperature discrimination lead to anomalous findings suggested by galvanometric techniques. For example, galvanometric techniques suggest that the resistance of preganglionic fibers is so great that it is possible for extensive enough sympathetic activity to be retained in lumbar and sacral dermatomes during spinal anesthesia to provide thoracic sensory anesthesia and lumbar levels of motor blockade following injection of local anesthetic into the subarachnoid space at the L_2 level of origin of the last and most caudad preganglionic fibers.

The pharmacologic explanation for the existence of differential blockade of preganglionic sympathetic fibers remains to be agreed on. This phenomenon is related to two others: nerve fiber size and concentration of local anesthetic in CSF. Sensitivity of nerve fibers to the blocking effect of local anesthetics is often, though not invariably, inversely related to nerve fiber size: the larger the nerve fiber, the less the sensitivity, and, in general, the smaller the nerve fiber, the greater the sensitivity. One does not see large motor fibers blocked with resulting somatic muscle paralysis during spinal anesthesia in the absence of sensory anesthesia. Also, as indicated above, gradients of concentration of local anesthetics exist in CSF that coincide with levels of differential sensory blockade. Indeed, it is possible to produce cutaneous vasodilation, that is, sympathetic denervation, without any change in peripheral sensory ability, by injecting into the subarachnoid space very dilute concentrations of local anesthetic (Nathan, 1979). Varying the concentration of local anesthetic injected makes it possible to intentionally produce, for diagnostic and therapeutic purposes, differential blockade not only of sympathetic fibers, but also of other types of nerves (Maxson, 1938; Sarnoff and Arrowood, 1946, 1947; Arrowood and Sarnoff, 1948; Tuohy, 1952; Landau, et al., 1960; McCollum and Stephen, 1964; Ghia, et al., 1979).

Differential sensitivity also may be related to factors other than pharmacologic sensitivity. For example, is the ventral or dorsal location of spinal nerve roots within the subarachnoid space a determinant of sensitivity to local anesthetics? If so, is this merely a reflection of ventral and dorsal differences in concentration of local anesthetic in CSF, especially when hyperbaric solutions are used and the patient is in the supine position?

The clinical significance of the fact that the level of preganglionic sympathetic denervation extends beyond the dermatomal level of pinprick anesthesia is that, when combined with the autonomic motor supply to various parts of the body (indicated in Table 1.7) and the autonomic sensory innervation (in Table 1.8), and, in view of the diffuse peripheral response to preganglionic denervation, then even "low" spinal anesthesia may be associated with considerable sympathetic paralysis. For example, a concentration of anesthetic agent may be present in the spinal fluid at the 11th thoracic vertebral level that will produce sympathetic denervation of the pelvic viscera and the lower limbs, yet the somatic sensory loss may not extend above the first lumbar segment. Even with a low sensory blockade there may frequently be some degree of concomitant sympathetic denervation if the concentration of local anesthetic at the second lumbar level is sufficient to block sympathetic fibers. Also, with "saddle anesthesia" obtained by slowly injecting a hyperbaric solution at the third lumbar interspace with the patient sitting, there may well be enough turbulence created within the subarachnoid space to carry the small amount of anesthetic necessary to block sympathetic fibers up to the second lumbar level. This may happen frequently, and there can be no real assurance that "saddle block" or, for that matter, any spinal anesthetic can invariably be given without some sympathetic paralysis. The slight degrees of sympathetic involvement that may accompany "saddle anesthesia" are neither normally apparent nor of clinical significance, but they may assume real importance in patients in hemorrhagic shock whose cardiovascular systems tolerate poorly any degree of sympathetic paralysis. On the other hand, as mentioned above (p. 18), during regression of spinal anesthesia it is possible, because of anatomic reasons, for sympathetic blockade to wear off before there is complete return of sensory function in the lower extremity and in the perineum.

In the same manner, sensory anesthesia to the seventh thoracic segment as for appendectomy is usually be associated with block of the sympathetic nerves to the fifth thoracic segment or higher. In such a case there is sympathetic denervation of the abdominal viscera and partial denervation of some of the thoracic organs. Spinal anesthesia high enough for upper abdominal surgery (e.g., cholecystectomy, gastrectomy) usually involves preganglionic sympathetic paralysis to the first thoracic level. There will then be a complete sympathetic block.

The extensive sympathetic innervation of the upper extremities shown in Table 1.7 serves as still another example of how extensive the impairment of sympathetic function may be during spinal anesthesia. Stimulation of any thoracic anterior root, from the second to the tenth inclusive, produces changes in skin resistance (a function of sympathetic activity) in the upper extremity (Ray, et al., 1943). Preganglionic block at these levels depresses autonomic activity in the arms. Since sensory paralysis to the mid-thoracic level is frequently obtained with spinal anesthesia, the autonomic innervation to the arms is impaired in such cases even though this may not be clinically apparent.

The knowledge that the level of sympathetic denervation extends further cephalad than does sensory (or motor) denervation during spinal anesthesia was used in the deliberate induction of hypotension ("hypotensive spinal") with vasodilation (Gillies, 1953; Griffiths and Gillies, 1948; Greene, 1952; Greene, et al., 1954) to decrease operative blood loss and to facilitate certain types of surgery in the years prior to the introduction of trimethaphan, hexamethonium, nitroprusside, nitroglycerin, and other vasodilators. Hypotensive spinal anesthesia was aimed at paralyzing the entire sympathetic outflow up to the first thoracic segment without producing an equally high blockade of sensory and motor nerves. At the time when complete preganglionic sympathetic block was achieved by this anesthetic technique, sensory anesthesia usually extended to the second or third thoracic segments, yet somatic motor nerves were blocked only to the fourth or fifth thoracic level.

Though not included in Table 1.7, we should mention the role of the sympathetic nervous system in production of CSF by the choroid plexus. There is ample histochemical, ultrastructural, and functional evidence that the mammalian choroid plexus is sympathetically innervated (Edvinsson, et al., 1974; Lindvall, et al., 1978; Herbst, et al., 1979; Nathanson, 1979). Adrenergic nerve fibers from the cervical sympathetic chain supply not only arterioles within the choroid plexus but also choroidal secretory epithelial cells. Their function is inhibitory. Cervical sympathetic stimulation decreases the normal rate of cerebrospinal fluid production by 32% (about 9.5% of total spinal fluid is normally replaced every minute). Surgical sympathectomy increases the rate of production by 33% over a period of 1–2 hr (Lindvall, et al., 1978). Total sympathetic block during T_3 sensory levels of spinal anesthesia would therefore be expected to be associated with an increase in the rate of production of CSF. The clinical significance of this remains to be determined, but spinal anesthesia would be expected to be associated with an increase, not a decrease in spinal fluid production. Postspinal headaches are due to decreased volume of CSF, but this is the result of increased loss of spinal fluid through the dural puncture, not decreased formation of spinal fluid by the choroid plexus. The increase in CSF pressure observed in experimental animals following stimulation of the cervical sympathetic nerves (Dorigotti and Glässer, 1972) occurs too rapidly to be due to changes in spinal fluid production. It probably represents changes in cerebral blood flow.

Information is lacking on the effects of spinal anesthesia on the rate of absorption of CSF within the spinal subarachnoid space. It seems unlikely that spinal anesthesia increases the rate of resorption of spinal fluid and thus contributes to a decrease in spinal fluid volume associated with postspinal headaches, especially several days after anesthesia, which is when postspinal headaches usually start.

One wonders if the expected increase in rate of production of CSF that may be associated with spinal anesthesia might contribute to development of tachyphylaxis by washing out or diluting local anesthetic in CSF.

Finally, spinal anesthesia predictably protects patients with spinal cord lesions at or above the T_6 level from the severe hypertension precipitated by operations performed in areas below T_6. This action is hardly surprising in view of the sympathetic denervation produced by spinal anesthesia. Spinal anesthesia is, however, no better and no worse than general anesthesia in protecting paraplegic patients from such hypertensive crises (Lambert, et al., 1982). The ability of spinal anesthesia to block mass sympathetic reflex activity in paraplegic patients also provides strong evidence of the extent to which sympathetics are blocked during spinal anesthesia.

Effects of Spinal Anesthesia on the Parasympathetic Nervous System

Spinal anesthesia has no effects on the cranial portions of the parasympathetic nervous system. Paralysis of parasympathetic fibers as they cross the subarachnoid space from their points of origin in the second, third, and fourth sacral segments occurs, however, with practically all spinal anesthetics. This has little effect on physiologic function except as related to the genital organs and the lower portion of the urinary tract. Because parasympathetic fibers are of small diameter and are thus particularly sensitive to the effects of local anesthetics, and because the concentration of local anesthetics is usually greatest in the caudad portions of the subarachnoid space, parasympathetic blockade may be prolonged well into the postoperative period. Since these fibers innervate the muscles of micturition, inability to void following spinal anesthesia is often related to continued block of parasympathetic motor function even when the anesthesia has otherwise apparently worn off. The residual paralysis of the parasympathetically innervated muscles involved in voiding becomes of special concern when normovolemic patients are overhydrated during spinal anesthesia as a means for prophylaxis or treatment of intraoperative hypotension. The resultant increase in urinary output in the presence of neurologic paralysis of the muscles of micturition often necessitates bladder catheterization.

Effects of Spinal Anesthesia on Afferent Sensory Nerves

Sensory anesthesia following injection of local anesthetics is primarily the result of two simultaneous pharmacologic effects: block of dorsal root ganglia (Frumin, et al., 1953, 1954) and block of sensory afferent dorsal spinal nerve roots. The former are probably more sensitive to the effects of local anesthetics than the latter. Both are, however, more resistant to the effects of local anesthetics than are efferent preganglionic sympathetic fibers. This explains the zone of differential sympathetic block which extends cephalad to the level of sensory blockade during hyperbaric spinal anesthesia. Both dorsal root ganglia and dorsal spinal nerve roots are also more sensitive to the effects of local anesthetics than are efferent somatic motor fibers. This explains the zone of differential motor block-ade which extends caudal to the level of sensory blockade during hyper-baric spinal anesthesia (p. 47).

The sensitivities of different sensory fibers to local anesthetics, due either to block of dorsal root ganglia or to block of dorsal spinal nerve roots are, however, often difficult to determine in humans during spinal anesthesia. They are especially difficult to determine by measuring the sequence in which the fibers are blocked during induction of spinal anes-thesia. Events move too rapidly to allow the subtle distinctions to be made that are necessary to accurately separate when different sensory modalities are blocked. Assessments of zones of differential blockade of sensory fibers after a stable level had become established are not only difficult to perform under clinical conditions, but also they may be con-founded by anatomic differences in the points of origin in the spinal cord of different nerves innervating the same peripheral cutaneous area analogous to the differences in points of origin of sympathetic and sen-sory fibers innervating the toes (p. 18).

To the above complexities can be added the fact, already alluded to above, that different types of sensory afferent fibers have different sensi-tivities to local anesthetics during clinical spinal anesthesia.

Yet another consideration in measurements of effects of spinal anes-thesia on somatic sensory fibers under clinical conditions is that the re-sults of testing can differ depending on the stimuli used as well as on how the stimuli are applied. Quantitative sensory tests developed during a study of epidural anesthesia (Arendt-Nielsen, et al., 1990 a) showed, when applied to a study of spinal anesthesia (Arendt-Nielsen, 1990 b), that argon laser pulses with output power ranging from 50 mW to 3.5 W (the latter being of an intensity short of that causing burns) could elicit pain in dermatomes anesthetic to pinprick. As the authors suggest, pain evoked by laser pulses may have the advantage of providing nociceptive stimuli closer to stimuli associated with a surgical incision than do stimuli provided by pinprick, and thus may provide more realistic estimates of the extent of operative anesthesia. Another advantage of laser pulses is that they avoid the technical problem inherent in using pinpricks as sensory stimuli: how does one dissociate sense of touch from that of pain when a sharp pin is applied to the skin?

Arendt-Nielsen, et al., also found that the number of stimuli applied to the same dermatome affected the ability of patients to perceive pain. Stimulation of a dermatome with ten needles elicited pain in a der-matome that was anesthetic to stimulation using one needle. As the authors note, this observation can be explained by the fact that spatial summation of afferent stimuli can affect thresholds to painful stimuli, a fact described many years ago by Sherrington (1907) and Hardy and Oppel (1937). Spatial summation of afferent stimuli may be why surgical incisions may be felt in dermatomes anesthetic to pinprick stimuli.

The preceding discussion indicates that dermatomal zones of differential sensory anesthesia develop during clinical spinal anesthesia but that the complexities involved in determining peripheral cutaneous pain thresholds are so great that simple stimuli widely used to measure these thresholds (temperature, pinprick, light touch) are not necessarily reliable as indicative of dermatomal levels of anesthesia so profound that a surgical incision will not be felt. There has been no systematic clinical study defining the exact relation, if any, between dermatomal anesthesia to surgical incision and dermatomal anesthesia to temperature, pinprick, or light touch. Clinical observation suggests that the segmental level for surgical anesthesia (skin incision) during hyperbaric spinal anesthesia may lie caudad to levels of anesthesia as reflected by the three most frequently used tests mentioned above. Since the segmental level of anesthesia to light touch lies below levels of anesthesia to temperature and pinprick, this suggests that light touch may be more useful than temperature or pinprick under clinical conditions as an index of where the segmental level of surgical anesthesia is. The prudent anesthesiologist may aim at providing patients having spinal anesthesia with dermatomal levels of light touch anesthesia one or two dermatomes above the dermatome in which the incision is to be made in preference to relying solely on levels of anesthesia to temperature or pinprick.

A caveat should be mentioned with regard to measures of sensory input such as peripheral vibratory sense and proprioception during recovery from (or during induction of) spinal anesthesia. They may not be accurate indices of differential sensitivity to local anesthetics of fibers in the subarachnoid space. Sensory pathways innervating structures beneath the skin are not the same as those that innervate overlying skin. Sensory anesthesia to pinprick in the skin overlying the external malleolus of the ankle in the presence of unimpaired vibratory sense does not necessarily prove the existence of differential blockade in the subarachnoid space. Sensory innervation of the bone enters the cord at a different level than does the sensory innervation of overlying skin. One could be blocked without the other, without proving the existence of differential blockade within the subarachnoid space. Analogous to this difference between dermatomal and mesenchymal segmental levels of sensory innervation is the better known but much greater difference between dermatomal and endodermal segmental levels of sensory innervation. Afferent sensory innervation of abdominal viscera is so different from sensory innervation of the overlying skin that, for example, surgical anesthesia at the T_{10} dermatomal level is adequate for a McBurney incision for an appendectomy, but sensory innervation of the appendix and the attached mesentery requires that at least a T_{4-6} level of dermatomal anesthesia be provided.

Pain due to a tourniquet during an otherwise satisfactory spinal anesthesia has been the subject of a host of studies and articles after first being reported by Cole in 1952. The popularity of tourniquet pain as a topic in the anesthetic literature is due perhaps as much to the enigma of its neuroanatomic, neurophysiologic, or neuropharmacologic basis as to the frequency with which it creates the clinically awkward situation when successful spinal anesthesia suddenly becomes a failed spinal anesthesia. Factors that have been implicated in onset of pain due to an inflated tourniquet on the lower extremity during satisfactory operative levels of spinal anesthesia include duration of inflation of the tourniquet, the amount of local anesthetic injected, the sensory level of anesthesia, the local anesthetic used, baricity of the anesthetic solution, and addition of vasoconstrictors or narcotics to the local anesthetic solution. Clinical impressions to the contrary, there is apparently no relation between the length of time the tourniquet is inflated and the incidence of tourniquet pain (Rocco, *et al.*, 1985; Bridenbaugh, *et al.*, 1986). On the other hand, the greater the amount, that is, dose, of local anesthetic used to produce the spinal anesthesia, the lower the incidence of pain (Egbert and Deas, 1962) when different doses are associated with equal sensory levels of anesthesia. This finding probably reflects the fact that an increase in dose produces a greater concentration of local anesthetic in CSF and, therefore, a more prolonged and intense degree of neural blockade. On the other hand, there is no relation between sensory level of spinal anesthesia and the occurrence of tourniquet pain when the sensory level is at or above about T_9 (de Jong and Cullen, 1963; Bonnet, *et al.*, 1988; Bridenbaugh, *et al.*, 1986). This suggests the possibility that at least some afferent fibers transmitting impulses arising from the site of the tourniquet bypass the neural blockade in the subarachnoid space by traveling cephalad in the paravertebral sympathetic chain to enter the cord at a level above the level of sensory anesthesia (de Jong, 1962; de Jong and Cullen, 1963). This in turn raises the possibility that the zones of differential sensory blockade that exist craniad to the dermatomal level of surgical anesthesia (pp. 15–18; 33–34) may be involved in the appearance of tourniquet pain unrelated to sensory level of anesthesia as estimated by pinprick. This possibility is supported by the observation that while the level of pinprick anesthesia does not correlate with the occurrence of tourniquet pain, the level of anesthesia to light touch does (Rocco, *et al.*, 1985).

With regard to the role of the local anesthetic itself in the development of tourniquet pain, Concepcion, *et al.* (1988) found that 15 mg of bupivacaine and 15 mg of tetracaine were associated with a statistically significant difference (25% and 60%, respectively) in the incidence of tourniquet pain, despite equal sensory levels of anesthesia. This local anesthetic dependency of the frequency of tourniquet pain may be explained on the basis of two factors. First, small A-delta and C fibers transmitting, respectively, fast and slow pain represent the neural pathway by which nociceptive impulses from the site of the tourniquet are conducted to the spinal cord. Second, there exists a differential sensitivity of C fibers to the blocking effects of bupivacaine and tetracaine. This involves sensitivity to frequency-dependent conduction, such that bupivacaine produces greater blockade than tetracaine (Strichartz and Zimmermann, 1984). Equal concentrations of bupivacaine and tetracaine in higher thoracic CSF fluid decrease equally over time, but a point is reached at which, though the concentrations are still equal, the concentration of tetracaine is no longer sufficient to block C fibers, while the same concentration of bupivacaine can (Stewart, *et al.*, 1988). Attractive though such an explanation may be, the origin of tourniquet pain may involve more than pressure and pain produced by the tourniquet (Hagenouw, *et al.*, 1986). Indeed, multivariate causes of tourniquet pain may make unitary explanations for its occurrence impossible. It has been reported, for example, that glucose injected intrathecally increases the incidence of tourniquet pain by some (Bridenbaugh, *et al.*, 1986) though not by others (Bonnet, *et al.*, 1988).

Another interesting but clinically benign neurophysiologic phenomenon that can be seen with considerable frequency when deliberately sought out is the appearance of nonpainful phantom limb sensations (Khurana, *et al.*, 1979). These sensations consist of the feeling that, shortly after induction of spinal anesthesia, one or both lower extremities lie in a position different than that in which the extremity actually is. Most often the position in which the phantom limb lies is similar to or even the same as the position in which the limb was at the time of onset of motor blockade. Twenty-four percent of the patients studied by Prevoznik and Eckenhoff (1964) whose legs were at right angles to the trunk at the onset of motor blockade continued to feel that their lower limbs were still in that position after the legs had been straightened out. Similarly, Khurana, *et al.* (1979) found that none of 50 patients given spinal anesthesia who were in the supine position with legs stretched out in the neutral position experienced phantom limb sensations but that 83% of 30 patients whose thighs were flexed on the abdomen at the onset of motor blockage developed phantom limb sensations. The incidence was 80% in patients who were in the lithotomy position as the anesthesia set. Straightening the legs out immediately after the intrathecal injection should be used to avoid this curious but sometimes unsettling phenomenon.

To be differentiated from the nonpainful phantom limb sensation during spinal anesthesia is the acute precipitation by spinal anesthesia of often exquisitely severe pain in the phantom limb of an amputee (Davis, 1958; Harrison, 1951; Leatherdale, 1956; Mackenzie, 1983; Moore, 1946; Murphy and Anandaciva, 1984; Sellick, 1985). The pain can suddenly appear in a patient with a previously totally asymptomatic amputation stump, even 40 years after the amputation. Pain in a previously painful amputation stump can also be worsened by spinal anesthesia. The pain associated with spinal anesthesia can be in either the stump or in a phantom limb. Painful phantom limbs have not been reported in nonamputees.

How and why spinal anesthesia can elicit either a phantom limb sensation in a normal patient, or precipitate acute phantom limb pain in a previously pain-free amputee is as obscure as is the etiology of phantom limb pain in the absence of spinal anesthesia. The consensus is that central mechanisms are involved in both instances. The how and why of nonpainful phantom limb sensations in nonamputees is probably related to a "memory pattern" of positional sense normally established in a closed neuronal circuit within the spinal cord. This closed circuit is normally continuously altered by input from the periphery. In the absence of peripheral input following induction of spinal anesthesia, the closed circuit, no longer modified, becomes self-perpetuating. The resulting repetitive pattern is interpreted as persistence of the position of the limb. The how and why of the acute precipitation of a painful phantom limb sensation in a previously asymptomatic patient is more difficult to define in view of the concept developed by Melzack (1971) that normally the brainstem reticular system inhibits transmission throughout the somatic sensory system. Amputation with loss of sensory input from the amputated extremity decreases the inhibitory effect of the reticular system and sets the stage for neural activity that is self-perpetuating and able to recruit neuronal activity in neighboring structures. This theory leads to the hypothesis that regional anesthesia, by altering total sensory input, would decrease the self-perpetuating neuronal activity and so relieve pain perceived as coming from the amputated limb. But spinal anesthesia does not relieve preexisting phantom limb pain. It may precipitate it if previously absent. Alternatively, perhaps sensory input from the periphery may normally have a general inhibitory effect on afferent input into the cord from other peripheral areas. With blockade of inhibitory input from a number of peripheral areas induced by spinal anesthesia, previously inhibited painful stimuli from the amputated extremity would then enter the cord without being attenuated.

When acute phantom limb pain does occur during spinal anesthesia, intravenous calcitonin may relieve it (Fiddler and Hindman, 1991), as may intravenous thiopental (Koyama, et al., 1988), other barbiturates and opioids.

Amputation stump neuromas that are painful even in the absence of tactile or other stimuli, are to be differentiated from spontaneously occuring phantom limb pain, even though neurophysiologically the two entities may be related. Spinal anesthesia does not aggravate neuromas or precipitate pain in an amputation stump. Spinal anesthesia may not, though, relieve pain in an amputation stump if the pain has been present long enough to have a central projection, that is pain which is unaffected by peripheral sensory denervation.

Effects of Spinal Anesthesia on Somatic Motor Nerves

Somatic motor nerves are, principally because of their large size, the most resistant of all fibers in the subarachnoid space to the effects of local anesthetics. Since larger motor fibers are more resistant to the effects of local anesthetics than are smaller sensory fibers, a level of somatic motor paralysis develops which is more caudad than the level of sensory block. Walts, et al. (1964) employed an electromyophone to determine the level of intercostal muscle activity in 33 patients during hyperbaric tetracaine spinal anesthesia. They found the average level of motor paralysis to be $T_{6.2}$ at a time when sensory levels averaged $T_{4.4}$. A similar zone of differential blockade between motor and sensory levels averaging about two spinal segments was also observed by Freund, et al. (1967) using electromyographic techniques. Because of this zone of differential motor blockade, the phrenic nerves usually remain unaffected by even mid-cervical levels of lumbar spinal anesthesia.

Though a zone of differential motor blockade classically develops during operative surgical anesthesia, the effect of differential spinal anesthesia on somatic motor function is more complex. Landau, et al. (1960), for example, administered differential procaine spinal anesthetics to 6 normal patients and to 12 patients with various types of chronic spasticity. This allowed them to block differentially fusimotor (A-gamma) fibers. They found that tendon reflexes were abolished at a time when muscle strength and proprioception (A-alpha and A-beta) were unimpaired. The selective blockade of the small ventral root fibers which constitute the efferent innervation of muscle spindle tension receptors explains the paradox first noted by Sarnoff and Arrowood (1947) that abdominal, knee kick, and ankle jerk reflexes are abolished during differential spinal anesthesia at a time when position sense, vibratory sense, and motor power remain unimpaired.

An interesting though rare response of somatic muscles to spinal anesthesia is the development of clonus. Fox, et al. (1979), reported a case in which myoclonus of both lower extremities occurred as the sensory level of anesthesia regressed from T_8. Myoclonus started when the sensory level had receded to T_{12} on one side, and to L_2 on the other side. It became most marked when the sensory level was L_2 on both sides. Myoclonus ceased when the sensory level had regressed to L_5.

Nadkarni and Tondare (1982) and Moorthy and Dierdorf (1990) reported similar cases in which transitory bilateral plantar flexion with bursts of clonic contractions of muscles of the lower extremities and abdomen also developed during regression of spinal anesthesia. Differing from the preceding reports is the elderly patient described by Watanabe, et al. (1987) who developed lower extremity myoclonus on two occasions during onset of, not during recovery from, spinal anesthesia. The myoclonus continued, though lessened in severity, for 70 min during spinal anesthesia adequate for a 2½-hr abdominal operation.

The etiology of the myoclonus in the patient reported by Nadkarni and Tondare (1982) was ascribed by the authors to increased spinal cord irritability associated with cord ischemia produced by the epinephrine injected with the local anesthetic to prolong the duration of the spinal anesthesia. Measurements of spinal cord blood flow during spinal anesthesia with local anesthetics plus epinephrine (pp. 53–54) fail, however, to support this explanation. Cord blood flow does not decrease during spinal anesthesia when epinephrine is added. A more likely explanation for the clonus is differential rates of recovery of spinal cord nerve roots and intracordal nerve tracts during regression of spinal anesthesia. The concentration of local anesthetics in the spinal cord during spinal anesthesia is greater posteriolaterally than anteriorly (p. 11). As the concentration of anesthetic in the cord decreases during regression of anesthesia, continued blockade of inhibitory neurons in posterolateral columns might persist beyond the time when anesthetic concentrations in anterior motor columns have decreased below effective anesthetic concentrations, thus resulting in clonus. On the other hand, the periodic leg movements observed on two occasions in the patient described by Watanabe, et al. (1987) were exactly the same both as the videotaped myoclonus their patient had during normal sleep in the author's laboratory (and confirmed electromyographically) and as repeatedly seen at home by the patient's wife. This case represents true sleep myoclonus, normal for this patient, regardless of its cause or precipitating factor, and, even more astonishing, persisting during spinal anesthesia.

Effects of Spinal Anesthesia on the Cord

Although the primary site of action of local anesthetics injected into the subarachnoid space is on nerve roots, such agents also affect the cord itself. Clinical evidence indicates that this does not, as postulated (Urban, 1973) result in temporary chemical transection of the cord. Forbes and Roizen (1978), for example, found, in 53 of 63 instances in which levels of anesthesia were assessed during regression of predominately unilateral anesthesia and in 116 of 117 instances in which levels were determined during regression of bilateral anesthesia, that the distribution of cutaneous anesthesia on the trunk followed nerve root dermatome patterns, not the pattern expected if the cord itself had been extensively anesthetized. Similarly, during segmental spinal anesthesia (Kamsler, et al., 1952) with blockade of mid-thoracic sensory nerve roots, nerve function distal to the completely anesthetized thoracic areas could still be demonstrated. Motor blockade is absent caudad to the thoracic area in which there is both sensory anesthesia and motor blockade. Nor is central transmission of pain impulses arising from an operative site below the level of the segmental thoracic anesthesia always blocked. Finer sensations, including light touch and temperature discrimination in areas below the level of thoracic segment anesthesia are not conducted past such a segmental spinal anesthesia, even though pain impulses still may be transmitted centrally, indicate that segmental spinal anesthesia may affect transmission of impulses within some, but not all tracts within the cord.

The possibility that spinal anesthesia can affect neural function within the spinal cord itself is supported by histologic evidence that local anesthetics are present in the cord during spinal anesthesia (pp. 11–13) and by the observation that under certain circumstances local anesthetics injected intrathecally can produce morphologic changes in the cord (Lundy, et al., 1933; Co Tui, et al., 1944; Adams, et al., 1974). Finally, that extremely low concentrations of procaine in CSF are capable of depressing nerve activity within the cord was demonstrated many years ago by Rudin, et al. (1951), is additional evidence that spinal cord function can be affected by spinal anesthesia. As Rudin, et al. showed in animals, as little as 0.1 mg per ml of procaine in spinal fluid during epidural anesthesia is sufficient to produce depression of the cord matter. Oscillating cord potentials, probably generated by cord gray matter, were suppressed at such minimal concentrations of procaine that sympathetic preganglionic fibers in the subarachnoid space, very sensitive to local anesthetics, were not blocked. Also, Dohi, et al. (1979), found that the intravenous injection of 2.5, 5, and 10 mg·kg^{-1} lidocaine in cats produced dose-related suppression of spontaneous activity as well as activity induced by peripheral stimuli in nociceptive neurons in Rexed lamina V. That this depressant effect on nociceptive receptors was seen with very low plasma levels, 3.6 ± 0.7 (SEM) μg·ml^{-1}, indicates the high sensitivity of these neurons to local anesthetics.

Further evidence of the effects of spinal anesthesia on the spinal cord under clinical conditions can be derived from studies of the effect of spinal anesthesia on cerebrocortical electrical potentials evoked by peripherally applied stimuli. Lund, et al. (1987), for example, found in 12 patients that bupivacaine spinal anesthesia with mean sensory (pinprick) levels of denervation at T$_9$ and with mean motor blockade of 1.3 (Bromage scale) was associated with statistically significant decreases in, but not elimination of, the amplitude of somatosensory evoked potentials recorded from the cortex following stimulation in the L_1 and S_1 dermatomes. There was no correlation in this study between the level of pinprick anesthesia and the magnitude of depression of the amplitude of the evoked responses. In the same patients there was a statistically significant increase in latency of evoked responses following stimuli at L_1 but not at S_1. Arendt-Nielsen, et al. (1990 a, b), also found in patients that, 20 min after injection of bupivacaine intrathecally, amplitudes of evoked cerebral potentials produced by stimulation by a single pinprick and by argon laser decreased 42% when the stimuli were in the L_1 dermatome and 31% when at the S_1 level. Latencies of evoked responses were also prolonged. Decreases in amplitude of evoked potentials were still present 60 and 120 min following injection.

The findings by Lund, et al. and Arendt-Nielsen, et al. demonstrate that during spinal anesthesia peripheral nociceptive stimuli applied to surgically anesthetized areas can produce measurable, though altered, electrical responses in the cerebral cortex in spite of the fact that the cutaneous stimuli (pinprick and argon laser beam) are no longer felt in the dermatome in which the stimuli have been applied. This finding implies that there may exist dissociation of conscious awareness of peripheral noxious stimuli and transmission to the brain of the stimuli during spinal anesthesia. It does not necessarily follow that spinal anesthesia is normally associated with cerebral bombardment by peripherally generated noxious stimuli during surgery and that complete blockade of afferent somatic sensory impulses cannot and does not occur during spinal anesthesia.

Given the fact that spinal anesthesia, even with pinprick levels at the C_8 level, does not affect central conduction times (Lang, et al., 1990), the above observed changes in latency times and amplitudes of cortical responses to peripheral stimuli during spinal anesthesia (Lund, et al., 1987; Arendt-Nielsen, et al., 1990 a, b) must be ascribed to extracranial effects of spinal anesthesia. The latter could involve (a) partial blockade of somatic sensory stimuli at the level of somatic sensory afferent nerves in the subarachnoid space with unaltered transmission of peripherally derived action potentials within the spinal cord; (b) no blockade at all of somatic sensory afferent fibers within the subarachnoid space but with inhibition of afferent impulses within the cord itself; or (c) a combination of both (a) and (b). Possibilities (b) and (c) are unlikely in view of the overwhelming evidence that the primary, even though perhaps not the only, site of action of local anesthetics in CSF lies within the subarachnoid space between the pia and dura matter. This conclusion is supported by data presented in a study by Lang, et al. (1989) in which it was shown that spinal anesthesia can totally block cerebrocortical responses to peripheral stimuli applied to anesthetized dermatomes and that, even when peripheral stimuli no longer evoke cerebrocortical responses, transmission of impulses within the cord is still possible. In this study, six patients with chronic pain were given diagnostic high spinal anesthetics to a sensory (pinprick) level of T_{1-2}. Before induction of spinal anesthesia, electrical stimulation of the posterior tibial nerve produced pain and the expected cortical evoked potentials. During spinal anesthesia, stimulation of the posterior tibial nerve produced no pain and no cortical evoked potentials. Before induction of spinal anesthesia, direct electrical stimulation of spinal cord by an electrode placed in the dorsal midline of the epidural space at T_9 or T_8 also produced cortical evoked responses. During T_{2-3} levels of sensory anesthesia stimulation of the cord at T_{8-9} continued to produce cerebral evoked responses (albeit these responses had reduced amplitude and increased latencies).

The fact that in the study by Lang, et al. (1989) cortical evoked responses to peripheral stimuli applied in anesthetized dermatomes were completely blocked by spinal anesthesia while, in the papers by Lund, et al. and Arendt-Nielsen, et al., peripheral stimuli in pinprick anesthetized areas still produced evoked, albeit altered, responses is probably related to differences in these studies in concentrations of local anesthetic in spinal fluid at the site where the peripheral nerve being stimulated entered the subarachnoid space. This is not completely certain, though, because the relative potencies of the local anesthetics used in these studies have not been adequately defined in patients. Lang, et al. (1989) used 100 mg (2 ml of 5%) articain to produce T_{2-3} levels of pinprick anesthesia. Lund, et al. used 15–20 mg (3.0–4.0 ml of 0.5%) bupivacaine, while Arendt-Nielsen, et al. used 17.5 mg (3.5 ml of 0.5%) bupivacaine to achieve pinprick levels of anesthesia to T_9 and T_{10}.

Decreases in blood flow to the spinal cord during spinal anesthesia might theoretically be associated with ischemia within the cord severe enough to impair neuronal function, either transiently or even permanently. Measurements of cord blood flow during spinal anesthesia are thus of physiologic and clinical importance.

The effects, if any, of spinal anesthesia on blood flow to the spinal cord might involve one or more of four mechanisms: (a) direct effects of local anesthetics on cord blood vessels; (b) indirect effects of local anesthetics on spinal cord vessels secondary to their disruption of autonomous spinal cord vascular innervation; (c) the effects of vasoconstrictors injected to prolong the duration of anesthesia; and (d) the effects of combining local anesthetics with vasoconstrictors.

In a study in dogs of the effects of intrathecal tetracaine on spinal cord blood flow, Kozody, et al. (1985 a) found that while the injection of saline into the lumbar subarachnoid space had no significant effect on spinal cord or dural blood flow, the injection of 20 mg tetracaine was associated with significant increases in both lumbosacral spinal cord blood flow and lumbosacral and thoracic dural blood flow 20 and 40 min after injection.

Porter, *et al.* (1985), on the other hand, found in similar studies that tetracaine induced no statistically significant change in cord blood flow, results also reported by Dohi, *et al.* (1987).

When lidocaine, instead of tetracaine, was injected intrathecally, Kozody, *et al.* (1985 b) found no significant change in spinal cord blood flow, nor did Porter, *et al.* (1985), or Dohi, *et al.* (1984). Porter, *et al.* (1985) also found that intrathecal metycaine had no effect on blood flow to the cord.

The above findings indicate that, though tetracaine may increase spinal cord blood flow, lidocaine and metycaine have no effect. In contrast, Crosby (1985) found that bupivacaine decreased spinal cord blood flow in rats by 27%–34%. Reasons for the difference in the findings of Kozody, Porter, and Dohi, *et al.* on the one hand and those of Crosby on the other hand are not clear. Reasons might include possible local vasoconstrictive effects of bupivacaine in contrast to either no effect or to local vasodilatory effects of other local anesthetics, to species differences, to differences in methods used to measure cord blood flow, and to differences in experimental design. Interestingly, Crosby also found that regional glucose utilization in the spinal cord decreased following intrathecal injection of bupivacaine. The decrease in glucose utilization was less than the decrease in blood flow. Perhaps deafferentation of the cord by intrathecal bupivacaine may have so decreased neural activity, and thus metabolic demands in the spinal cord, that glucose utilization decreased. This explanation would seem more likely than the hypothesis that the decrease in cord blood flow induced by bupivacaine resulted in spinal cord ischemia so great as to restrict delivery of metabolic substrates to the cord in amounts needed to maintain normal energy consumption. A decrease in spinal cord glucose utilization has also been reported by Cole, *et al.* (1990), who found that the spinal cord and intracranial metabolic responses to somatosensory stimulation in the rat decreased during tetracaine spinal anesthesia in contrast to the increase seen during general (halothane) anesthesia.

The above studies of effects of intrathecal local anesthetics on spinal cord blood flow indicate that neither direct effects of the local anesthetics on spinal cord vasculature, nor sympathetic denervation of spinal cord vessels are routinely associated with decreases in spinal cord blood flow so great as to produce either transitory or prolonged ischemic changes in spinal cord function. The possibility remains, however, that spinal cord vascular autoregulatory mechanisms are so affected by intrathecal local anesthetics that systemic physiologic perturbations may affect blood flow to the spinal cord. This issue was addressed in dogs by Dohi, *et al.* (1987). They found, as mentioned above, that the intrathecal injection of tetracaine had no effect on spinal cord blood flow during normal ventilation. They found also that modest decreases in arterial blood pressure during spinal anesthesia were unaccompanied by changes in blood flow to the spinal cord. They furthermore found that spinal anesthesia had no significant effect on the increase in cord blood flow produced by acute hypercapnia (arterial carbon dioxide pressure ($PaCO_2$) = 57 mmHg). Before spinal anesthesia, cord blood flow increased from baseline, normocapnic levels of 31.8 ± 8.1 ml·100 g^{-1}·min^{-1} (mean ± SD) to 39.9 ± 6.0 ml·100 g^{-1}·min^{-1} during the hypercapnia, a statistically significant increase. During spinal anesthesia cord blood flow also increased, from 26.8 ± 9.0 to 34.2 ± 13.0 mg·100 g^{-1}·min^{-1}, also a statistically significant increase but not significantly different than seen in the absence of spinal anesthesia. Dohi, et al. (1987) found that the effects of acute blood loss (20% of estimated blood volume) on spinal cord blood flow were also similar before and after spinal anesthesia in dogs. In the absence of spinal anesthesia, spinal blood flow averaged 27.9 ± 6.3 ml·100 g^{-1}·min^{-1} before, and 26.7 ± 6.7 ml·100 g^{-1}·min^{-1} after, induction of this degree of acute hypovolemia. During spinal anesthesia, corresponding values were 30.6 ± 14.6 before and 24.1 ± 14.6 ml·100 g^{-1}·min^{-1} after acute hypovolemia. The autoregulatory mechanisms controlling spinal blood flow were, thus, moderately decreased, but not eliminated by spinal anesthesia in the presence of acute hypovolemia adequate to decrease mean arterial blood pressure from 110 ± 13 to 66 ± 8 mmHg. The absence of any correlation between mean arterial pressure and cord blood flow in the presence of normovolemic hypotension produced by spinal anesthesia (Porter, et al., 1985) indicates that moderate levels of arterial hypotension during clinical spinal anesthesia are unlikely to be associated with physiologically inimical decreases in blood flow to the spinal cord.

The above data are from studies in which vasoconstrictors were not injected intrathecally along with the local anesthetics to prolong the duration of anesthesia. What, however, are the effects of vasoconstrictors on spinal cord blood flow when administered alone or when administered with local anesthetics? Kozody, et al. (1984) found in dogs that the intrathecal injection of neither saline plus 200 μg epinephrine nor 5 mg phenylephrine had any statistically significant effect on spinal cord blood flow in the absence of spinal anesthesia. When 200 μg epinephrine was injected intrathecally with lidocaine, the delayed spinal cord hyperemia and the dural hyperemia seen when lidocaine alone was injected without epinephrine were eliminated, but otherwise epinephrine had no effect on cord blood flow (Kozody, et al., 1985 b). In dogs given tetracaine spinal anesthetics, the addition of epinephrine similarly eliminated the increase in spinal and dural blood flow seen when tetracaine was given without epinephrine, but the epinephrine did not decrease cord blood flow below preanesthetic levels (Kozody, et al., 1985 a). Porter, et al. (1985) and Dohi, et al. (1987) also found that neither 100, 300, nor even

500 μg of epinephrine alone (in the absence of any local anesthetic) had any significant effect on spinal cord blood flow in dogs when injected intrathecally. It seems unlikely that epinephrine injected intrathecally to prolong spinal anesthesia has adverse effects on blood flow to the spinal cord.

Though epinephrine has no effect on spinal cord blood flow, clonidine, an alpha$_2$-adrenergic receptor agonist with some mild alpha$_1$-adrenergic agonist properties also, does significantly reduce spinal cord blood flow of rats when injected intrathecally alone, without local anesthetics. Whether this effect is mediated entirely by direct subarachnoid effects of clonidine, or whether systemic effects of clonidine are also involved, is presently not clear (Crosby, et al., 1990). Phenylephrine (Neosynephrine), a pure alpha$_1$-adrenoceptor agonist, differs from epinephrine, a mixed alpha$_1$- and alpha$_2$-agonist, in that it significantly decreases spinal cord blood flow in concentrations greater than 0.2% when administered to dogs intrathecally alone, without a local anesthetic, while epinephrine has no such effect (Dohi, et al., 1984). When phenylephrine is injected with lidocaine, there is also a prompt decrease in spinal cord blood flow that persists for 60–90 min. These findings with phenylephrine stand in contrast both with the absence of changes in cord blood flow when lidocaine alone is injected intrathecally (Dohi, et al., 1984) and with the effects of epinephrine on spinal cord blood flow when injected intrathecally with lidocaine.

The preponderance of experimental data in animals indicates that spinal anesthesia with or without epinephrine has no significant adverse effects on spinal cord blood flow, but whether this applies equally well to other vasoconstrictors or alpha$_2$-agonists, including clonidine, remains to be clarified.

Finally, a clinically important effect of spinal anesthesia on the spinal cord concerns the modulation or perhaps even the elimination of the intracordal hyperexcitability created by repetitive bombardment by noxious afferent stimuli coming from the periphery during surgery (Woolf, 1983; Cook, et al., 1987; Woolf and Wall, 1987). The salutary effects of blocking afferent impulses from an operative site have long been advocated as a means to decrease both shock (Crile, 1913) and postoperative pain whether the operative site is injected (Owen, et al., 1985; Patel, et al., 1983), sprayed (Sinclair, et al., 1988), or irrigated (Blades and Ford, 1950; Gibbs, et al., 1988) with local anesthetics. The ability of spinal anesthesia, along with other methods for blocking afferent noxious stimuli, to decrease postoperative pain, has been quantitated in a study (Tverskoy, et al., 1990) of 36 patients undergoing inguinal herniorrhaphy under either spinal anesthesia, general anesthesia (thiopental, halothane, nitrous oxide), or general anesthesia combined with infiltration of the site of incision with bupivacaine before the incision was made.

The severity of postoperative pain elicited by pressure on the site of incision using an algometer, the severity of pain produced by movement, and the severity of constant incisional pain all were measured 24 hr, 48 hr, and 10 days postoperatively. Local anesthetic, either by infiltration or by intrathecal injection, significantly decreased the severity of all three types of pain. Within 24 hr constant incisional pain had essentially disappeared when local anesthetics were used in the incision or with spinal anesthesia. Times from end of the operation to patients' first request for analgesics were also significantly prolonged by local anesthetics: 64 min in patients having general anesthesia, 212 min in patients having spinal anesthesia, and 515 min in patients having general anesthesia plus local anesthetic infiltration. Spinal anesthesia was less effective than general plus local anesthesia, but both were more effective in management of postoperative pain than was general anesthesia. Though outcome in terms of postoperative complications and time to postoperative return to normal mobility remain to be quantified in future studies, regional anesthesia, including spinal anesthesia, has much to offer as a method for decreasing postoperative pain. Spinal anesthesia might be particularly helpful in instances in which type and site of surgery make incisional infiltration impractical.

The potentiation of the analgesic effects of narcotics administered epidurally or intrathecally by local anesthetics is not discussed here for reasons stated in the Preface.

Effects of Spinal Anesthesia on the Brain

The effects of spinal anesthesia on the brain may best be considered by dividing the subject into the following three arbitrary parts even though a certain amount of overlap inevitably results: first, cerebral blood flow; secondly, function of the brainstem; and, finally, cerebral cortical function.

Cerebral Blood Flow during Spinal Anesthesia

Cerebral blood flow is governed by two main factors: mean arterial blood pressure and local resistance to blood flow in cerebral vessels. Spinal anesthesia could theoretically influence cerebral blood flow by altering either blood pressure or cerebrovascular resistance, or both. Since spinal anesthesia is characterized by preganglionic sympathetic blockade, it is well to start by determining whether sympathetic block in itself will alter cerebral blood flow.

It is known that preganglionic sympathetic axons passing over the upper two thoracic white *rami communicantes* send fibers to the stellate and superior cervical sympathetic ganglia. From these ganglia, postganglionic fibers ascend intracranially not only along with the vertebral and basilar arteries, but also with the middle meningeal and internal carotid arteries (White, *et al.*, 1952). There remains doubt however, as to the role of these postganglionic sympathetic fibers in determining the caliber of cerebral vessels. Fog (1937) was one of the first to emphasize that pial vessels are not subject to significant control by vasomotor nerves. It is now generally accepted that sympathetic nerves to cranial vessels have little or no effect on cerebral blood flow in humans, even though they may affect cerebral circulation in certain experimental animals (James, *et al.*, 1969; Tkachenko, *et al.*, 1969; Dorigotti and Glässer, 1972). Studies of cerebral blood flow before and after stellate ganglion block have almost invariably shown that such a procedure has no significant effect on cerebral blood flow. Harmel, *et al.* (1949) studied 13 normotensive and hypertensive patients before and after bilateral stellate ganglion block. The average cerebral blood flow before block was 49 ml·100 g^{-1}·min^{-1}, while after the block it was 48 ml·100 g^{-1}·min^{-1}. In 19 patients, including normal controls, Scheinberg (1950) found that the cerebral blood flow averaged 57 ± 2.2 ml·100 g^{-1}·min^{-1} before unilateral stellate block. The corresponding figure after the block was 54 ± 3.3 ml·100 g^{-1}·min^{-1}. Naffziger and Adams (1950) studied 15 patients, all presumably with intracranial disease, before and after unilateral stellate block. In 14 patients, there was no change, but in 1 patient the cerebral blood flow increased from 45 to 88 ml·100 g^{-1}·min^{-1} following the block. This increase was of such magnitude as to raise the question of laboratory or technical errors. The only report disagreeing with the results mentioned above is that of Shenkin, *et al.* (1951). These authors found an increase of borderline statistical significance in cerebral blood flow following bilateral surgical excision of the stellate ganglia. In seven patients, all with cerebral pathology, the cerebral blood flow increased from control values of 45.6 to 55.6 ml·100 g^{-1}·min^{-1} following operation. This increase was accompanied by a decrease in cerebrovascular resistance, a change that was not reported by Harmel, *et al.*, or by Scheinberg.

The quantitative data therefore indicate that, by and large, interruption of sympathetic impulses at the stellate ganglion has little if any effect on cerebral blood flow. This leads to the conclusion that blockade of preganglionic sympathetic fibers going to the cervical sympathetic chain during high spinal anesthesia will in itself have no appreciable or significant effect on blood flow to the brain.

During high spinal anesthesia other factors, besides possible block of sympathetic fibers going to the stellate ganglion, influence cerebral blood flow. Chief among these is the arterial hypotension that may accompany such anesthesia. As mentioned above, cerebral blood flow is directly related to cerebrovascular resistance. Arterial blood pressure is, however, one of the main determinants of cerebrovascular resistance. As arterial blood pressure decreases, there is usually a reflex decrease in cerebrovascular resistance so that cerebral blood flow remains relatively unchanged (Shenkin, et al., 1948). Precisely how decreases in arterial pressure produce decreases in cerebrovascular resistance remains unexplained, but the result is that there exists no direct relationship between cerebral blood flow and arterial pressure. A 20% decrease in blood pressure does not, for example, always result in a 20% decrease in cerebral blood flow. Certain drugs may have a preferential effect on the caliber of cerebral vessels so that when they are administered, cerebrovascular resistance is no longer related to arterial blood pressure (Shenkin, 1951), but they are the exception. The majority of drugs that decrease blood pressure also decrease cerebrovascular resistance.

The effects of spinal anesthesia on cerebral blood flow were first reported by Kety, et al. in 1948 and 1950. These investigators studied 17 patients prior to, and during differential spinal sympathetic block produced by the technic of Sarnoff and Arrowood (1946). All patients had essential hypertension. The mean arterial blood pressure averaged 155 mmHg before spinal anesthesia was induced. Control values of cerebral blood flow and cerebrovascular resistance were 52 ml·100 g^{-1}·min^{-1} and 3.1 units, respectively. Following differential spinal sympathetic block in the supine position, the mean arterial blood pressure decreased to 115 mmHg, cerebral blood flow was reduced to 46 ml·100 g^{-1}·min^{-1}, and cerebrovascular resistance decreased to 2.6 units. All these changes were statistically significant. Kleinerman, et al. in 1958 reported on the effects of surgical spinal anesthesia on cerebral blood flow. They studied nine nonoperative, normotensive subjects with spinal levels high enough to produce plethysmographically demonstrable increases in finger blood flow (i.e., sensory levels to T_3 and above). During the period of anesthesia there were statistically significant decreases in mean arterial blood pressure (from 92.5 to 63.4 mmHg). However, because there were also significant decreases in cerebrovascular resistance (from 2.1 to 1.5 units), there was no change in cerebral blood flow. Blood flow to the brain averaged 44.6 ml·100 g^{-1}·min^{-1} before spinal anesthesia and 46.1 ml·100 g^{-1}·min^{-1} during anesthesia. These same investigators also studied 4 patients with essential hypertension. Mean arterial blood pressure in these four patients decreased from 158 mmHg before, to 79 mmHg during anesthesia, changes that were accompanied by decreases in cerebrovascular resistance (from 3.5 to 2.1 units). The latter changes were, however, proportionately less than the former, with the result that cerebral blood flow decreased from 46.5 to 37.5 ml·100 g^{-1}·min^{-1}. These results, together with those obtained by Kety, et al., confirm the findings of the majority of those who have investigated the effects of sympatholytic and ganglionic blocking agents and techniques on cerebral blood flow. As arterial pressure decreases during spinal anesthesia, cerebrovascular resistance decreases. However, it is apparent from these studies that normotensive patients react quantitatively differently than do hypertensive patients. In normotensive patients Kleinerman, *et al.* found that cerebrovascular resistance and blood pressure decreased proportionately so that there was no decrease in cerebral blood flow and, in fact, a modest increase. On the other hand, the 17 hypertensive patients studied by Kety, *et al.*, as well as the 4 hypertensive patients reported by Kleinerman, *et al.*, failed to exhibit a direct relationship between arterial pressure and cerebral resistance comparable to that found in normotensive subjects. At a time when the 17 patients of Kety, *et al.* showed an average decrease in mean arterial pressure of 26%, there was a concurrent decrease of 12% in cerebral blood flow. In the four hypertensive patients reported by Kleinerman, *et al.*, a 50% decrease in mean arterial pressure was accompanied by a 17% decrease in blood flow to the brain. During spinal anesthesia normotensive patients are, therefore, better able to maintain cerebral blood flow in the face of arterial hypotension than are hypertensive patients.

No further studies on the effects of spinal anesthesia on cerebral blood flow in humans have been carried out in the many years since those cited above were published. This is so despite the availability of substantially more sophisticated noninvasive techniques for measurement of cerebral blood flow in patients, especially regional cerebral blood flow. Perhaps the original data on global cerebral blood flow during spinal anesthesia in humans need not be repeated; the studies were performed so well in the first place. It is a pity, nevertheless, that those who have experience with, and equipment available for, measuring regional cerebral blood flow have not applied them to patients. Such measurements of regional cerebral blood flow would be especially useful in patients with cardiovascular or cerebrovascular disease during spinal anesthesia with its frequently associated decreases in blood pressure. The same can be said with regard to the paucity of data on cerebral blood flow in animals published in recent decades. Sivarajan, *et al.* reported in 1975 that in monkeys cerebral blood flow remains within normal limits during hypotension associated with spinal anesthesia and that the percentage of cardiac output going to the brain is not changed during spinal anesthesia. Dohi, *et al.* (1984, 1987) confirmed that during spinal anesthesia in dogs, too, there is no correlation between cerebral blood flow and mean arterial blood pressure, which remained above 80 mmHg. Furthermore, neither phenylephrine injected into the lumbar space of dogs alone or with lidocaine (Dohi, *et al.*, 1984), nor intrathecal epinephrine in amounts as great as 500 μg (Dohi, *et al.*, 1984; Porter, *et al.*, 1985) had any significant effect on cerebral blood flow. Again, while studies of global cerebral blood flow in animals are useful, so, too, would be studies of regional cerebral blood flow.

No data have been published on the effects of spinal anesthesia on cerebrovascular autoregulation in humans as affected by changes in oxygen or carbon dioxide concentrations, abnormal core temperatures, or the administration of various cerebrovascularly active drugs.

It is not surprising that the normotensive patients studied by Kleinerman, et al. (1958) showed no significant changes in cerebral metabolism during spinal anesthesia, in view of the fact that cerebral blood flow remained unaffected because of autoregulation. Neither cerebral oxygen consumption nor cerebral glucose utilization were affected by the anesthesia. We know, however, from clinical experience that if the blood pressure decreases low enough with spinal anesthesia, evidence of inadequate cerebral circulation appears (p. 64). Even though decreases in blood pressure during spinal are normally not accompanied by proportionate decreases in the amount of blood flow to the brain, severe arterial hypotension is certain to be associated with clinically and physiologically significant and dangerous decreases in blood flow. Cerebral vasodilation, even when maximal, will be unable to maintain adequate blood flow to the brain when the blood pressure has decreased below a certain critical level. In normotensive humans the lower limit of cerebral autoregulation is reached when mean arterial pressure is in the range of 60–70 mmHg. Below this level cerebral blood flow decreases as mean arterial pressure decreases further. This can be compensated for by an increase in oxygen extraction, but when mean arterial pressure is 35–40 mmHg, even this compensatory mechanism fails and cerebral hypoxia ensues. In hypertensive patients with a resting mean arterial pressure of 146 mmHg, Strandgaard, et al., (1973) found that the lower limit of cerebral autoregulation was reached as blood pressure was decreased by trimethaphan to approximately 120 mmHg. Cerebral hypoxia, as evidenced by dizziness, somnolence, and hyperventilation, appeared when mean arterial pressure was approximately 102 mmHg (73% of the resting level). In normotensive subjects signs of cerebral hypoxia did not appear until trimethaphan decreased mean arterial pressure to 40 mmHg (66% of the resting level). Similarly, Finnerty, et al. (1953, 1957) found in unanesthetized patients that when the cerebral blood flow decreased below an average value of 35 ml·100 g^{-1}·min^{-1} due to hexamethonium, there was onset of signs and symptoms of cerebral ischemia. In normal patients the mean arterial pressure necessary to provide this critical blood flow to the brain was found to be about 30–40 mmHg. In patients with malignant hypertension, the critical level was 100–110 mmHg.

Data such as these probably apply during spinal anesthesia. As a clinical rule of thumb it is best to assume that in the supine position, levels of mean arterial pressure below 55 mmHg during spinal anesthesia are associated with decreases in cerebral blood flow in normal patients frequently enough that they should be avoided (Morris, et al., 1953; Finnerty, et al., 1957). In patients with hypertension or with arteriosclerotic changes involving cerebral vessels, the blood pressure should, however, be maintained considerably above this in order to assure adequate cerebral blood flow (Shanbrom and Levy, 1957).

While cerebral blood flow is relatively unaffected by changes in blood pressure or sympathetic tone, it responds with exquisite sensitivity to alterations in arterial carbon dioxide tension. Increases in carbon dioxide tension above normal levels of 40 mmHg are associated with prompt and striking increases in cerebral blood flow. Decreases below 40 mmHg are accompanied by equally prompt and pronounced decreases in flow. The possibility exists that the sympathetic denervation of spinal anesthesia may affect cerebral blood flow by altering the sensitivity of cerebral vessels to changes in carbon dioxide tension when blood pressure is unchanged. This possibility has not been examined during spinal anesthesia, but it has been studied by Galindo (1964) in experimental animals during high epidural block. In 15 anesthetized (thiopental) dogs, Galindo found that a 75.0% increase in arterial carbon dioxide tension was associated with a 78.5% increase in internal carotid blood flow before epidural block, but that an 82.5% increase in arterial carbon dioxide tension during epidural block was accompanied by an increase in blood flow averaging only 10.8%. These data suggest that sympathetic blockade may alter the response of internal carotid flow to increases in carbon dioxide tension. However, the possibility exists that the local anesthetic agent employed for the epidural anesthesia (1% lidocaine) affected the results following its vascular absorption. Therefore, further studies under more controlled conditions are warranted before it can be concluded that spinal anesthesia has a comparable effect. Better quantitated is the observation that when arterial pressure is reduced by ganglionic blocking agents to the point where cerebral hypoxia ensues, the hyperventilation caused by cerebral ischemic hypoxia produces no further diminution of cerebral blood flow (Strandgaard, et al., 1973). Reactivity of cerebral vessels to changes in carbon dioxide tension is markedly reduced or abolished when cerebral blood flow is low enough to be associated with cerebral hypoxia but this apparently occurs independently of sympathetic nervous system activity.

Regardless of the relationship between arterial blood pressure and cerebral blood flow under laboratory experimental conditions, if severe arterial hypotension does develop during clinical spinal anesthesia, a moderate head-down position should be employed in order to maintain as great a cerebral blood flow as possible. Not only will the head-down position increase cardiac output, and so raise the systemic pressure, but it will also slightly increase the intraluminal pressure in cerebral arteries by gravity alone. Extreme head-down positions are to be avoided in such instances because the resulting increase in venous pressure may have a deleterious effect on cerebral capillary blood flow in the presence of arterial hypotension. The head-up position should never be employed in the presence of hypotension due to spinal anesthesia.

Effects of Spinal Anesthesia on the Brainstem

A frequently encountered adage in clinical anesthesia states that local anesthetics injected into the lumbar subarachnoid space must at all costs be prevented from ascending into the ventricular system. The implication is not only that local anesthetics used for spinal anesthesia can and do enter the ventricles, but that when there, they can produce direct depression of vital centers in the brainstem. This sequence of events is often used to explain both cardiac and respiratory arrest during spinal anesthesia. The theory deserves careful consideration, for if medullary paralysis due to direct action of local anesthetics on the brainstem is a potential danger during spinal anesthesia, then all steps should be taken to prevent its occurrence. Such steps would include use of the head-up position when inadvertently high levels of anesthesia are obtained with hyperbaric solutions.

Although the above theory was proposed intermittently for many years on clinical grounds by many anesthetists (Pitkin, 1928; Sise, 1929; Hill, 1951; Hill and Macdonald, 1933), it was Co Tui's work in the early 1930s (Co Tui and Standard, 1932; Co Tui, 1934, 1936) that provided an experimental basis for it. Co Tui demonstrated that the intracisternal injection of procaine in dogs caused simultaneous respiratory paralysis and hypotension. He hypothesized that these effects were due to direct medullary paralysis. Downward diffusion of the local anesthetic into the cervical subarachnoid space, where it could paralyze the phenic nerves and cause respiratory arrest leading to cardiac arrest, was not prevented in these experiments. The intracisternal dose of procaine required to produce these results was 60–70 mg in dogs weighing 17–20 kg. Forty milligrams of procaine injected into the cisterna magna did not produce respiratory paralysis. Co Tui also demonstrated that the injection of 75 mg. of procaine (2.5 ml. of a 3% solution) into the fourth ventricle of a dog produced respiratory paralysis and death. On the basis of these experiments, Co Tui came to the conclusion that direct medullary paralysis could occur during spinal anesthesia and that the paralysis was the result of depression of the brainstem by the drugs used to produce spinal anesthesia.

These early observations on ventilatory responses following the topical application of local anesthetics to the brainstem have since been followed by studies under more controlled conditions. Mitchell, *et al.* (1963) described an area on the ventrolateral surface of the medulla of experimental animals which is sensitive to changes in pH and carbon dioxide tension, and which is depressed following perfusion with artificial CSF containing 0.1% procaine. Since 0.1% procaine applied to this area produced apnea regardless of the level of alveolar carbon dioxide tension, and since 5% procaine placed in the fourth ventricle did not affect respiration, these authors suggested that the major portion of the respiratory response to carbon dioxide originates in this area on the ventrolateral medulla sensitive to changes in hydrogen ion concentration. On the other hand, Cozine and Ngai (1967) found that while 1% procaine applied to the ventrolateral aspect of the medulla of cats did decrease ventilation, apnea occurred in only 1 of 36 animals. Cozine and Ngai found that topical local anesthetic was a respiratory depressant to the extent that it shifted the carbon dioxide-ventilation curve to the right, a finding also reported by Rosenstein, *et al.* (1968). They concluded that the medullary surface chemoreceptors are only one of several central mechanisms which respond to changes in hydrogen ion concentration. On this basis, complete apnea would not be expected to result even if an effective concentration of local anesthetic were present about the medulla. Indeed this is what Haranath and Venkatakrishna-Bhatt found (1968 a, b). Perfusion of 1% procaine or injection of as much as 40 mg lidocaine into the cerebral ventricles of conscious dogs produced paresis of the limbs, vomiting, defecation, and sometimes loss of consciousness, but respiration was not depressed, it increased. Loeschke and Koepchen (1958 a, b), while reporting similar results in experimental animals, concluded that procaine in the CSF affected neither the respiratory nor the vasomotor centers. They did find, however, that procaine in ventricular CSF could block afferent fibers from peripheral chemo- and pressoreceptors to these centers. The centers themselves, however, were unaffected.

Undoubtedly local anesthetics can have a depressant effect if applied directly to the brainstem in high enough concentrations and in great enough volumes. Whether the concentration of local anesthetic in ventricular fluid during spinal anesthesia ever becomes great enough to produce medullary paralysis is, however, most unlikely on the basis of experimental and clinical observations. For example, Vehrs (1931, 1934) reported that the maximum concentration of procaine that could be present about the brainstem of dogs without producing respiratory changes averaged 1.0%, with a range from 0.50–1.25%. Vehrs found, however, that injection of 2 ml of 3.33% procaine into the cisterna magna resulted in such dilution of the procaine by CSF that the resulting concentration about the brainstem was less than 1.0%, and so produced no effect on respiration even though, again, total sensory anesthesia resulted. This was confirmed by Johnston and Henderson (1932) who found that injection of either 1.0 ml of 5% procaine or 0.5 ml of 10% procaine into the cisterna magna of dogs produced variable results. In some, there was no effect on blood pressure or respiration, in others there was a rise in blood pressure, while in some there was descent of the drug into the cervical subarachnoid space to produce intercostal and phrenic paralysis. The authors also injected the same volumes and concentrations of procaine into the fourth ventricle of dogs. This produced transient changes in blood pressure and respiration due to the pressure of the injected fluid, but no significant or prolonged effect on the nerve centers of the brainstem. Thompson (1934) not only confirmed the above, but emphasized again the important role played by concentration of the anesthetic agent. He found that the injection of 1.0 ml or either a 1.0% or a 1.5% solution of procaine into the lateral ventricle of a dog produced no change in respiration but was associated with a slight decrease in blood pressure and bradycardia. Injecting 1.0 ml of a 2.5% solution into the lateral ventricle produced entirely different results. This amount of procaine produced respiratory arrest for 15–30 min, severe bradycardia, and a marked decrease in blood pressure. Thompson concluded that while local anesthetics could depress the brainstem, it was doubtful if such ever occurred during spinal anesthesia under clinical conditions. He further emphasized this by taking 1.0-ml samples of cisternal fluid from dogs made apneic by the injection of 150 mg of procaine into the lumbar subarachnoid space and injected the 1.0 ml of cisternal fluid into the lateral ventricles of normal dogs with no effect on blood pressure, pulse, or respiration of the recipient animals. Irwin, et al. (1955) also demonstrated the large amounts of local anesthetic needed to produce respiratory arrest. In their studies on respiration in dogs, they found that 5 mg of procaine per kilogram of body weight (as a 2.5% solution) had to be injected intracisternally in order to produce respiratory arrest. Such concentrations of local anesthetic agents as are necessary to produce respiratory or cardiovascular effects by direct topical action are, of course, considerably in excess of those concentrations which depress the brainstem if present in the blood perfusing the brain (Jolly and Steinhaus, 1956).

Clinical experience confirms that the concentration of local anesthetic in ventricular fluid during spinal anesthesia is not great enough to produce medullary depression. The injection in humans of local anesthetics into the cisterna magna (Vehrs, 1931, 1934), or the cervical subarachnoid space (Tait and Caglieri, 1900), although hardly advised, produces complete sensory anesthesia, but is not attended by evidence of medullary paralysis if the patient is managed properly (Chapter 2). Similarly, the intentional production of "total spinal anesthesia" with drugs injected via the lumbar subarachnoid space, though also hardly recommended, provides surgical anesthesia of the head, neck, and upper extremities without signs of medullary depression if, again, the patient is properly managed (Payne, 1901; Jonnesco, 1909; Pauchet, 1920; Babcock, 1928; Koster, 1928; Koster and Kasman, 1929; Wright, 1930). Even the inadvertent injection into the subarachnoid space of massive doses of local anesthetic (e.g., 60 mg of dibucaine and 60 mg of procaine (Jones, 1953)) is attended by physiologic changes that can best be explained without hypothesizing medullary paralysis. In clinical practice there is no evidence to indicate that spinal anesthesia high enough to allow intra-abdominal surgery is accompanied by concentrations of local anesthetic in ventricular fluid great enough to depress either the respiratory center or the vasomotor center. Among 22 patients each given 150 mg of procaine in the lumbar subarachnoid space while in the Trendelenburg position, the concentration of procaine in fluid removed from the cisterna magna has been found to be less than 0.02 mg·ml^{-1} in 14. In the remaining 8 patients, cisternal procaine levels ranged from 0.06 to 0.21 mg·ml^{-1} (Koster, *et al.*, 1938). Concentrations such as those in cisternal fluid are, as we have already seen, inadequate to produce medullary paralysis under experimental conditions. Any local anesthetic that might actually reach the cisterna magna during spinal anesthesia is also, of course, more likely to spread laterally into the cerebral subarachnoid space than to ascend against the flow of CSF through the foramina of Magendie and Luschka to the fourth ventricle.

Respiratory arrest and cardiovascular collapse do occur with high spinal anesthesia. In some instances they are due to paralysis of medullary nerve centers. But such paralysis is not attributable to the direct action of the spinal drug on the brainstem. The paralysis is instead a result of *inadequate medullary blood flow* secondary to extreme arterial hypotension. The commonest cause of decreased cerebral blood flow during the hypotension of spinal anesthesia is the head-up position. The head-up position is employed in such cases with the mistaken concept that unless the head is elevated, the local anesthetic agent will ascend high enough to produce medullary paralysis. Such cannot and will not occur. Anoxic paralysis of the brainstem will, however, result if the head is raised. Elevation of the head or use of reverse Trendelenburg position is one of the most frequent preventable causes of sudden death during spinal anesthesia.

Effects of Spinal Anesthesia on Cerebral Cortical Function

The effects of spinal anesthesia on cerebral cortical function can be divided into two groups: those that are transitory, lasting only for the duration of the anesthesia; and those that persist for variable periods of time into the postoperative period.

The main evidence suggesting that spinal anesthesia may have an effect on cerebral cortical function during the period of anesthesia is based on two clinical phenomena. First, patients given high spinal anesthesia frequently either lapse into what appears to be normal sleep or may actually lose consciousness (Koster and Kasman, 1929; Vehrs, 1934; Jones, 1953; Huvos, *et al.*, 1962). Second, if patients with high spinal anesthesia are given an inhalation anesthetic such as nitrous oxide-oxygen, very low concentrations of anesthetic gases are required to maintain unconsciousness (Greene, 1952). A discussion of the immediate effect of spinal anesthesia on cerebral cortical function, therefore, becomes a discussion of the etiology of this clinically observed sedation.

Theoretically the local anesthetic agent used to produce spinal anesthesia could appear in the cerebral subarachnoid space and, by acting directly on the cerebral cortex, result in somnolence. As already discussed, concentrations of procaine as high as 0.21 mg·ml$_{-1}$ have been found in spinal fluid in the cisterna magna during high spinal anesthesia (Koster, *et al.*, 1938). From the cisterna magna local anesthetics could migrate laterally into the cerebral subarachnoid space. There are several objections, however, to this as an explanation of the depressed cerebral cortical activity. First, there is considerable uncertainty concerning the effects of local anesthetic agents applied directly to the cerebral cortex. When carried to cortical cells by the blood stream, most local anesthetics appear to irritate, rather than to depress, the cerebral cortex. Hyperactivity progressing to seizure activity is characteristic of the central nervous system reaction to most, although not all, local anesthetics absorbed into the vascular system in toxic amounts. But following their direct application to the cerebral cortex, convulsions are infrequent. When procaine solutions are accidentally dropped on the cerebral cortex during craniotomies performed under local anesthesia, or when local anesthetics are directly applied to the cerebral cortex of experimental animals (Dereymaker and Sorel, 1967), there is a striking lack of response. Such applications are usually associated with neither excitation nor depression. Certainly failure of noxious stimuli to elicit cortical evoked responses when applied peripherally in areas rendered anesthetic by spinal anesthesia (pp. 49–51) does not represent direct depression of cerebral cortical function produced by local anesthetics in intracranial CSF. The blockade of somatosensory evoked responses in the cerebral cortex during spinal anesthesia represents primarily blockade of somatic afferent impulses within the spinal subarachnoid space. Though local anesthetics within the substance of the spinal cord may modulate transmission of impulses in spinal cord tracts (p. 51), spinal anesthesia is not associated with effects on intracranial transmission (Lang, *et al.*, 1990).

On the basis of the above-mentioned clinical observations it is unlikely that the somnolence associated with high spinal anesthesia is the result of local anesthetics in the cerebral subarachnoid space. Laboratory studies substantiate this. Although local anesthetics decrease rates of oxygen utilization by nerve tissue when present in concentrations great enough to alter normal nerve function, the somnolence observed in patients given a total sympathetic block by differential spinal anesthesia (Sarnoff and Arrowood, 1946) is not associated with a decrease in cerebral oxygen consumption (Kety, *et al.*, 1950). These observations of both Sarnoff and Arrowood and of Kety, *et al.*, emphasize that the depressed level of consciousness during spinal anesthesia is not due to decreased utilization of oxygen, and that even if local anesthetic were in the cerebral subarachnoid space, it does not influence cerebral metabolism. Actually, concentrations as high as 0.46% procaine have no effect on the rate of oxygen consumption by resting cortical cells (Geddes and Quastel, 1956). If, as seems most likely, depression of cortical cellular activity by procaine must include decreased oxygen utilization, then the concentration of 0.46% required to lower oxygen consumption by cerebral cortical cells is further evidence that local anesthetics in the cerebral subarachnoid space during spinal anesthesia have little or no clinically significant actions. The fact that 0.21% procaine is the highest concentration recorded for procaine in cisternal fluid during spinal anesthesia (Koster, *et al.*, 1938) makes it unlikely that similar or even lower concentrations in the cerebral subarachnoid space have any important action.

But there is also another major objection to the theory that the somnolence of high spinal anesthesia is due to the direct action of the local anesthetic on cerebral cells. This objection is based on the fact that there is little relationship between cortical activity and consciousness. Dandy, for example, showed as early as 1946 that neither bilateral excision of the cerebral cortex in dogs nor unilateral resection in humans affected consciousness. Even bilateral ligation of the anterior cerebral arteries in humans does not alter consciousness, provided the blood supply to the corpus callosum is not impaired. Penfield (1950) and Jefferson (1944), among others, agreed with Dandy that normal cortical activity is not a prerequisite of consciousness. Consciousness is, instead, probably more related to the functional activity of the reticular activating system in the brainstem (French, *et al.*, 1953; Davis, *et al.*, 1957). Therefore, even if concentrations of local anesthetics in the cerebral subarachnoid space during spinal anesthesia were great enough to depress cerebral cortical activity directly, the relationship of such depression to the somnolence of high spinal anesthesia would remain doubtful.

A second possible explanation, therefore, for the somnolence or even loss of consciousness during high spinal anesthesia involves the effect of anesthesia on the reticular activating system. Although, as mentioned above, it is highly unlikely that concentrations of local anesthetics can appear in the ventricular system during spinal anesthesia great enough to depress the vasomotor or respiratory centers, concentrations may be present which would depress the reticular activating system. In view of the fact that different types of nerve fibers are blocked by different concentrations of local anesthetic agents, and in view of the fact that synapses are more susceptible than are axons (Larrabee and Posternak, 1952), it is quite possible that an area as rich in synapses as the reticular activating system could be depressed by concentrations of local anesthetics that have no effect on the respiratory or vasomotor centers. This is probably the explanation for the observation that when 2.5% procaine is applied to the brainstem of experimental animals, there is loss of consciousness without respiratory or vascular collapse (Koster and Kasman, 1929). This is also probably the explanation for the loss of consciousness in humans following intracisternal injection of procaine (Vehrs, 1931).

It has also been suggested that total sensory deafferentation resulting from high spinal block produces alterations in consciousness (Stovner, 1957). This theory is based on the hypothesis that wakefulness is the result of bombardment of the central nervous system by afferent stimuli. Complete removal of all afferent impulses would then theoretically result in sleep. *Complete* deafferentation of the brain does not occur with high spinal anesthesia, of course. Even during total spinal anesthesia the optic and auditory nerves are still functional (Jonnesco, 1909). So also are various afferent visceral nerves. Furthermore, it is unlikely that there is no intrinsic activity of the central nervous system independent of afferent stimuli. Nevertheless, it is a widely observed clinical fact that the higher the level of spinal anesthesia, the more frequent and more pronounced drowsiness becomes. It is not unlikely that somatic sensory input to the central nervous system plays at least some role in maintaining the normal state of awareness. The observation that drowsiness occurs without the development of characteristic electroencephalographic sleep patterns during spinal anesthesia (Huvos, *et al.*, 1962) emphasizes that the drowsiness of high spinal anesthesia is not true sleep. Although deafferentation may contribute to some degree to the somnolence of high spinal anesthesia, the fact that during differential spinal block patients become somnolent despite absence of significant sensory impairment (Sarnoff and Arrowood, 1946) speaks against it as the sole cause.

High spinal anesthesia could also produce somnolence secondary to alterations in cerebral hemodynamics. It has long been recognized that arterial hypotension can produce alterations in electroencephalographic activity (Beecher, *et al.*, 1938; Dow, 1938). Beecher, *et al.*, for example, found that the electroencephalographic changes with hypotension produced by hemorrhage or cardiac tamponade were "indistinguishable from those caused by an increase in depth of anesthesia." If the blood pressure were lowered sufficiently, the recorded activity of the cortex disappeared. Since arterial blood pressure is such a major determinant of cerebral blood flow, it might be assumed that the decrease in electroencephalographic activity during arterial hypotension is the result of diminished blood flow to the brain resulting in an anoxic paralysis of cortical cells. However, the problem is more complex than this, as has been demonstrated by the work of Schallek and Walz (1954). These authors found that intravenous hexamethonium would produce changes in the electroencephalograms of dogs, but that the changes were related more to the rate at which the arterial pressure decreased rather than to the level to which it decreased. In addition, Stone, *et al.* (1955) found that humans given hexamethonium became quiet and sedated when the arterial blood pressure was decreased even though there were no simultaneous changes in cerebral blood flow. Although it is dangerous to draw comparisons between the effects on cerebral cortical function of spinal anesthesia and drugs such as hexamethonium, it is evident that the relationship between cerebral cortical function and blood pressure depends upon more than changes in cerebral blood flow. It appears likely that hypotension in itself can result in depressed levels of consciousness even though unattended by significant changes in cerebral blood flow. Undoubtedly hypotension, especially in its more severe forms, can also cause changes in cerebral blood flow which result in decreased cortical activity. Such cerebral depression would be additive to that produced by hypotension itself. In a given instance it would be impossible to determine under clinical conditions whether hypotension, decreased blood flow to the brain, or both were contributing to the sedation so often associated with high spinal anesthesia.

In summary, spinal anesthesia, especially when reaching high dermatomal levels, may be attended by decreased states of consciousness which are best ascribed to concurrent changes in either arterial blood pressure or cerebral blood flow. The clinical impression that the degree of somnolence during high spinal anesthesia can be altered by changing the blood pressure (elevation of the legs or use of vasopressors such as methoxamine which have no direct central effect) supports this hypothesis. In some cases, however, high levels of spinal anesthesia may also be associated with direct depression of the reticular activating system which would also contribute to the somnolence. It is doubtful whether either deafferentation or direct depression of the cerebral cortex during high spinal anesthesia contribute to any great extent to the observed decrease in cerebral cortical activity.

In addition to changes in cerebral cortical activity which may be observed during spinal anesthesia, changes in cerebral function may also be present after the anesthesia has worn off. These changes in cerebral cortical function appearing after or persisting beyond the duration of anesthesia may be so extremely subtle that they can be detected only by the use of complicated psychological tests. Or they may be so pronounced that they are apparent even to nonmedical personnel. As an example of the less readily detectable changes in cortical function, the results of the study by Greene, *et al.* (1954) in 25 patients given hypotensive spinal anesthesia may be quoted. The patients in this study were subjected to a battery of psychomotor tests delicate enough to detect not only qualitative changes so often associated with organic brain disease, but also quantitative changes in performance, motivation, and memory. The tests were performed preoperatively and 2–4 weeks postoperatively. Postoperatively, 5 of 25 patients showed consistent signs of mental impairment both by clinical signs and by the quantitative tests. Two additional patients showed mental impairment, but the evaluation was made questionable by associated severe depressive reactions. And, finally, two patients showed impairment by quantitative tests but with no clinical signs. Only two of the patients showed mental changes marked enough to be noticed by the medical and nursing staff in charge.

It is impossible to say whether these findings were due to the hypotension, to the spinal anesthesia, or to the general stress of surgery and anesthesia. Certainly the hypotension may have been an important etiologic factor. Nilsson (1953), using the extremely sensitive flicker-fusion test as a measure of cortical function, found that 6 of 15 patients made hypotensive with hexamethonium showed postoperative abnormalities suggesting cerebral damage. But some of the changes reported following hypotensive spinal anesthesia could also represent manifestations of the long recognized and well established syndrome of psychosis following operations performed under spinal (Bianchi, 1921) or general anesthesia (Cobb and McDermott, 1938; Abeles, 1938) regardless of whether hypotension developed or not. Postoperative mental impairment is not limited to patients developing hypotension. This is indicated by the preliminary study on control patients done by Greene, *et al.* (1954). Although insufficient numbers of patients were studied to draw definite conclusions, 2 of 11 patients having major surgery performed under normotensive spinal anesthesia showed postoperative mental impairment. Chung, *et al.* (1987) found a similarly low incidence of postoperative mental impairment in a study of geriatric patients, as did Rollason, *et al.* (1971), who also found there to be no difference in elderly patients in incidence or severity of mental impairment regardless of whether hypotension during low spinal was or was not corrected by a vasopressor. Low frequencies of postoperative mental impairment were related in the above paper by Chung, *et al.*, and in the paper by Bigler, *et al.* (1985), to very low amounts of opioids and sedatives administered pre- and intraoperatively and to, among other factors, age, type of operation, and type and frequency of perioperative medication. Though spinal anesthesia without perioperative sedatives and narcotics is associated (in carefully controlled clinical studies) with less postoperative mental impairment than is seen following general anesthesia (Bigler, *et al.*, 1985; Chung, *et al.*, 1987), the significance of this in terms of clinical outcome remains to be proven: in a large, prospective study of patients having hip surgery, no difference was seen in long-term survival between spinal and general anesthesia (Valentin, et al., 1986). The same lack of difference in postoperative mortality was reported by Davis, et al. (1987). In their study, the 28-day mortality was 6.6% with spinal anesthesia, and 5.9% with general anesthesia.

Memory is infrequently affected by spinal anesthesia even in patients premedicated with barbiturates and a narcotic (Gruber and Reed, 1968). Transient amnesia has, however, been reported following uneventful spinal anesthesia (Dykes, et al., 1972), and is especially likely to occur when the amounts of intra- and postoperative sedatives, opioids, and anxiolytics increase.

In addition to relatively subtle changes, severe and permanent impairment of cerebral function may follow spinal anesthesia (Noble, 1946; Kral, 1951; Hampton and Little, 1953; Gillies, 1953; Courville, 1954). These impairments invariably represent organic brain damage, including that seen as a result of severe intra-anesthetic hypoxemia or ischemic hypoxia following cardiac arrest. This type of brain damage can, of course, be found following any type of anesthesia in which cerebral hypoxia develops. The morphologic changes that follow severe impairment of cerebral blood flow during spinal anesthesia have been described by Courville (1954). They consist of necrosis of the intermediate cellular lamina of the cerebral cortex, patchy necrosis of the globus pallidus, degeneration of the myelinated nerve fibers of the cerebral white matter, and partial destruction of cerebellar Purkinje fibers. Similar but less extensive histologic changes are probably also present in patients who have recovered from cardiac arrest but who are left with permanent neurologic damage.

Severe, permanent impairment of cerebral function can also be seen perioperatively in association with spinal anesthesia that is due to cerebrovascular accidents (intracerebral hemorrhage or cerebral arterial thrombosis) or even herniation of the uncus against the tentorium (Eerola, et al., 1981; Mantia, 1981; Siegle, et al., 1982; Welch, 1959). Uncal herniation can certainly be directly related to spinal anesthesia, but the relationship between postoperative cerebrovascular accidents and spinal anesthesia is almost always temporal, that is, casual, not causal. Although theoretically extreme hypotension might set the stage for cerebral arterial thrombosis, while extreme hypertension following overdose of vasopressor administered to correct hypotension might precipitate intracerebral hemorrhage, credible case reports to substantiate such possibilities have not been published. It is worth remembering that cerebrovascular accidents are also seen in association with lumbar puncture alone, without spinal anesthesia (Benzon, 1984; Edelman and Wingard, 1980; Pavlin, et al., 1979; Schube and Raskin, 1936).

Disorders of the cranial nerves, most frequently involving the abducens (VI), but also the trigeminal (V), facial (VII), and auditory (VIII) nerves, have been reported following, but not during, spinal anesthesia (Fog, *et al.*, 1990; King and Calhoun, 1987; Lee and Roberts, 1978; Phillips, *et al.*, 1969; Robles, 1968; Richer and Ritacca, 1989). Except perhaps for impairment of hearing, the genesis of these neural disorders is generally mechanical, not pharmacologic, as suggested by the frequency with which they are accompanied by postural postlumbar puncture headaches. The low cerebrospinal fluid pressure causing postdural puncture headaches also causes cranial contents to sag when the patient assumes the upright position. This sagging may cause pressure to be exerted on the cranial nerves at points where they are fixed by bony structures. The effect of decreased intracranial pressure on function of the ear is probably more complicated, involving vestibular and cochlear function as well as function of the auditory nerve itself (Fog, *et al.*, 1990).

Central pain is a phenomenon whose origin has been ascribed to projection of impulses from the sensory cortex rather than, as with most pain, projection of impulses from sites outside the intracranial portions of the central nervous system. Central pain can occur after prolonged, strong nociceptive input from the periphery. Central pain may also be seen after strokes. The latter is characteristically unilateral in peripheral distribution and is associated with pronounced dysesthesias and abnormal temperature sensitivity. Diagnostic spinal anesthesia has been suggested as a method for differentiating central pain from pain that is peripheral in origin, on the basis that if pain persists in the presence of a high level of sensory denervation produced by spinal anesthesia, then the pain must be central in origin. The validity of this concept has, however, been questioned by Crisologo, *et al.* (1991). They found that differential spinal anesthesia, as described by Arrowood and Sarnoff (1948), promptly, though only transiently, relieved the peripheral manifestations of pain central in origin in two of three patients who developed central pain after strokes. Crisologo, *et al.* concluded that the complete relief of peripheral pain in the two patients with central pain makes untenable the concept that high spinal anesthesia is of value in the diagnosis of poststroke central pain. The explanation of how and why spinal anesthesia relieves poststroke central pain is as obscure as the neurologic basis for this type of pain.

REFERENCES

ABELES, M. M.: Postoperative psychoses. Am. J. Psychiat. *94*: 1187, 1938.
ADAMS, H. J., MASTRI, A. R., EICHOLZER, A. W., AND KILPATRICK, G.: Morphological effects of intrathecal etidocaine and tetracaine in rabbit spinal cord. Anesth. Analg. *53*: 904, 1974.

ARENDT-NIELSEN, L., ØBERG, B., AND BJERRING, P.: Quantitative assessment of extradural bupivacaine analgesia. Br. J. Anaesth. 65: 633, 1990 a.

ARENDT-NIELSEN, L., ANKER-MØLLER, E., BJERRING, P., AND SPANGSBERG, N.: Onset phase of bupivacaine analgesia assessed quantitatively by laser stimulation. Br. J. Anaesth. 65: 639, 1990 b.

ARROWOOD, J. G., AND SARNOFF, S. J.: Differential spinal block. V. Use in the investigation of pain following amputation. Anesthesiology 9: 614, 1948.

BABCOCK, W. W.: Spinal anesthesia: An experience of 24 years. Am. J. Surg. 5: 571, 1928.

BAKER, C. E., BERRY, R. L., ELSTON, R. C., AND THE LOCAL ANESTHETICS FOR NEURALGIA STUDY GROUP: Effect of pH of bupivacaine on duration of repeated sciatic nerve blocks in the albino rat. Anesth. Analg. 72: 773, 1991.

BEECHER, H. K., McDONOUGH, F. K., AND FORBES, A.: Effects of blood pressure changes on cortical potentials during anesthesia. J. Neurophysiol. 1: 324, 1938.

BENGTSSON, M.: Changes in skin blood flow and temperature during spinal analgesia evaluated by Doppler flowmetry and infrared thermography. Acta Anaesthesiol. Scand. 28: 625, 1984.

BENGTSSON, M., LÖFSTRÖM, J. B., AND MALMQVIST, L.-Å.: Skin conductance during spinal analgesia. Acta Anaesthesiol. Scand. 29: 67, 1985.

BENGTSSON, M., NILSSON, G. E., AND LÖFSTRÖM, J. B.: The effect of spinal anaesthesia on skin blood flow evaluated by laser Doppler flowmetry. Acta Anaesthesiol. Scand. 27: 206, 1983.

BENZON, H. T.: Intracerebral hemorrhage after dural puncture and epidural blood patch: nonpostural and noncontinuous headache. Anesthesiology 60: 258, 1984.

BIANCHI, G.: Psicosi allucinatoria acuta consecutiva ad atto operativo con rachianestesia in alcoolista. Policlinico 28: 1459, 1921.

BIGLER, D., ADELHOJ, B., PETRING, O. U., PEDERSON, N. D., BUSCH, P., AND KALHKE, P.: Mental function and morbidity after acute hip surgery during spinal and general anaesthesia. Anaesthesia 40: 672, 1985.

BLADES, B., AND FORD, W. B.: A method for control of postoperative pain. Surg. Gynecol. Obstet. 91: 524, 1950.

BONNET, F., ZOZIME, J. P., MARCANDORO, J., BUISSON, B., TOUBOUL, C., AND SAADA, M.: Tourniquet pain during spinal anesthesia: hyperbaric vs. isobaric tetracaine. Reg. Anesth. 13: 29, 1988.

BRIDENBAUGH, P. O., HAGENOUW, R. R. P. M., GIELEN, M. J. M., AND ESTRÖM, H. H.: Addition of glucose to bupivacaine spinal anesthesia increases incidence of tourniquet pain. Anesth. Analg. 65: 1181, 1986.

BRIDENBAUGH, P. O., MOORE, D. C., AND BRIDENBAUGH, L. D.: Capillary PO_2 as a measure of sympathetic blockade. Anesth. Analg. 50: 26, 1971.

BRILL, S., AND LAWRENCE, L. B.: Changes in temperature of the lower extremities following the induction of spinal anesthesia. Proc. Soc. Exp. Biol. Med. 27: 728, 1930.

BROMAGE, P. R., PETTIGREW, R. T., AND CROWELL, D. E.: Tachyphylaxis in epidural analgesia. I. Augmentation and decay of local anesthesia. J. Clin. Pharmacol. 9: 30, 1969.

BRULL, S. J., AND GREENE, N. M.: Time courses of differential sensory blockade during spinal anesthesia with hyperbaric tetracaine or bupivacaine. Anesth. Analg. 69: 342, 1989.

CHAMBERLAIN, D. P., AND CHAMBERLAIN, B. D. L.: Changes in skin temperature of the trunk and their relationship to sympathetic blockade during spinal anesthesia. Anesthesiology 65: 139, 1986.

CHUNG, F., MEIER, R., LAUTENSCHLAGER, E., CARMICHAEL, F. J., AND CHUNG, A.: General or spinal anesthesia: Which is better in the elderly? Anesthesiology 67: 422, 1987.

COBB, S., AND McDERMOTT, N. T.: Postoperative psychosis. Med. Clin. North Am. 22: 569, 1938.

COHEN, C. A., AND KALLOS, T.: Failure of spinal anesthesia due to subdural catheter placement. Anesthesiology 37: 352, 1972.

COHEN, E. N.: Distribution of local anesthetic agents in the neuraxis of the dog. Anesthesiology 29: 1002, 1968.

COHEN, E. N., LEVINE, D. A., COLLISS, J. E., AND GUNTHER, R. E.: The role of pH in the development of tachyphylaxis to local anesthetic agents. Anesthesiology 29: 994, 1968.

COLE, F.: Tourniquet pain. Anesth. Analg. 31: 63, 1952.

COLE, D. J., LIN, D. M., DRUMMOND, J. C., AND SHAPIRO, H. M.: Spinal tetracaine decreases central nervous system metabolism during somatosensory stimulation in the rat. Can. J. Anaesth. 37: 231, 1990.

CONCEPCION, M. A., LAMBERT, D. H., WELCH, K. A., AND COVINO, B. G.: Tourniquet pain during spinal anesthesia: A comparison of plain solutions of tetracaine and bupivacaine. Anesth. Analg. 67: 828, 1988.

CONVERSE, J. G., LANDMESSER, C. M., AND HARMEL, M. H.: Concentration of pontocaine hydrochloride in cerebrospinal fluid during spinal anesthesia and influence of epinephrine in prolonging sensory anesthetic effect. Anesthesiology 15: 1, 1954.

COOK, A. J., WOOLF, C. J., WALL, P. D., AND McMAHON, S. B.: Expansion of cutaneous receptive field of dorsal horn neurons following C-primary afferent fibre input. Nature 325: 151, 1987.

Co TUI, F. W.: The effect of pathologic states on the minimum lethal dose of procaine intracisternally. J. Pharmacol. Exp. Ther. 50: 51, 1934.

Co TUI, F. W.: Spinal anesthesia: The experimental basis of some prevailing clinical practices. Arch. Surg. 33: 825, 1936.

Co TUI, F. W., PREISS, A. L., BARCHAM, I., AND NEVIN, M. I.: Local nervous tissue changes following spinal anesthesia in experimental animals. J. Pharmacol. Exp. Ther. 81:209, 1944.

Co TUI, F. W., AND STANDARD, S.: Experimental studies on subarachnoid anesthesia: Paralysis of vital medullary centers. Surg. Gynecol. Obstet. 55: 290, 1932.

COURTNEY, K. R.: Mechanism of frequency-dependent inhibition of sodium currents in frog myelinated nerve by the lidocaine derivative GEA 968. J. Pharmacol. Exp. Ther. 195: 225, 1975.

COURTNEY, K. R., KENDIG, J. J., AND COHEN, E. N.: Frequency dependent conduction block: the role of nerve impulse pattern in local anesthetic potency. Anesthesiology 48: 111, 1978.

COURVILLE, C. B.: Case studies in cerebral anoxia. III. Structural changes in the brain after cardiac standstill during spinal anesthesia. Bull. Los Angeles Neurol. Soc. 19: 1942, 1954.

COVINO, B. G., AND VASSALLO, H. G.: Local Anesthetics: Mechanisms of Action and Clinical Use. New York: Grune & Stratton, 1976.

COZINE, R. A., AND NGAI, S. H.: Medullary surface chemoreceptors and regulation of respiration in the cat. J. Appl. Physiol. 22: 117, 1967.

CRILE, G. W.: The kinetic theory of shock and its prevention through anoci-association (shockless operation). Lancet ii: 7, 1913.

CRISOLOGO, P. A., NEAL, B., BROWN, R., McDANAL, J., AND KISSIN, I.: Lidocaine-induced spinal block can relieve central poststroke pain: Role of the block in chronic pain diagnosis. Anesthesiology 74: 184, 1991.

CROSBY, G.: Local spinal cord blood flow and glucose utilization during spinal anesthesia with bupivacaine in conscious rats. Anesthesiology 63: 55, 1985.

CROSBY, G., RUSSO, M. A., SZABO, M. D., AND DAVIES, K. R.: Subarachnoid clonidine reduces spinal cord blood flow and glucose utilization in conscious rats. Anesthesiology 73: 1179, 1990.

DANDY, W. E.: Location of conscious center in brain-corpus striatum. Bull. Johns Hopkins Hosp. 79: 34, 1946.

DAOS, F. G., AND VIRTUE, R. W.: Sympathetic block persistence after spinal or epidural anesthesia. J.A.M.A. *183*: 285, 1963.

DAVIS, F. M., WOOLNER, D. F., FRAMPTON, C., WILKINSON, A., GRANT, A., HARRISON, R. T., ROBERTS, M. T. S., AND THADAKA, R.: Prospective, multi-centre trial of mortality following general or spinal anaesthesia for hip fracture surgery in the elderly. Br. J. Anaesth. *59*: 1080, 1987.

DAVIS, H. S., COLLINS, W. F., RANDT, C. T., AND DILLON, W. H.: Effect of anesthetic agents on evoked central nervous system responses: Gaseous agents. Anesthesiology *18*: 634, 1957.

DAVIS, T.: Spinal analgesia. Anesthesiology *19*: 682, 1958.

DE JONG, R. H.: Tourniquet pain during spinal anesthesia. Anesthesiology *23*: 881, 1962.

DE JONG, R. H.: Phantom limb. Anesthesiology *25*: 742, 1964.

DE JONG, R. H.: Differential nerve block by local anesthetics. Anesthesiology *53*: 443, 1980.

DE JONG, R. H., AND CULLEN, S. C.: Theoretical aspects of pain: Bizarre pain phenomena during low spinal anesthesia. Anesthesiology *24*: 628, 1963.

DEREYMAKER, A., AND SOREL, L.: Experimental epilepsy and blood-brain barrier. Epilepsia *8*: 145, 1967.

DOHI, S., KITAHATA, L. M., TOYOOKA, H., OHTANI, M., NAMIKI, A., AND TAUB, A.: An analgesic action of intravenously administered lidocaine on dorsal-horn neurons responding to noxious thermal stimulation. Anesthesiology *51*: 123, 1979.

DOHI, S., MATSUMIYA, N., TAKESHIMA, R., AND NAITO, H.: The effects of subarachnoid lidocaine and phenylephrine on spinal cord and cerebral blood flow in dogs. Anesthesiology *61*: 238, 1984.

DOHI, S., TAKESHIMA, R., AND NAITO, H.: Spinal cord blood flow during spinal anesthesia in dogs: The effects of tetracaine, epinephrine, acute blood loss and hypercapnia. Anesth. Analg. *66*: 599, 1987.

DORIGOTTI, L., AND GLÄSSER, A. H.: Decrease in cerebrospinal fluid pressure induced by cervical sympathetic stimulation. Pharmacol. Res. Commun. *4*: 151, 1972.

DOUGLAS, W. W., AND MALCOLM, D. J.: The effect of localized cooling on conduction in cat nerves. J. Physiol. *130*: 53, 1955.

DOW, R. S.: Electrical activity of cerebellum and its functional significance. J. Physiol. *94*: 67, 1938.

DRIPPS, R. D.: A comparison of the malleable needle and catheter techniques for continuous spinal anesthesia. N.Y. State J. Med. *50*: 1595, 1950.

DYKES, M. H. M., SEARS, B. R., AND CAPLAN, L. R.: Transient global amnesia following spinal anesthesia. Anesthesiology *36*: 615, 1972.

EDVINSSON, L., NIELSEN, K. C., OWMAN, C., AND WEST, K. A.: Adrenergic innervation of the mammalian choroid plexus. Am. J. Anat. *139*: 299, 1974.

EDELMAN, J. D., AND WINGARD, D. W.: Subdural hematomas after lumbar puncture. Anesthesiology *52*: 166, 1980.

EEROLA, M., KAUKINEN, L., KAUKINEN, S.: Fatal brain lesion following spinal anaesthesia. Acta Anaesthesiol. Scand. *25*: 115, 1981.

EGBERT, L. D., AND DEAS, T. C.: Cause of pain from a pneumatic touniquet during spinal anesthesia. Anesthesiology *23*: 287, 1962.

FASSOULAKI, A., DRASNER, K., AND EGER, E. I., II: Is chronic ethanol associated with tolerance to intrathecal lidocaine in the rat? Anesth. Analg. *70*: 489, 1990.

FELDER, D. A., LINTON, R. R., TODD, D. P., AND BANKS, C.: Changes in the sympathectomized extremity with anesthesia. Surgery *29*: 803, 1951.

FIDDLER, D. S., AND HINDMAN, B. J.: Intravenous calcitonin alleviates spinal anesthesia-induced phantom limb pain. Anesthesiology *74*: 187, 1991.

FINK, B. R.: Mechanisms of differential axial blockade in epidural and subarachnoid anesthesia. Anesthesiology *70*: 851, 1989.

FINK, B. R., AND CAIRNS, A. M.: Differential peripheral axon block with lidocaine: Unit studies in the cervical vagus nerve. Anesthesiology 59: 182, 1983.

FINK, B. R., AND CAIRNS, A. M.: Differential slowing and block of conduction by lidocaine in individual afferent myelinated and unmyelinated axons. Anesthesiology 60: 111, 1984.

FINK, B. R., AND CAIRNS, A. M.: Diffusional delay in local anesthetic block in vitro. Anesthesiology 61: 555, 1984.

FINK, B. R., AND CAIRNS, A. M.: Differential margin of safety in conduction in individual peripheral axons. Anesthesiology 63: 65, 1985.

FINK, B. R., AND CAIRNS, A. M.: Lack of size-related differential sensitivity to equilibrium conduction block among mammalian myelinated axons exposed to lidocaine. Anesth. Analg. 66: 948, 1987 a.

FINK, B. R., AND CAIRNS, A. M.: Differential use-dependent (frequency-dependent) effects in single mammalian axons: Data and clinical considerations. Anesthesiology 67: 477, 1987 b.

FINNERTY, F. A., JR., GUILLAUDEU, R. L., AND FAZEKAS, J. F.: Cardiac and cerebral hemodynamics in drug induced postural hypotension. Circ. Res. 5: 34, 1957.

FINNERTY, F. A., JR., WITKIN, L., AND FAZEKAS, J. F.: Acute hypotension and cerebral hemodynamics. M. Ann. District of Columbia 22: 115, 1953.

FOG, M.: Cerebral circulation: the reaction of the pial arteries to a fall in blood pressure. Arch. Neurol. Psychiatry 37: 351, 1937.

FOG, J., WANG, L. P., SUNBERG, A., AND MUCCHIANO, C.: Hearing loss after spinal anesthesia is related to needle size. Anesth. Analg. 70: 517, 1990.

FORBES, A. R., AND ROIZEN, M. F.: Does spinal anesthesia anesthetize the spinal cord? Anesthesiology 48: 440, 1978.

FORD, D. J., RAJ, P. P., SINGH, P., REGAN, K. M., AND OHLWEILER, D.: Differential peripheral nerve block by local anesthetics in the cat. Anesthesiology 60: 28, 1984.

FOREGGER, R.: Surface temperatures during anesthesia. Anesthesiology 4: 392, 1943.

FOX, E. J., VILLANUEVA, R., AND SCHUTTA, H. S.: Myoclonus following spinal anesthesia. Neurology 29: 379, 1979.

FRANZ, D. N., AND PERRY, R. S.: Mechanisms for differential block among single myelinated and non-myelinated axons by procaine. J. Physiol. 236: 193, 1974.

FRENCH, J. D., VERZEANO, M., AND MAGOUN, H. W.: Neural basis of anesthetic state. Arch. Neurol. Psychiatry 69: 519, 1953.

FREUND, F. G., BONICA, J. J., WARD, R. J., AKAMATSU, T. J., AND KENNEDY, W. J., JR.: Ventilatory reserve and level of motor block during high spinal and epidural anesthesia. Anesthesiology 28: 834, 1967.

FRUMIN, M. J., SCHWARTZ, H., BURNS, J. J., BRODIE, B. B., AND PAPPER, E. M.: Sites of sensory blockade during segmental spinal and segmental peridural anesthesia in man. Anesthesiology 14: 576, 1953.

FRUMIN, M. J., SCHWARTZ, H., BURNS, J., BRODIE, B. B., AND PAPPER, E. M.: Dorsal root ganglion blockade during threshold segmental spinal anesthesia in man. J. Pharmacol. Exp. Ther. 112: 387, 1954.

GALINDO, A.: Hemodynamic changes in the internal carotid artery produced by total sympathetic block (epidural anesthesia) and carbon dioxide. Anesth. Analg. 43: 276, 1964.

GALINDO, A., AND WITCHER, T.: Blockade of sensory and motor pathways by bupivacaine, etidocaine, and lidocaine. Reg. Anesth. 7: 7, 1982.

GASSER, H. S., AND ERLANGER, J.: Role of fiber size in establishment of nerve block by pressure or cocaine. Am. J. Physiol. 88: 581, 1929.

GEDDES, I. C., AND QUASTEL, J. H.: Effects of local anesthetics on respiration of rat brain cortex in vitro. Anesthesiology 17: 666, 1956.

GHIA, J. N., TOOMERY, T. C., MAO, W., DUNCAN, G., AND GREGG, J. M.: Towards an understanding of chronic pain mechanisms: Use of psychologic tests and a refined differential spinal block. Anesthesiology 50: 20, 1979.

GIASI, R. M., D'AGOSTINO, E., AND COVINO, B. G.: Absorption of lidocaine following sub-arachnoid and epidural administration. Anesth. Analg. *58*: 360, 1979.

GIBBS, P., PURUSHOTHAM, A., AULD, C., AND CUSCHIERI, R. J.: Continuous wound perfusion with bupivacaine for postoperative pain. Br. J. Surg. *75*: 923, 1988.

GILLIES, J.: Hypotension in anaesthesia. Br. Med. J. *I*: 504, 1953.

GISSEN, A. J., COVINO, B. G., AND GREGUS, J.: Differential sensitivities of mammalian nerve fibers to local anesthetic agents. Anesthesiology 53: 467, 1980.

GISSEN, A. J., COVINO, B. G., AND GREGUS, J.: Differential sensitivities of fast and slow fibers in mammalian nerve. II. Margin of safety for nerve transmission. Anesth. Analg. *61*: 561, 1982 a.

GISSEN, A. J., COVINO, B. G., AND GREGUS, J.: Differential sensitivity of fast and slow fibers in mammalian nerve. III. Effect of etidocaine and bupivacaine on fast/slow fibers. Anesth. Analg. *61*: 570, 1982 b.

GORDH, T.: Analysis of the sensation of warmth in the lower extremities as the primary effect in spinal anesthesia. Reg. Anesth. 2: 5, 1977.

GREENE, N. M.: Hypotensive spinal anesthesia. Surg. Gynecol. Obstet. *95*: 331, 1952.

GREENE, N. M.: The pharmacology of local anesthetic agents with special reference to their use in spinal anesthesia. Anesthesiology 16: 573, 1955.

GREENE, N. M.: The area of differential block during spinal anesthesia with hyperbaric tetracaine. Anesthesiology 19: 45, 1958.

GREENE, N. M.: Blood levels of local anesthetics during spinal and epidural anesthesia. Anesth. Analg. *56*: 357, 1979.

GREENE, N. M.: Preganglionic sympathetic blockade in man: a study of spinal anaesthesia. Acta Anaesthesiol. Scand. 25: 463, 1981.

GREENE, N. M.: A new look at sympathetic denervation during spinal anesthesia. Anesthesiology 65: 137, 1986.

GREENE, N. M., BUNKER, J. P., KERR, W. S., VON FELSINGER, J. M., KELLER, J. W., AND BEECHER, H. K.: Hypotensive spinal anesthesia: respiratory, metabolic, hepatic, renal, and cerebral effects. Ann. Surg. *140*: 641, 1954.

GRIFFITHS, H. W. C., AND GILLIES, J.: Thoraco-lumbar splanchnicectomy and sympathec-tomy: anaesthetic procedure. Anaesthesia 3: 134, 1948.

GRODINSKY, M., BEBER, M., AND BARKER, C. P.: Test for presence of novocaine in nervous tissue. Science 77: 450, 1933.

HAGENOUW, R. R. P. M., BRIDENBAUGH, P. O., VAN EGMOND, J., AND STUEBING, R.: Tourniquet pain: A volunteer study. Anesth. Analg. 65: 1175, 1986.

HAMPTON, L. J., AND LITTLE, D. M.: Complications associated with the use of "controlled hypotension" in anesthesia. Arch. Surg. 67: 549, 1953.

HARANATH, P. S. R. K., AND VENKATAKRISHNA-BHATT, H.: Studies on cinchocaine and lido-caine administered into cerebral ventricles of conscious and anesthetized dogs. Indian J. Med. Res. 56: 217, 1968.

HARDY, J. D., AND OPPEL, T. W.: Studies in temperature sensation. III. The sensitivity of the body to heat and the spatial summation of end organ responses. J. Clin. Invest 16: 533, 1937.

HARMEL, M. H., HAFKENSCHIEL, J. H., AUSTIN, G. M., CRUMPTON, C. W., AND KETY, S. S.: The effect of bilateral stellate ganglion block on the cerebral circulation in normotensive and hypertensive patients. J. Clin. Invest. 28: 415, 1949.

HARRISON, G.: Phantom limb pain occurring during spinal analgesia. Anaesthesia 6: 115, 1951.

HEAVENER, J. E., AND DE JONG, R. H.: Lidocaine blocking concentrations for B- and C-nerve fibers. Anesthesiology 40: 228, 1974.

HELRICH, M., PAPPER, E. M., BRODIE, B. B., FINK, M., AND ROVENSTINE, E. A.: The fate of intrathecal procaine and the spinal fluid level required for surgical anesthesia. J. Pharma-col. Exp. Ther. *100*: 78, 1950.

HERBST, T. J., RAICHLE, M. E., AND FERRENDELLIJ. A.: β-adrenergic regulation of adenosine 3',5'-monophosphate concentration in brain microvessels. Science 204: 330, 1979.

HILL, E. F.: Spinal anaesthesia. Br. J. Anaesth. 23: 15, 1951.

HILL, E. F., AND MACDONALD, A. D.: Observations on experimental spinal anesthesia. J. Pharmacol. Exp. Ther. 47: 151, 1933.

HOWARTH, F.: Studies with a radioactive spinal anaesthetic. Br. J. Pharmacol. 4: 333, 1949.

HUVOS, M. C., GREENE, N. M., AND GLASER, G. H.: Electroencephalographic studies during acute subtotal sensory denervation in man. Yale J. Biol. Med. 34: 592, 1962.

IRWIN, R. L., STONE, J. E., DRAPER, W. B., AND WHITEHEAD, R. W.: Urine secretion during diffusion respiration following apnea inducted by intracisternal injection of procaine hydrochloride. Anesthesiology 16: 665, 1955.

JAMES, I. M., MILLAR, R. A., AND PURVES, J. J.: Observations on the extrinsic neural control of cerebral blood flow in the baboon. Circ. Res. 25: 77, 1969.

JEFFERSON, G.: Nature of concussion. Br. Med. J. 1: 1, 1944.

JOHNSTON, J. F. A., AND HENDERSON, V. E.: An experimental inquiry into spinal anesthesia. Anesth. Analg. 11: 78, 1932.

JOLLY, E. R., AND STEINHAUS, J. E.: The effect of drugs injected into limited portions of the cerebral circulation. J. Pharmacol. Exp. Ther. 116: 273, 1956.

JONES, R. G. G.: A complication of epidural technique. Anaesthesia 8: 242, 1953.

JONNESCO, T.: Remarks on general spinal anaesthesia. Br. Med. J. 2: 1396, 1909.

KAMSLER, P. M., DABBS, H., AND SOUTHWORTH, J. L.: Regional spinal anesthesia utilizing the continuous spinal technic of Tuohy. Anesthesiology 13: 397, 1952.

KETY, S. S., KING, B. D., HAFKENSCHIEL, J. H., HORVATH, S. M., AND JEFFERS, W. A.: The cerebral circulation in essential hypertension and effects of differential spinal sympathetic block. J. Clin. Invest. 27: 543, 1948.

KETY, S. S., KING, B. D., HORVATH, S. M., JEFFERS, W. A., AND HAFKENSCHIEL, J. H.: The effects of acute reduction in blood pressure by means of differential spinal sympathetic block on the cerebral circulation of hypertensive patients. J. Clin. Invest. 29: 402, 1950.

KHURANA, S., SINGH, C. V., CHHABRA, B., AND KAMBRA, G. L.: Phantom limb sensation under subarachnoid and epidural analgesia: A comparative clinical study of two hundred cases. Can. Anaesth. Soc. J. 26: 114, 1979.

KIM, J. M., LASALLE, A. D., AND PARMLEY, R. T.: Sympathetic recovery following lumbar epidural and spinal analgesia. Anesth. Analg. 56: 352, 1977.

KING, R. A., AND CALHOUN, J. H.: Fourth cranial nerve palsy following spinal anesthesia. J. Clin. Neuro-ophthalmology 7(1): 20, 1987.

KIRNÖ, K., KUNIMOTO, M., LUNDIN, S., ELAM, M., AND WALLIN, B. G.: Can galvanic skin response be used as a quantitative estimate of sympathetic nerve activity in regional anesthesia? Anesth. Analg. 73: 138, 1991.

KITAHARA, T., KURI, S., AND YOSHIDA, J.: The spread of drugs used for spinal anesthesia. Anesthesiology 17: 205, 1956.

KLEINERMAN, J., SANCETTA, S. M., AND HACKEL, D. B.: Effects of high spinal anesthesia on cerebral circulation and metabolism in man. J. Clin. Invest. 37: 285, 1958.

KOSTER, H.: Spinal anesthesia, with special reference to its use in surgery of the head, neck and thorax. Am. J. Surg. 5: 554, 1928.

KOSTER, H., AND KASMAN, L. P.: Spinal anesthesia for the head, neck and thorax; its relation to respiratory paralysis. Surg. Gynecol. Obstet. 49: 617, 1929.

KOSTER, H., SHAPIRO, A., AND LEIKENSOHN, A.: Concentration of procaine in the cerebrospinal fluid of the human being after subarachnoid injection. Arch. Surg. 37: 603, 1938.

KOSTER, H., SHAPIRO, A., AND LEIKENSOHN, A.: Spinal anesthesia: procaine concentration changes at site of injection in subarachnoid anesthesia. Am. J. Surg. 33: 245, 1936.

KOSTER, H., SHAPIRO, A., WARSHAW, R., AND MARGOLICK, M.: Removal of procaine from the cerebrospinal fluid during anesthesia. Arch. Surg. 39: 682, 1939.

KOYAMA, K., WATANABE, S., TSUNETO, S., TAKAHASHI, H., AND NAITO, H.: Thiopental for phantom limb pain during spinal anesthesia. Anesthesiology 69: 598, 1988.

KOZODY, R., PALAHNIUK, R. J., AND CUMMING, M. O.: Spinal cord blood flow following subarachnoid tetracaine. Can. Anaesth. Soc. J. 32: 23, 1985 a.

KOZODY, R., SWARTZ, J., PALAHNIUK, R. J., BIEHL, D. R., AND WADE, J. G.: Spinal cord blood flow following subarachnoid lidocaine. Can. Anaesth. Soc. J. 32: 472, 1985 b.

KOZODY, R., PALAHNIUK, R. J., WADE, J. G., AND CUMMING, M. O.: The effect of subarachnoid epinephrine and phenylephrine on spinal cord blood flow. Can. Anaesth. Soc. J. 31: 503, 1984.

KRAL, V. A.: Neuropsychiatric sequelae of cardiac arrest during spinal anaesthesia; one year follow-up of case. Can. Med. Assoc. J. 64: 138, 1951.

KROIN, J. S., PENN, R. D., LEVY, F. E., AND KERNS, J. M.: Effect of repetitive lidocaine infusion on peripheral nerve. Exp. Neurol. 94: 166, 1986.

KÜSTNER, H., AND EISSNER, W.: Quantitative Untersuchungen über das Verhalt des Novokains im Liquor. Münch. Med. Wsckr. 7: 622, 1930.

LAMBERT, D. H., DEANE, R. S., AND MAZUZAN, J. E., JR.: Anesthesia and the control of blood pressure in patients with spinal cord injury. Anesth. Analg. 61: 344, 1982.

LANDAU, W. M., WEAVER, R. A., AND HORNBEIN, T. F.: Fusimotor nerve function in man. Arch. Neurol. 3: 10, 1960.

LANG, E., KRAINICK, J. E., AND GERBERSHAGEN, H. U.: Spinal cord transmission of impulses during high spinal anesthesia as measured by cortical evoked potentials. Anesth. Analg. 69: 15, 1989.

LANG, E., ERDMANN, K., AND GERBERSHAGEN, H. U.: High spinal anesthesia does not depress central nervous system function as measured by central conduction time and somatosensory evoked potentials. Anesth. Analg. 71: 176, 1990.

LARRABEE, M. G., AND POSTERNAK, J. M.: Selective action of anesthetics on synapses and axons in mammalian sympathetic ganglia. J. Neurophysiol. 15: 91, 1952.

LEATHERDALE, R. A.: Phantom limb pain associated with spinal analgesia. Anaesthesia 11: 249, 1956.

LEE, J. O., AND ROBERTS, R. B.: Paresis of the fifth cranial nerve following spinal anesthesia. Anesthesiology 49: 217, 1978.

LEVY, J. H., ISLAS, J. A., GHIA, J. N., AND TURNBULL, C. A.: A retrospective study of the incidence and causes of failed spinal anesthetics in a university hospital. Anesth. Analg. 64: 705, 1985.

LINDVALL, M., EDVINSSON, L., AND OWMAN, C.: Histochemical, ultrastructural, and functional evidence for a neurogenic control of CSF production from the choroid plexus. Adv. Neurol. 20: 111, 1978.

LIPPERT, P., HOLTHUSEN, H., AND ARNDT, J. O.: Tachyphylaxis to local anesthetics does not result from reduced drug effectiveness at the nerve itself. Anesthesiology 70: 71, 1989.

LIPSCHITZ, E., DAVIS, D. L., AND FOLDES, F. F.: Disappearance of tetracaine from subarachnoid space. Fed. Proc. 12: 342, 1953.

LOESCHKE, H. H., AND KOEPCHEN, H. P.: Beeinflussung von Atmung und Vasomotorik durch Einbringen von Novocaine in die Liquorräume. Pflugers Arch. Ges. Physiol. 266: 611, 1958 a.

LOESCHKE, H. H., AND KOEPCHEN, H. P.: Versuch zur Lokalisation des Angriff-sortes der Atmungs-und Kreisaufwirkung von Novocain im Liquor cerebrospinalis. Pflugers Arch. Ges. Physiol. 266: 628, 1958 b.

LÖFSTRÖM, J. B., MALMQVIST, L.-Å., BENGTSSON, M.: Can the "sympathogalvanic reflex" (skin conductance response) be used to evaluate the extent of sympathetic block during spinal analgesia? Acta Anaesthesiol. Scand. 28: 578, 1984.

LORENTE DE NÓ, R., AND CONDOURIS, G. A.: Decremental conduction in peripheral nerve. Integration of stimuli in the neuron. Proc. Natl. Acad. Sci. USA 45: 592, 1959.

LUND, C., SEGMAR, P., HANSEN, O. B., AND KEHLET, H.: Effect of intrathecal bupivacaine on somatosensory evoked potentials following dermatomal stimulation. Anesth. Analg. 66: 809, 1987.

LUNDIN, S., WALLIN, G., AND ELAM, M.: Intraneural recording of muscle sympathetic activity during epidural anesthesia in humans. Anesth. Analg. 69: 788, 1989.

LUNDY, J. S., ESSEX, H. E., AND KERNOHAN, J. W.: Experiments with anesthetics: lesions produced in spinal cord of dogs by dose of procaine HCl sufficient to cause permanent and fatal paralysis. J.A.M.A. 101: 1546, 1933.

MACKENZIE, N.: Phantom limb pain during spinal anaesthesia. Anaesthesia 38: 886, 1983.

MANCHIKANTI, L., HADLEY, C., MARKWELL, S. J., AND COLLIVER, J. A.: A retrospective analysis of failed spinal anesthetic attempts in a community hospital. Anesth. Analg. 66: 363, 1987.

MANTIA, A. M.: Clinical report of the occurrence of an intracerebral hemorrhage following post-lumbar puncture headache. Anesthesiology 55: 684, 1981.

MAXSON, L. H.: Spinal Anesthesia. Philadelphia: The J. B. Lippincott Co., 1938.

McCOLLUM, D. E., AND STEPHEN, C. R.: The use of graduated spinal anesthesia in the differential diagnosis of pain in the back and lower extremities. South. Med. J. 57: 410, 1964.

MEIJER, J., deLANGE, J. J., AND ROS, H. H.: Skin pulse wave monitoring during lumbar epidural and spinal anesthesia. Anesth. Analg. 67: 356, 1988.

MELZACK, R.: Phantom limb pain: Implications for treatment of pathologic pain. Anesthesiology 35: 409, 1971.

MEYER, J., AND NOLTE, H.: Liquorkonzentration von Bupivacaine nach subduraler Applikation. Reg. Anaesth. 1: 38, 1978 (Suppl. to Anaesthesist 27: 5, 1978).

MILES, J. E.: Phantom limb syndrome occurring during spinal anesthesia; relationship to etiology. J. Nerv. Ment. Dis. 123: 365, 1956.

MILLER, G. L., AND DISCUSSANTS OF HIS LETTER TO THE EDITOR. Reg. Anesth. 6: 122, 1981.

MITCHELL, R. A., LOESCHCKE, H. H., MASSION, W. H., AND SEVERINGHAUS, J. W.: Respiratory responses mediated through superficial chemosensitive areas on the medulla. J. Appl. Physiol. 18: 523, 1963.

MOORE, B.: Pain in amputation stump associated with spinal anaesthesia. Med. J. Aust. 2: 645, 1946.

MOORE, R. A., BULLINGHAM, R. E. S., McQUAY, H. J., HAND, C. W., ASPEL, J. B., ALLEN, M. C., AND THOMAS, D.: Dural permeability to narcotics: In vitro determination and application to extradural administration. Br. J. Anaesth. 54: 1117, 1982.

MOORTHY, S. S., AND DIERDORF, S. F.: Restless legs during recovery from spinal anesthesia. Anesth. Analg. 70: 337, 1990.

MÖRCH, E. T., ROSENBERG, M. K., AND TRUANT, A. T.: Lidocaine for spinal anaesthesia. A study of the concentration in spinal fluid. Acta. Anaesthesiol. Scand. 1: 105, 1957.

MORRIS, G. C., JR., MOYER, J. H., SNYDER, H. B., AND HAYNES, B. W., JR.: Vascular dynamics in controlled hypotension: study of cerebral and renal hemodynamics and blood volume changes. Ann. Surg. 138: 706, 1953.

MUNHALL, R. J., SUKHANI, R., AND WINNIE, A. P.: Incidence and etiology of failed spinal anesthetics in a university hospital. Anesth. Analg. 67: 843, 1988.

MURPHY, J. P., AND ANANDACIVA, S.: Phantom limb pain and spinal anaesthesia. Anaesthesia 39: 188, 1984.

NADKARNI, A. V., AND TONDARE, A. S.: Localized clonic convulsions after spinal anesthesia with lidocaine and epinephrine. Anesth. Analg. 61: 945, 1982.

NAFFZIGER, H. C., AND ADAMS, J. E.: Role of stellate block in various intracranial pathological states. Arch. Surg. 61: 286, 1950.

NATHAN, P. W.: Observations on sensory and sympathetic function during intrathecal analgesia. J. Neurol. Neurosurg. Psychiatry 39: 114, 1979.

NATHAN, P. W., AND SEARS, T. A.: Some factors concerned in differential nerve block by local anesthetics. J. Physiol. 157: 565, 1961.

NATHANSON, J. A.: β-Adrenergic-sensitive adenylate cyclase in secretory cells of choroid plexus. Science 204: 843, 1979.

NILSSON, E.: The application of a method for the investigation of cerebral damage following anaesthesia using controlled hypotension: a preliminary communication. Br. J. Anaesth. 25: 24, 1953.

NOBLE, A. B.: Cerebral anoxia complicating spinal anesthesia. Can. Med. Assoc. J. 54: 378, 1946.

ORR, J. E., LOWE, G. D. O., NIMMO, W. S., WATSON, R., AND FORBES, C. D.: A haemorrheological study of lignocaine. Br. J. Anaesth. 58: 306, 1986.

OWEN, H., GALLOWAY, D. J., AND MITCHELL, K. G.: Analgesia by wound infiltration after surgical excision of benign breast lumps. Ann. R. Coll. Surg. Engl. 67: 114, 1985.

PAINTAL, A. S.: A comparison of the nerve impulses of mammalian non-medullated nerve fibers with those of the smallest diameter medullated fibres. J. Physiol. 193: 523, 1967.

PATEL, J. M., LANZAFAME, R. J., WILLIAMS, J. S., MULLEN, B. V., AND HINSHAW, J. R.: The effect of incisional infiltration of bupivacaine hydrochloride upon pulmonary functions, atelectasis and narcotic need following elective cholecystectomy. Surg. Gynecol. Obstet. 157: 338, 1983.

PAUCHET, V.: Spinal anesthesia. Am. J. Surg. 34: 1, 1920.

PAVLIN, D. J., MCDONALD, J. S., CHILD, B., AND RUSCH, V.: Acute subdural hematoma—an unusual sequela to lumbar puncture. Anesthesiology 51: 338, 1979.

PAYNE, R.: Subarachnoid injection of cocaine as a general anesthetic for operations upon the head. Trans. Am. Laryngol. Rhinol. Otol. Soc. 7: 215, 1901.

PENFIELD, W., AND RASMUSSEN, T.: The Cerebral Cortex of Man: A Clinical Study of Localization of Function. New York: The Macmillan Company, 1950.

PFLUG, A. E., AASHEIM, G. M., AND FOSTER, C.: Sequence of return of neurological function and criteria for safe ambulation following subarachnoid block (spinal anaesthetic). Can. Anaesth. Soc. J. 25: 133, 1978.

PHILLIPS, O., EBNER, H., NELSON, A. T., AND BLACK, M. H.: Neurologic complications following spinal anesthesia with lidocaine: A prospective review of 10,440 cases. Anesthesiology 30: 284, 1969.

PITKIN, G. P.: Controllable spinal anesthesia. Am. J. Surg. 5: 537, 1928.

PORTER, S. S., ALBIN, M. S., WATSON, W. A., BUNEGIN, L., AND PANTOJA, G.: Spinal cord and cerebral blood flow responses to subarachnoid injection of local anaesthetics with and without epinephrine. Acta Anaesthesiol. Scand. 29: 330, 1985.

PREVOZNIK, S. J., AND ECKENHOFF, J. E.: Phantom sensations during spinal anesthesia. Anesthesiology 25: 767, 1964.

RAY, B. S., HINSEY, J. C., AND GEOHEGAN, W. A.: Observations on the distribution of the sympathetic nerves to the pupil and upper extremity as determined by stimulation of the anterior roots in man. Ann. Surg. 118: 647, 1943.

RAYMOND, S. A., STEFFENSON, S. C., GUZINO, L. D., AND STRICHARTZ, G. R.: The role of length of nerve exposed to local anesthetics in impulse blocking action. Anesth. Analg. 68: 563, 1989.

RICHER, S., AND RITACCA, D.: Sixth nerve palsy after lumbar anesthesia. Optometry Vision Sci. 66(5): 320, 1989.

ROBLES, R.: Cranial nerve paralysis after spinal anesthesia. Northwest Med. 67: 845, 1968.

ROCCO, A. G., RAYMOND, S. A., MURRAY, E., DHINGRA, U., AND FREIBERGER, D.: Differential spread of touch, cold and pinprick during spinal anesthesia. Anesth. Analg. 64: 917, 1985.

ROE, C. F., AND COHN, F. L.: Sympathetic blockade during spinal anesthesia. Surg. Gynecol. Obstet. 136: 265, 1973.

ROLLASON, W. N., ROBERTSON, G. S., CORDINER, C. M., AND HALL, D. J.: A comparison of mental function in relation to hypotensive and normotensive anaesthesia in the elderly. Br. J. Anaesth. 43: 561, 1971.

ROSENBERG, P. H., AND HEINONEN, E.: Differential sensitivity of A and C nerves to long-acting local anaesthetics. Br. J. Anaesth. 55: 163, 1983.

ROSENBERG, P. H., HEINONEN, E., JANSSON, S.-E., AND GRIPENBERG, J.: Differential nerve block by bupivacaine and 2-chloroprocaine. Br. J. Anaesth. 52: 1183, 1980.

ROSENSTEIN, R., McCARTHY, L. E., AND BORISON, H. L.: Respiratory effects of ethanol and procaine injected into the cerebrospinal fluid of the brainstem of cats. J. Pharmacol. Exp. Ther. 162: 174, 1968.

RUDIN, D. O., FREMONT-SMITH, K., AND BEECHER, H. K.: Permeability of dura mater to epidural procaine in dogs. J. Appl. Physiol. 3: 388, 1951.

SARGENT, W. W., BRADLEY, W. E., AND VAN BERGEN, F. H.: An electrophysiologic evaluation of the spinal fluid exchange technic in diminishing spinal anesthesia. Anesth. Analg. 50: 748, 1971.

SARNOFF, S. J., AND ARROWOOD, J. G.: Differential spinal block. Surgery 20: 150, 1946.

SARNOFF, S. J., AND ARROWOOD, J. G.: Differential spinal block. III. The block of cutaneous and stretch reflexes in the presence of unimpaired position sense. J. Neurophysiol. 10: 205, 1947.

SCHALLEK, W., AND WALZ, D.: Effects of drug-induced hypotension on electroencephalogram of dog. Anesthesiology 15: 673, 1954.

SCHEINBERG, P.: Cerebral blood flow in vascular disease of the brain, with observations on the effects of stellate ganglion block. Am. J. Med. 8: 139, 1950.

SCHUBE, P. G., AND RASIN, N.: Cerebral hemorrhage following lumbar puncture. J. Nerv. Ment. Dis. 84: 636, 1936.

SCURLOCK, J. E., MEYMARIS, E., AND GREGUS, J.: The clinical character of local anaesthetics: A function of frequency-dependent conduction block. Acta Anaesthesiol. Scand. 22: 601, 1978.

SECHZER, P. H.: Subdural space in spinal anesthesia. Anesthesiology 24: 869, 1963.

SELLICK, B. C.: Phantom limb pain and spinal anesthesia. Anesthesiology 62: 801, 1985.

SHANBROM, E., AND LEVY, L.: The role of systemic blood pressure in cerebral circulation in carotid and basilar artery thromboses. Am. J. Med. 23: 197, 1957.

SHENKIN, H. A., CABIESES, F., AND VAN DEN NOORDT, G.: The effect of bilateral stellectomy upon the cerebral circulation of man. J. Clin. Invest. 30: 90, 1951.

SHENKIN, H. A., SCHEUERMAN, W. G., SPITZ, E. B., AND GROFF, R. A.: The effects of change in position upon the cerebral circulation in man. Am. J. Med. Sci. 216: 714, 1948.

SHERRINGTON, C. S.: The Integrative Action of the Nervous System, New Haven, Yale University Press, 1907.

SIEGLE, J. H., DEWAN, D. M., AND JAMES, F. M., III: Cerebral infarction following spinal anesthesia for cesarean section. Anesth. Analg. 61: 390, 1982.

SINCLAIR, D. M.: Failure of 4 successive spinal anaesthetics. S. Afr. Med. J. 47: 1984, 1973.

SINCLAIR, R., CASSUTO, J., HÖGSTRÖM, S., LINDÉN, I., FAXÉN, A., HEDNER, T., AND EKMAN, R.: Topical anesthesia with lidocaine aerosol in the control of postoperative pain. Anesthesiology 68: 895, 1988.

SISE, L. F.: Spinal anesthesia fatalities and their prevention. N. Engl. J. Med. 200: 1071, 1929.

SIVARAJAN, M., AMORY, D. W., LINDBLOOM, L. E., AND SCHWETTMAN, R. S.: Systemic and regional blood-flow changes during spinal anesthesia in the Rhesus monkey. Anesthesiology 43: 78, 1975.

SMITH, S. M., AND REES, V. L.: The use of prolonged continuous spinal anesthesia to relieve vasospasm and pain in peripheral embolism. Anesthesiology 9: 229, 1970.

STAIMAN, A., AND SEEMAN, P.: Conduction-blocking concentrations of anesthetics increase with nerve axon diameter: studies with alcohol, lidocaine and tetrodotoxin on single myelinated fibers. J. Pharmacol. Exp. Ther. *201*: 340, 1977.

STARK, P., GERGS, P., AND NOLTE, H.: Die pH-Veranderungen des Liquor spinalis durch Bupivacain. Anaesthesist *26*: 395, 1977.

STEWART, A., LAMBERT, D. H., CONCEPCION, M. A., DATTA, S., FLANAGAN, H., MIGLIOZZI, R., AND COVINO, B. G.: Decreased incidence of tourniquet pain during spinal anesthesia with bupivacaine: a possible explanation. Anesth. Analg. *67*: 833, 1988.

STONE, H. H., MACKRELL, T. N., AND WECHSLER, R. L.: The effect on cerebral circulation and metabolism in man of acute reductions in blood pressure by means of intravenous hexamethonium bromide and head-up tilt. Anesthesiology *16*: 168, 1955.

STOVNER, J.: Sub-total spinal analgesia. Anaesthesia *12*: 463, 1957.

STRANDGAARD, S., OLESEN, J., SKINHØJ, E., AND LASSEN, N. A.: Autoregulation of brain circulation in severe arterial hypertension. Br. Med. J. *1*: 507, 1973.

STRICHARTZ, G., AND ZIMMERMANN, M.: An explanation for pain originating from tourniquets during regional anesthesia. Reg. Anesth. *9*: 4, 1984.

STRONG, O. S., AND ELWYN, A.: *Human Neuroanatomy*. First Edition. Williams and Wilkins Co., Baltimore, 1943.

TAIT, D., AND CAGLIERI, G.: Experimental and clinical notes on the subarachnoid space. J.A.M.A. *35*: 6, 1900.

THOMPSON, K. W.: Spinal anesthesia: an experimental study. Surg. Gynecol. Obstet. *58*: 852, 1934.

TKACHENKO, B. I., KRASILNIKOV, V. G., POLENOV, S. A., AND CHERNJAVSKAJA, G. V.: Responses of resistance and capacitance vessels at various frequency electrical stimulation of sympathetic nerves. Experientia *25*: 38, 1969.

TRUENT, A. P., AND LANZONI, V.: The effect and distribution of local anesthetics in the normal and desheathed nerve. Fed. Proc. *11*: 397, 1952.

TUCKER, G. T., BOYES, R. N., BRIDENBAUGH, P. O., AND MOORE, D. C.: Binding of anilide-type local anesthetics in human plasma. II. Complications in vivo, with special reference to transplacental distribution. Anesthesiology *33*: 304, 1970.

TUOHY, E. G.: The adaptations of continuous spinal anesthesia. Anesth. Analg. *31*: 372, 1952.

TVERSKOY, M., COZACOV, C., AYACHE, M., BRADLEY, E. L., AND KISSIN, I.: Postoperative pain after inguinal herniorrhaphy with different types of anesthesia. Anesth. Analg. *70*: 29, 1990.

URBAN, B. J.: Clinical observations suggesting a changing site of action during induction and recession of spinal and epidural anesthesia. Anesthesiology *39*: 496, 1973.

VALENTIN, N., LOMHOLT, B., JENSEN, J. S., HEJGAARD, N., AND KREINER, S.: Spinal or general anaesthesia for surgery of the fractured hip? A prospective study of mortality in 578 patients. Br. J. Anaesth. *58*: 284, 1986.

VEHRS, G. R.: Heart beat and respiration in total novocaine analgesia. Northwest Med. *30*: 256, 1931.

VEHRS, G. R.: *Spinal Anesthesia: Technic and Clinical Application*. St. Louis: The C.V. Mosby Co., 1934.

WALTS, L. F., KOEPKE, G., AND MARGULES, R.: Determination of sensory and motor levels after spinal anesthesia with tetracaine. Anesthesiology *25*: 634, 1964.

WATANABE, S., SAKAI, K., ONO, Y., SEINO, H., AND NAITO, H.: Alternating periodic leg movement induced by spinal anesthesia in an elderly male. Anesth. Analg. *66*: 1031, 1987.

WEISKOPF, R. B.: Unexplained failure of a continuous spinal anesthetic. Anesthesiology *33*: 114, 1970.

WELCH, K.: Subdural hematoma following spinal anesthesia. Arch. Surg. *79*: 49, 1959.

WHITE, J. C., SMITHWICK, R. H., AND SIMEONE, F. A.: *The Autonomic Nervous System*. Third Edition. New York: The Macmillan Co., 1952.

WILDSMITH, J. A. W., BROWN, D. T., PAUL, D., AND JOHNSON, S.: Structure-activity relationships in differential nerve block at high and low frequency stimulation. Br. J. Anaesth. 63: 444, 1989.

WILDSMITH, J. A. W., GISSEN, A. J., GREGUS, J., AND COVINO, B. G.: Differential nerve blocking activity of amino-ester local anaesthetics. Br. J. Anaesth. 57: 612, 1985.

WILDSMITH, J. A. W., GISSEN, A. J., TAKMAN, B., AND COVINO, B. G.: Differential nerve blockade: esters vs. amides and the influence of pKa. Br. J. Anaesth. 59: 379, 1987.

WOOLF, C. J.: Evidence for a central component of post-injury pain hypersensitivity. Nature 306: 686, 1983.

WOOLF, C. J., AND WALL, P. D.: The brief and the prolonged facilitatory effects of unmyelinated afferent input on the rat spinal cord are independently influenced by peripheral nerve injury. Neuroscience 17: 1199, 1986.

WRIGHT, A. D.: Spinal analgesia with special reference to operations above diaphragm. Proc. Roy. Soc. Med. 24: 5–12, 1930–1931.

CHAPTER 2

The Cardiovascular System

The effects of spinal anesthesia on the cardiovascular system are the result of preganglionic sympathetic block produced by the local anesthetic agent injected in the subarachnoid space. Neither the local anesthetic agent itself nor vasoconstrictors injected into the subarachnoid space to prolong duration of anesthesia have any systemic cardiovascular effects following their absorption by the vascular system (Bonica, *et al.*, 1966, Greene, 1979; Feldman, *et al.*, 1984). A possible exception to this statement has been the recent demonstration of a decrease in diastolic blood pressure associated with administration of 150 μg of the alpha-2 agonist clonidine during hyperbaric tetracaine spinal in humans (Bonnet, *et al.*, 1989) or with the intrathecal administration of 5 μg in rats (Finch, *et al.*, 1980; Yasouka and Yaksh, 1983). But even these findings have not been confirmed by previous studies that investigated the motor and sensory effects of intrathecally administered clonidine. Such studies failed to report any significant hemodynamic changes in animals (Mensink, *et al.*, 1987; Bedder, *et al.*, 1986) or in humans (Racle, *et al.*, 1987 and Bonnett, *et al.*, 1989). The systemic cardiovascular responses to intrathecal injection of clonidine certainly need clarification under clinical conditions, but otherwise the generalization that local anesthetics or vasoconstrictors administered intrathecally lack direct effects on the cardiovascular system is accurate, even despite the significant increases in free norepinephrine levels that have been noted in the cerebrospinal fluid following addition of norepinephrine to spinal dibucaine (Goto, *et al.*, 1988) or to epidural mepivacaine (Goto, *et al.*, 1990). Properly administered spinal anesthesia has justifiably been termed a pharmacologic "bargain" (Anderson, 1966), because the extent of anesthesia produced per milligram of drug administered so vastly exceeds that obtained with any other regional anesthetic technique.

Inasmuch as the cardiovascular changes are, therefore, related to the cephalad distance to which the local anesthetic spreads in the subarachnoid space and, thus to the extent of preganglionic sympathetic denervation (Chapter 1), the degree to which spinal anesthesia alters normal hemodynamic function varies considerably from patient to patient. In some, there is little sympathetic block, and so, few vascular changes. In others, the sympathetic denervation is more extensive or even complete, and the vascular changes are profound. Spinal anesthesia has few direct effects on function of organs aside from those caused by alterations in blood flow, and different organs react differently to sympathetic denervation and changes in perfusion. It is, therefore, desirable to consider the cardiovascular effects of spinal anesthesia in some detail and to formulate certain basic principles to serve as points of reference for further discussion. Specifically, although an oversimplification of the multiple changes that it induces by virtue of its associated sympathectomy, spinal anesthesia results in some degree of blood pressure reduction. Thus, to understand the physiologic adaptations of the body in response to the reduction in blood pressure, a brief review of hemodynamic parameters and their interrelationships is beneficial, starting with arterial blood pressure as a measurement of the status of the cardiovascular system. Mean arterial pressure (MAP; i.e., the average blood pressure during a cardiac cycle) is dependent on cardiac output (CO) and peripheral resistance (or systemic vascular resistance (SVR)) (Figure 2.1).

Reduction in MAP, such as that induced by sympathetic denervation, may be due to a reduction in CO, SVR, or both. In turn, CO depends on heart rate (HR) and ventricular stroke volume (SV), with SV in turn being determined by the amount of blood returning to the heart (preload), the resistance against which the left ventricle must contract (afterload), and the intrinsic myocardial performance (contractility) (Figure 2.1). Although the mathematical formulas in Table 2.1 are useful as guidelines, one must realize the complexity of the relationships between these

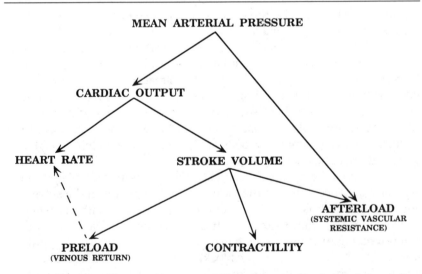

Figure 2.1. Factors that determine arterial blood pressure and their interrelationships.

Table 2.1.
Hemodynamic Parameters

Formula	Units	Normal Range
MAP = DP + ⅓ (SP − DP)	mmHg	80–120
MAP = CO × SVR	mmHg	80–120
CO = HR × SV	$L·min^{-1}$	4–8
CI = CO/BSA	$L·min^{-1}·m^{-2}$	2–5
SV = CO/HR × 1000	$ml·beat^{-1}$	60–90
SI = SV/BSA	$ml·beat^{-1}·m^{-2}$	40–60
SVR = (MAP − CVP) 80/CO	$dynes·sec·cm^{-5}$	900–1500
TPR = MAP × 1322/CO × 0.06 [a]	$dynes·sec·cm^{-5}$	900–1500

Abbreviations: BSA, body surface area; CI, cardiac index; CO, cardiac output; DP, diastolic pressure; HR, heart rate; MAP, mean arterial pressure; SI, stroke index; SP, systolic pressure; SV, stroke volume; SVR, systemic vascular resistance; TPR, total peripheral resistance.
[a] Conversion factor for CO (in $L·mm^{-1}$) into $ml·sec^{-1}$.

cardiovascular parameters. Thus, for instance, preload not only determines SV but can also influence (HR) as well as contractility by altering the degree of ventricular stretch. The following section deals with the effects that spinal anesthesia exerts on the cardiovascular parameters.

Arterial and Arteriolar Circulation (Afterload)

Afterload is a measure of the resistance against which the ventricle must eject blood. It is therefore easiest to define afterload as the stress within the wall of the ventricle generated during systole. The amount of ventricular wall stress or tension (T_w) generated during systole depends on the volume of the ventricular chamber (i.e., radius of the chamber, r), the pressure in the system (i.e., intraventricular pressure, P), and the ventricular wall thickness (h). This relationship is expressed by LaPlace's law:

$$T_w = \frac{Pr}{2h} \text{ (in dynes·cm}^{-2})$$

Spinal anesthesia decreases afterload because immediately following sympathetic denervation, normal arteries and arterioles dilate. There are many ways of demonstrating this vasodilation (Butterworth, *et al.*, 1987; Butterworth, *et al.*, 1986; Cabalum, *et al.*, 1979; Taivainen, 1991). The rate of perfusion of saline into a peripheral artery increases 40–200 percent after the induction of spinal anesthesia (Burch and Harrison, 1931). The increase in pulse volume demonstrable plethysmographically during spinal anesthesia (Neumann, *et al.*, 1945; Sancetta, *et al.*, 1952; Kleinerman, *et al.*, 1958; Rawson, 1959) is also evidence of vasodilation. As measured in the toes, the pulse volume becomes three times greater than control values after induction of low spinal anesthesia and six times greater after a high block. In the absence of an increase in cardiac SV, such increases in pulse volume can be explained only on the basis of vasodilation. de Marees, *et al.* (1976) in their studies of effects of spinal anesthesia on hemodynamic function found, for example, that the vasodilation produced by spinal anesthesia increased blood flow to the calf, from 9.7 to 10.9 ml/100 ml tissue. Not only is the pulse volume changed, but the contour of the peripheral arterial pulse wave is altered as well. The arterial pulse wave normally shows a dicrotic notch or incisura high on the descending limb. Following induction of spinal anesthesia, the dicrotic notch is lower on the descending limb (Eather, *et al.*, 1949), and it may even approach the diastolic level of the wave. This change is pathognomonic of arterial and arteriolar vasodilation.

Although spinal anesthesia produces peripheral vasodilation, there are significant quantitative and qualitative differences in the way various arteries and arterioles from different parts of the body react following blockade of their sympathetic innervation. Vascular changes in one organ system do not necessarily reflect similar changes in others. Cronenwett *et al.* (1983) in studies of the effect of sympathetic denervation on muscle and skin blood flow of dogs found that while sympathectomy induced no change in the muscle capillary blood flow and decreased skin capillary flow from 28 to 13 ml·min^{-1} per 100 g, total extremity blood flow nevertheless increased from 7 to 30 ml·min^{-1}. The increase was due to redistribution of blood flow through arteriovenous anastomoses. In contrast to capillaries, the arteriovenous anastomoses have little intrinsic muscle tone. Therefore, even minimal decreases in the level of sympathetic innervation resulted in a marked increase in the blood flow through them.

It is impossible to make generalized deductions concerning the reaction of arterial vessels after studying only one type of vessel. The response of cutaneous vessels of the hand to sensory stimuli, epinephrine, temperature, and exercise is entirely different from that of vessels in the muscles of the forearm (Grant and Pearson, 1938; Kunkel, *et al.*, 1939; Abramson and Ferris, 1940; Wenger, *et al.*, 1986; Cronenwett, *et al.*, 1983). Cutaneous vessels of the hands react differently even from those of the feet (Abramson, *et al.*, 1939). Differences in response also persist following sympathetic denervation, and for this reason the changes in arteries and arterioles resulting from spinal anesthesia are impossible to predict accurately (Davis, *et al.*, 1989 a). The only possible generalization is that no arteries or arterioles become constricted following their preganglionic sympathetic denervation by spinal blockade. In one organ (e.g., the skin), vasodilation is more pronounced than in another (e.g., skeletal muscle). Although vasodilation may be minimal or absent in certain areas, the general response of vessels is to dilate following sympathectomy. Cannon's "Law of Denervation" states that denervated structures may develop hypersensitivity to agonists (Cannon and Rosenblueth, 1949). The possibility that vasoconstriction could occur during spinal anesthesia, as suggested by Cannon and Rosenblueth, is purely theoretical and most unlikely. Peripheral neuroeffector systems do exhibit increased sensitivity to stimuli following denervation. This is most marked after sympathectomy; a week or more must elapse after sympathetic denervation, however, before the hypersensitivity attains measurable importance (Griffin, et al., 1954; Cooper, et al., 1956; Barcoft and Swan, 1953). There is no evidence to indicate that, during the acute pharmacologic sympathectomy of spinal anesthesia, effector organs such as smooth muscles of arteries respond abnormally to stimulation.

Vasodilation of arteries and arterioles during spinal anesthesia results in diminished resistance to the flow of blood in the periphery. This is in accordance with Poiseuille's law which states that the resistance to laminar flow of a liquid varies inversely to the fourth power of the radius of the lumen through which the liquid is flowing. One quantitative index of resistance to blood flow is the total peripheral vascular resistance (TPR) calculated as:

$$TPR = MAP \text{ (in mmHg)} \cdot \frac{1332}{CO} \text{ (in ml·sec}^{-1})$$

where 1332 is the constant applied to convert TPR to dynes·sec·cm^{-5}. Measured in this fashion, TPR consists of two components: peripheral vascular tone, which is determined by the diameter of the peripheral vessels through which arterial blood flows, and resistance, which is determined by viscosity (under conditions of laminar flow) (pp. 173–175). This formula, however, ignores the contribution of central venous pressure (CVP) (i.e., pressure measured at the junction of superior vena cava and right atrium) to resistance of the system. Systemic vascular resistance (SVR) takes into account the importance of CVP, since SVR is the change in pressure divided by flow:

$$SVR = (MAP - CVP) \cdot \frac{80}{CO}$$

In the clinical setting, however, the contribution of CVP is relatively minor, and especially so during spinal anesthesia. Therefore, the difference between SVR and TPR is minimal. Thus, TPR is used to define vascular resistance (afterload). The resistance is a function of hematocrit (HCT) and shear rate. If hematocrit changes, TPR changes in the same direction (though not linearly) even though total peripheral vascular tone may remain unchanged. If HCT remains constant, TPR increases if cardiac output decreases, since viscosity varies inversely with velocity gradient (i.e., shear rate). Vascular resistance as generally measured and reported in the literature often fails to differentiate between changes in arterial or arteriolar diameter (i.e., based on Poiseuille's law) and changes ascribable to alterations in blood viscosity (pp. 173–175). Because the latter are quantitatively a substantially less important determinant of TPR in vivo than the former, TPR is thus a useful, if not always qualitatively entirely accurate, indication of changes in arterial and arteriolar diameters. But the concept of TPR as a measure of vasodilation on the arterial side of the circulation carries with it yet further caveats. Since different parts of the circulation undergo varying degrees of vasodilation following sympathetic denervation, measuring changes in *total* peripheral resistance obviously gives no indication of the amount of *regional* vasodilation. A more important limitation is the fact that measurements of resistance to flow, whether determined in particular peripheral areas or as TPR, do not reflect changes in the caliber of arteries and arterioles with mathematical precision. Normally, 60 percent of TPR is precapillary in origin, and the remaining 40 percent is derived from the postarteriolar bed (Dale and Richards, 1918–1919; Krogh, 1929; Landis, 1934; Fisch, *et al.*, 1950). Following arteriolar dilation, the postarteriolar bed represents a proportionately greater part of TPR, and the percentage of TPR arising from resistance to flow through the arterioles decreases (Haddy and Gilbert, 1956). Under such circumstances, the major resistance to flow shifts more distally, and the TPR usually decreases, though not in proportion to the degree of arteriolar dilation.

Despite these limitations of the value of TPR as a measure of arterial vessel caliber, estimations of TPR during spinal anesthesia do serve as a general guide to the degree of vascular tone of the peripheral arteries and arterioles. Without prior administration of vasopressors, TPR decreases with spinal anesthesia. The extent to which it is reduced can be roughly correlated with the extent of sympathetic block as determined by the cephalad level of sensory anesthesia. With sensory levels of anesthesia at T_{10} and below, TPR usually shows no statistically or physiologically significant change (Samii, *et al.*, 1979). Not only is the percentage of the peripheral arterial circulation denervated too low to affect TPR appreciably, but also compensatory vasoconstriction may occur in sympathetically intact areas during low spinal anesthesia (p. 94). Using the direct Fick principle to measure CO, Sancetta, *et al.* (1952) determined TPR in 10 nonoperative patients, 5 with "low" spinal anesthesia (sensory level below T_4) and 5 with "high" spinals (sensory level above T_4). In four of the five patients with "low" spinal anesthesia levels, TPR decrease was between 1.6 and 7.2 units; in one, TPR increased by 0.7 units. The average change was a decrease of 13.5 percent. All of the five patients with "high" spinal anesthesia (i.e., probably with a complete sympathetic block) had an average decrease in TPR of 18.8 percent. In absolute units, the decreases ranged from 1.1 to 14.3 units. The same investigators (Sancetta, et al., 1953) also studied six operative patients with sensory levels of anesthesia from T_7 to T_{11}. The average decrease in TPR was 13.2 percent with decreases ranging from 2.5 to 11.4 absolute units; one patient showed an unexplained increase of 11.1 units. Among the total of 16 patients studied by this group of investigators, 14 showed a decrease and 2 showed an increase in total peripheral vascular resistance during spinal anesthesia. Using essentially the same methods, Pugh and Wyndham (1950) studied patients in the supine horizontal position before and after induction of spinal anesthesia with sensory blockade up to T_4 or T_6. Among the 12 patients suitable for measurement of TPR, the average decrease was approximately 11 percent. In two of their patients, there were increases in TPR of five and one percent; in the remaining 10 patients, TPR decreased. In three patients these decreases amounted to 33 percent, 17 percent, and 35 percent. Because of the limitations inherent in the technique of measuring peripheral resistance, the authors regarded only the decreases of 33 percent, 17 percent, and 35 percent as significant. It is nevertheless an important observation that 10 of their 12 patients showed decreases in TPR, and that the average decrease was 11 percent.

Analogous results (i.e., a decrease in TPR) were also obtained by Kleinerman, et al. (1958). These investigators found that TPR decreased 29 percent, from an average baseline value of 2.1 units, to 1.5 units during spinal anesthesia, a change associated with a level of anesthesia high enough to produce cutaneous vasodilation in the upper extremities. Other investigators (Li, et al., 1963), studying nonoperative patients with lower levels of spinal anesthesia (T_{5-6}) found that TPR decreased 14 percent, from 1650 ± 332 to 1416 ± 320 dyne·sec·cm^{-5}. Ward, et al. (1965), Bonica, et al. (1966), Kennedy, et al. (1968), and Kennedy, et al. (1970) found, in their studies of nonoperative patients, decreases in peripheral vascular resistance similar to those of Kleinerman and colleagues. More recently, de Angelis, et al. (1982) also found, in nine patients undergoing transurethral prostatectomy under spinal anesthesia, that the SVR index decreased 17 percent during surgery.

Eckenhoff, et al. (1948) confirmed in dogs the findings of significant decreases in TPR associated with spinal anesthesia, but the results reported by Rovenstine, et al. (1942) are quantitatively somewhat different. In seven nonoperative volunteers with sensory levels of anesthesia at T_4 to T_6 (i.e., with nearly complete sympathetic denervation), they found that the average decrease in TPR was only 3.7 percent. Only three of their subjects showed significant decreases. The explanation for the difference between these results, as well as those reported by Sobin (1949) on the one hand and other investigators on the other hand probably lies in the fact that Rovenstine, *et al.* determined CO by ballistocardiography, a method less accurate than use of the Fick principle. Johnson (1951) reported that only 4 of 10 patients showed decreases in total peripheral vascular resistance during high spinal anesthesia, but these results are invalidated for the purposes of the present discussion by the fact that all his patients were given 50 mg of ephedrine immediately prior to induction of anesthesia. Although not measured directly, a recent study (Runciman, *et al.*, 1984 b) also demonstrated a slight decrease in the peripheral vascular resistance induced by T_4 sensory spinal anesthesia in sheep.

The arterial and arteriolar vasodilation that follows sympathetic denervation during spinal anesthesia, and that is accompanied by changes in vascular resistance to blood flow, is rarely maximal. A certain intrinsic tone is autonomously maintained following vasomotor denervation. Theoretically, this residual tone might be explained on the basis of simultaneous denervation of vasodilator sympathetic fibers (Lewis and Pickering, 1931; Barcroft and Edholm, 1946; Symposium, 1966). If maximal arteriolar dilation occurs only as the result of stimulation of vasodilator sympathetic fibers, then paralysis of such fibers by spinal anesthesia would prevent complete dilation. It is partly for this reason that spinal anesthesia produces vascular responses that are different from those produced by alpha- or beta-adrenergic receptor blockers. Spinal anesthesia denervates both types of receptors simultaneously. Vasodilator fibers are, however, of little clinical significance in normal, resting humans (Warren, *et al.*, 1942; Sarnoff and Simeone, 1947; Frumin, *et al.*, 1953; Folkow, 1955), and they probably play little role in the prevention of maximal vasodilation following spinal anesthesia. The residual tone that persists after sympathetic denervation appears to represent simply an inherent property of all smooth muscle. That this residual tone can and does vanish under certain circumstances, with resultant complete vasodilation, is certain. Butterworth, *et al.* (1987) studied the effect of total spinal anesthesia on arterial and venous responses (i.e., vasomotion) to infusions of dopamine and dobutamine in dogs. In the absence of total spinal anesthesia, both dopamine and dobutamine decreased venous capacitance (i.e., increased venous return) in a dose-dependent manner. Furthermore, dobutamine decreased MAP in a dose-related fashion, but dopamine had no significant effects on it. During total spinal anesthesia, both dopamine and dobutamine produced greater dose-related decreases in venous capacitance than in the absence of spinal anesthesia. Dobutamine had no significant effect on the MAP during spinal anesthesia but dopamine increased it. The mechanisms by which spinal anesthesia prevents dobutamine from inducing hypotension beyond the hypotension induced by spinal anesthesia may include one of two possibilities, or a combination of both. The first possibility is that during total spinal anesthesia (i.e., total sympathectomy), the resting tone of arteriolar smooth muscle is removed entirely and, therefore, further relaxation by the beta-2 actions of dobutamine would not be possible. Alternatively, dobutamine also has weak alpha-1 receptor agonist activity (vasoconstriction) and during total sympathetic denervation, this weak alpha-1 activity of dobutamine may counterbalance the beta-2 receptor activated vasodilation (Fuchs, *et al.*, 1980; Leier and Unverferth, 1983; Ozaki, *et al.*, 1982). Other conditions under which the residual tone of sympathetically denervated smooth muscles on the arterial side of the circulation may be removed include those associated with abnormal accumulation of cellular metabolites or with decreased oxygen tension (Pappenheimer, 1952; Peters, *et al.*, 1990). Since it is often difficult to determine whether further vasodilation involves arteries, arterioles, or postarteriolar vessels, this phenomenon of "secondary" dilation is deferred until the physiology of the capillary circulation is discussed (pp. 95–101).

Though spinal anesthesia is characterized by peripheral vasodilation on the arterial side of the circulation, it must be emphasized that the extent to which the caliber of arteries and arterioles is modified or altered following denervation may vary considerably from patient to patient. This is one reason why all patients with similar degrees of sympathetic denervation do not show equal changes in either peripheral vascular resistance or in peripheral pulse volume (Sancetta, *et al.*, 1952). Young, robust patients are able to maintain this intrinsic tone better than older or cachectic patients. The extent to which this intrinsic tone maintains the normal size of arterial vessels during spinal anesthesia also varies from organ to organ. It is most effective in the renal (Smith, *et al.*, 1939; Assali, *et al.*, 1951) and splanchnic (Mueller, *et al.*, 1952) vessels, less so in those of striated muscle (Prinzmetal and Wilson, 1936; Barcroft, *et al.*, 1943; Barcroft and Edholm, 1946), and least effective in the skin vessels. Maintenance of residual arteriolar tone also depends on the circumstances under which the spinal anesthesia is given. Residual tone can be maintained in nonoperative patients who are resting quietly in the supine position to the extent that the lumina of the arteries and arterioles are relatively unchanged. This is shown by the fact that under laboratory conditions, even with extensive sympathetic block, there may be little or no decrease in peripheral resistance (Smith, *et al.*, 1939; Rovenstine, *et al.*, 1942). Under clinical conditions, when the patient may be apprehensive and subjected to changes of position and to surgical manipulation, this finely balanced intrinsic tone is interfered with to a greater extent, vasodilation occurs, and the peripheral vascular resistance decreases, resulting in profound changes throughout the cardiovascular system (Sancetta, *et al.*, 1953). The fact that this autonomous arterial tone is maintained so tenuously following sympathetic denervation is one reason for the frequent discrepancies between results of investigations into the physiology of spinal anesthesia conducted in the laboratory and those performed under clinical conditions.

When arterial and arteriolar dilation occurs in sympathetically denervated areas, simultaneous compensatory reflex vasoconstriction may take place in areas where the sympathetic nerve supply has remained unaffected. Such vasoconstriction is initiated by a decrease in arterial blood pressure, which, acting on the pressor receptors of the carotid sinus and aortic arch, causes increased sympathetic activity in areas where the sympathetic nerves are intact. This is detectable in the arms by decreases in skin temperature (Milwidsky and de Vries, 1948), by decreased volume of the pulse wave as determined plethysmographically (Foster, *et al.*, 1945; Neuman, *et al.*, 1945; Sancetta, *et al.*, 1952), and by decreased forearm blood flow (Berenyi, *et al.*, 1964). Upper extremity compensatory vasoconstriction does not develop during high spinal anesthesia when the concentration of the local anesthetic in spinal fluid in the high thoracic area is enough to interrupt preganglionic fibers to the arms. When there is reflex vasoconstriction in the upper limbs, alterations in TPR are of course, no longer directly proportional to the degree of arterial dilation produced in the anesthetized areas, thus limiting the value of total peripheral vascular resistance determinations as a measure of vasodilation. The effectiveness of this reflex vasoconstriction in preventing hypotension is, however, limited. As Pugh and Wyndham (1950) pointed out, the upper limbs of a 75-kg man have a tissue volume of 6500 ml, and at a normal flow rate of 3 ml of blood/100 ml of tissue/min, the total blood flow to the upper limbs is about 200 ml·min^{-1}. This is less than 5 percent of the total CO, and consequently the contribution of such a small area to the TPR must necessarily be relatively small. To be more effective in combatting hypotension, compensatory vasoconstriction should involve a mass of tissue with a relatively large blood flow such as the brain. However, compensatory cerebral vasoconstriction does not occur during spinal anesthesia.

Postarteriolar Circulation

The term "postarteriolar bed" refers to that portion of the vascular system that lies between the distal ends of the arterioles and the collecting venules. It is also referred to as the microvasculature. The physiology of the circulation in this area is of paramount importance, for tissue respiration and metabolic activity take place here. Spinal anesthesia affects this portion of the vascular system profoundly. Even though details of terminology used to describe postarteriolar microvascular structures vary among different authors, a useful, clear, and conceptually valid nomenclature was introduced by Chambers and Zweifach (Chambers and Zweifach, 1944, 1947; Zweifach, *et al.*, 1944; Chambers, 1948; Lee and Holze, 1950; Zweifach, 1954 a, b, 1957; Zweifach and Metz, 1955; Folkow and Mellander, 1964; Sobin and Tremer, 1966; Zweifach and Intaglietta, 1966; Luft, 1966; Burton, 1966). Other authors use different terms and have slightly differing hypotheses on the physiology of postarteriolar circulation. Such differences, however, are secondary compared to the importance of the concept that the postarteriolar circulation does not consist merely of passive tubelike vessels but instead, is made up of several types of vessels. These vessels are characterized by well-defined individual responses and functions having a complex interrelationship with each other and with the arterial and venous circulations.

The "parent" vessels from which most capillaries have their origin are prolongations of terminal arterioles called thoroughfare (or central) channels (Fig. 2.2). They can be traced through the postarteriolar bed until they merge with other similar channels and form collecting venules. The portion of a thoroughfare channel nearest the arteriole is encircled by a thin layer of muscle cells and is known as a metarteriole. The investing muscle fibers become progressively smaller and more sparse as the metarteriole progresses toward the venule, and ultimately the muscle disappears. That portion of the thoroughfare channel that is devoid of muscle fibers is designated the arteriovenous capillary. Arising at acute angles from the metarterioles are the true capillaries. At their point of origin, they are surrounded by muscle cells which form the precapillary sphincters. At a variable distance, the capillaries, which are purely endothelial vessels (Luft, 1966), rejoin the central channel at its venular end. There are, in addition, a certain number of capillaries with precapillary sphincters that arise directly from arterioles, as well as occasional short channels known as metarteriolar-venular anastomoses (A.V.A. in Fig. 2.2) which pass directly from metarterioles to venules without giving off capillaries. The muscular elements of the postarteriolar bed, limited to metarterioles and precapillary sphincters, are characterized by periodic and irregular phases of contraction and dilation. The activity of the precapillary sphincters is not necessarily synchronous with that of the metarterioles, the former often being constricted while the latter are dilated, or vice versa.

Capillary blood flow is normally regulated primarily by the vasomotor activity of the muscular components of the metarterioles and precapillary sphincters (Zweifach and Intaglietta, 1966). When maximally constricted, the precapillary sphincters completely occlude the flow of blood into the capillaries. The capillaries are then open but devoid of red cells which have drained into the venous end of the thoroughfare channels. Plasma may or may not, however, continue to flow through the capillar-

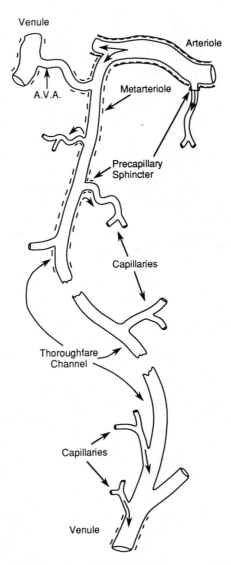

Figure 2.2. Diagram of the postarteriolar bed. AVA = metarteriolar-venular anastomoses. (Redrawn with permission from Chambers, R., and Zweifach, B. W.: Topography and function of the mesenteric capillary circulation. Am. J. Anat. 75: 173, 1944.)

ies. When the sphincters are completely relaxed, the flow of blood through the capillaries becomes so rapid that individual erythrocytes cannot be distinguished through the dissecting microscope (Chambers and Zweifach, 1944; Lee and Holze, 1950). The velocity of blood flow in the postarteriolar bed varies substantially. The less branching there is between a vascular channel and the parent artery, the greater is the velocity of flow. The greater the branching, that is, the more removed a vascular channel is from the parent artery because of branching, the slower the velocity of flow. This is illustrated in Figure 2.3, which relates arterial branching order to velocity of flow of erythrocytes (but not of whole blood or plasma). By the time blood reaches the capillaries, its velocity is even lower than indicated in Figure 2.3. Because capillary flow rates are influenced by tone of precapillary sphincters (Freis, *et al.*, 1957; Burton, 1966), and because mean velocity of erythrocytes is greater than that of plasma due to laminar flow (Freis, *et al.*, 1949), it is difficult to

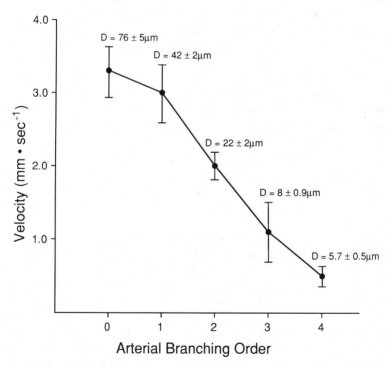

Figure 2.3. Red blood cell velocity in consecutive branches of bat wing arteries. Values above bars represent vessel diameters (D) in micrometers (mean ± SEM). (Redrawn with permission from Mayrowitz, H. N., Tuma, R. F., and Wiedeman, M. P.: Relationship between microvascular blood velocity and pressure distribution. Am. J. Physiol. *232*: H400, 1977.)

give a meaningful figure that will indicate average flow velocities in the postarteriolar bed. Lee and Holze (1950), however, found that in patent capillaries in the human conjunctiva erythrocytes flowed at a rate of 0.009 to 0.04 mm·sec^{-1}, with an average rate of flow of 0.026 mm·sec^{-1}. Since these capillaries averaged 0.065 mm in length, it took an average of 2 sec for an erythrocyte to flow through an open capillary. Zweifach and Intaglietta (1966) found that the velocity of flow in frog mesentery capillaries ranges from 0.17 to 0.91 μm·sec^{-1}.

The rhythmic vasomotion involving the postarteriolar bed also means that all capillaries do not contain blood at the same time. For those that do, the amount varies with the degree of relaxation of the precapillary sphincters. The amount of blood that passes through the true capillaries instead of directly to the venules through the thoroughfare channels thus depends on the number of open precapillary sphincters. Under normal conditions, a considerable portion of the blood goes straight through the intermediate arteriovenous shunts into the venous circulation.

The activity of the muscle fibers surrounding the metarterioles is similar to that of the precapillary sphincters. When maximally contracted, they reduce the diameter of the lumen of the metarteriole to 5–7 μm (Chambers and Zweifach, 1944).

Capillary blood flows and pressures are influenced not only by activity of precapillary sphincters and metarteriolar muscle fibers, but also by the efficiency of the venular outflow. Elevation of venous pressure causes an increase in intracapillary pressure, although usually the latter will remain 1–15 mmHg above the venular pressure (Eichna and Bordley, 1942; Fisch, et al., 1950; Friedland, et al., 1943; Bazett, 1947). Since position (i.e., gravity) affects venous pressure, it is apparent that position will also affect capillary pressure and blood flow independently of any effect that the change in position may have on arterial pressure (Landis, 1929–1931, 1934).

Changes in capillary size occur only secondarily to alterations in transmural, including intraluminal, pressures (Burton, 1966; Bohlen and Gore, 1977). Control of capillary blood flow is not related to ability of either the pericapillary Rouget cells or the endothelial cells of the capillaries themselves to contract. These structures have no function in regulating blood flow. Endothelial cells of capillaries do possess an inherent ability to change their form, but this does not represent true contractility nor is it a significant determinant of capillary flow. Because changes in capillary hemodynamics are secondary to changes in other portions of the cardiovascular system, it is inaccurate to use the terms "capillary constriction" or "dilation."

Intracapillary pressures are normally highly variable, depending on the tone of the muscular elements of the postarteriolar bed and on the

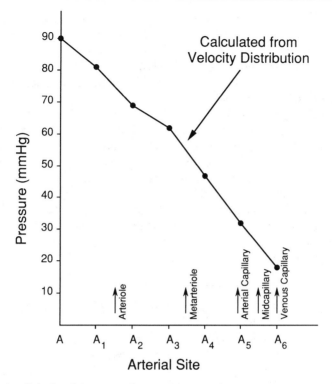

Figure 2.4. Calculated intravascular pressures in the microvasculature of the bat wing. (Adapted with permission from Mayrowitz, H. N., Tuma, R. F., and Wiedeman, M. P.: Relationship between microvascular blood velocity and pressure distribution. Am. J. Physiol. *232:* H400, 1977.)

efficiency of venous outflow. The pressure in the arterioles ranges from 21 to 75 mmHg, averaging about 52 mmHg (Landis, 1934; Eichna and Bordley, 1942; Mayrovitz, *et al.*, 1977). Thus, the pressure in the arteriolar end of a true capillary (Fig. 2.4) varies from 21 to 48 mmHg (average 32 mmHg), and in the venular end, from 6 to 18 mmHg (average 12 mmHg) (Landis, 1929–1931, 1934; Eichna and Wilkins, 1942; Fisch, *et al.*, 1950; Lee, 1957). As a result, there is a pressure gradient of about 20 mmHg between the two ends of the capillary. This moves blood through the capillary to the collecting venules where the pressure averages 14 mmHg (Eichna and Bordley, 1942). With the extreme vasoconstriction associated with some pathologic states or that follows an intravenous injection of epinephrine, the pressure in the capillary may decrease to levels as low as 7 mmHg (Eichna and Wilkins, 1942; Eichna, 1943). During maximal vasodilation, on the other hand, capillary pressure may rise to levels as high as 50 mmHg (Landis, 1934; Eichna and Wilkins, 1942; Eichna, 1943).

But under normal conditions the activity of smooth muscles of arterioles, metarterioles, and precapillary sphincters is such that there is no correlation between capillary pressure and systemic arterial pressure (Krogh, 1929; Marx and Schoop, 1956; Lee, 1957).

The intrinsic vasomotion of the postarteriolar vessels has long been recognized as being mediated by chemical, physical, and neural factors (Green and Kepchar, 1959; Cobbold, *et al.*, 1963). Thus, Fagrell, *et al.* (1980) studied the relationship between capillary blood flow velocity and hematocrit in human skin capillaries. They were able to observe periodic fluctuations of both capillary blood flow velocity (CBV) and relative HCT. The frequency of these fluctuations was 5–10 cycles·min^{-1}. The changes in CBV were almost always accompanied by changes in HCT. The authors concluded that normal vasomotion decreases the diameter of the arteriole until the erythrocytes are mechanically prevented from passing into the capillary. Although adjacent capillaries seem to have the same vasomotion pattern, variations often are seen (Figure 2.5) (Fagrell, *et al.*,

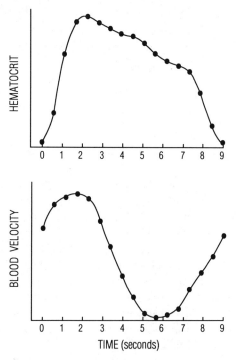

Figure 2.5. Mean capillary hematocrit and blood velocity during seven vasomotion cycles. (Redrawn with permission from Fagrell, B., Intaglietta, M., and Östergren, J.: Relative hematocrit in human skin capillaries and its relation to capillary blood flow velocity. Microvasc. Res. *20:* 327, 1980.)

1980). Rodgers, *et al.* (1984) used the technique of laser Doppler velocimetry to compare the patterns of cutaneous blood flow in the forearm of normal patients with those of patients with sickle cell disease. They observed that microcirculatory flow in patients with sickle cell disease was effected by synchronization of rhythmic flow in large domains of microvessels. The periodic flow that resulted was probably a compensatory mechanism to offset the deleterious altered rheology of sickled erythrocytes containing polymerized hemoglobin-S.

Chemical substances which produce vasodilation independently of neurogenic reflexes include metabolites such as carbon dioxide and lactic acid when present in abnormally high concentrations (Krogh, 1929; Folkow, 1949). Chien (1984), using the laser Doppler, reviewed the rheology of sickle cells and the associated microcirculatory changes. Vasomotion was the result of rhythmic contractions of microvascular smooth muscle that were modulated by the local tissue metabolic environment. Reduction in blood flow led to local metabolic changes that induced vasodilation; the resulting increase in blood flow reversed the metabolic changes that caused the vasodilation, thus resulting in vasoconstriction. Under normal physiologic conditions, periodic vasomotor activity takes place at the individual precapillary sphincters or at the terminal arterioles, and the extent of cyclic metabolic fluctuation is small.

Certain drugs such as histamine and acetylcholine, pyrogenic toxins, and some of the general anesthetic agents also produce postarteriolar vasodilation (Grant, 1929–1931; Landis, 1929–1931; Lewis and Landis, 1929–1931; Eichna and Wilkins, 1942; Chambers and Zweifach, 1944, 1947; Pappenheimer, 1952). Anoxia and decrease in pH similarly cause dilation in noninnervated vessels, even though they produce vasoconstriction in normally innervated vessels by means of centrally initiated reflexes (Krogh, 1929; Freeman, 1935; Folkow, 1949; Zweifach and Metz, 1955). Kim and Reed (1987) in their studies of changes in partial pressure of venous oxygen (P_vO_2) in cutaneous veins during regression of spinal anesthesia found that sympathetic denervation induced by spinal anesthesia increased P_vO_2 by opening of arteriovenous anastomoses in the cutaneous circulation. These changes in oxygenation were reversed by sympathetic recovery. Mechanical stimulation such as heavy direct trauma (Grant, 1929–1931; Chambers and Zweifach, 1944) increases intraluminal capillary pressures by producing vasodilation (Folkow, 1949). Heat (Lewis, 1929–1931; Landis, 1929–1931; Beecher, 1936; Eichna and Wilkins, 1942) also directly produces vasodilation. Physiologic and pharmacologic vasoconstrictors as well as light touch are some of the stimuli that can cause vasoconstriction independently of neural control.

The innervation of the smooth muscle in metarterioles and precapillary sphincters is sympathetic in origin. It serves to maintain intrinsic muscle tone and to control the complicated process of vasomotion. Sympathetic denervation results in cessation of vasomotion and produces relaxation of the muscular elements of the precapillary sphincters and metarterioles leading to vasodilation. The postarteriolar vasodilation that follows sympathetic denervation is not, however, maximal; as with arterioles, a certain degree of residual tone remains. That vasodilation is not complete is indicated by the following observations: first, vasodilation may be produced not only by interruption of sympathetic nerves, but also reflexly by immersion of a distant portion of the body in hot water. Such vasodilation may be measured by the resulting increases in skin temperature. When the lower extremities are placed in hot water, the reflex vasodilation occurring in the hands produces a greater increase in skin temperature of the hands than does sympathetic denervation of the hands (Lewis and Pickering, 1931; Sarnoff and Simeone, 1947). The vasodilation, therefore, is more complete in the former instance than in the latter. Second, drugs such as histamine produce more vasodilation in sympahetically denervated vessels than that produced by the denervation itself (Dale and Richards, 1918–1919). Third, reactive hyperemia persists after sympathetic denervation. If a normal extremity is deprived of its arterial circulation by a tourniquet, following restoration of the circulation, hyperemia occurs in the tissues distal to the point at which the tourniquet was applied. This reaction is due largely, though not entirely, to the accumulation of metabolites, to reduction in oxygen tension, and to alteration of the tissue pH during the ischemic period. But following sympathetic denervation, reactive hyperemia persists, producing a vasodilation above and beyond that produced by the sympathectomy itself (Folkow, 1949; Pappenheimer, 1952). These findings indicate that sympathectomized areas can and do have vascular responses, especially dilation, due to changes in cellular environment that are additive to the vascular changes produced by sympathectomy alone.

The fact that vasodilation is not maximal following sympathetic denervation is of considerable importance during spinal anesthesia. It means that vascular responses in excess of those produced by the anesthetic denervation can and do occur. For example, amyl nitrite and histamine cause further vasodilation during spinal anesthesia (Co Tui, 1934; Hilton, 1957). The same vasodilation can be observed when an abnormally high carbon dioxide concentration is present. An increase in carbon dioxide tension has two opposite actions on the normally innervated cardiovascular system; one, a direct (peripheral) effect of the carbon dioxide on the peripheral vessels resulting in vasodilation, the other, mediated centrally through the response of the vasomotor center to the increased carbon dioxide tension, produces peripheral vasoconstriction indirectly due to catecholamine release. In the presence of an intact sympathetic nervous system, the central effect outweighs the peripheral effect. Vasoconstriction takes place, vascular resistance increases, and the blood pressure increases. During spinal anesthesia, the sympathetic efferent nerves from the vasomotor center are blocked. Carbon dioxide accumulation then results in further vasodilation of sympathetically denervated vessels, with a consequent further decrease in arterial blood pressure (Seevers and Waters, 1932 a; Co Tui, 1936; Burstein, 1939; Payne, 1958).

The change in cardiovascular response to carbon dioxide retention produced by sympathetic denervation has also been illustrated by Galindo (1964) in studies of the effect of high epidural anesthesia in experimental animals. He found that the normal response to respiratory acidosis (75 percent increase in arterial carbon dioxide tension) consisted of an 18.5 percent increase in mean arterial blood pressure in intact dogs. In dogs with higher epidural anesthesia, comparable degrees of respiratory acidosis were associated with decreases in blood pressure below the level of hypotension resulting from the anesthesia alone. During epidural blockade in the presence of normal arterial carbon dioxide tension, arterial blood pressures averaged 31.5 percent below preanesthesia control levels. When respiratory acidosis was superimposed on epidural anesthesia, mean arterial blood pressure averaged 35.6 percent below control levels. Similarly, hypoxia or anoxia also augment the degree of vasodilation due to spinal anesthesia, because the normal vascular response to low oxygen tension is blocked. General anesthetics including potent inhalation agents, barbiturates, and most of the opioid analgesics also are capable of augmenting vasodilation of already denervated peripheral vessels. Thus, if anoxia or hypercarbia occur during spinal anesthesia, if tissue blood flow becomes insufficient to maintain normal cellular respiration and to remove cellular metabolites, or if vasodilating drugs, especially general anesthetic agents, are given, further vasodilation will occur. The degree of this vasodilation will be of greater magnitude than that already produced by the spinal block. The results of such alterations, involving both arterioles and the postarteriolar bed, can be profound, especially if tissue hypoxia is widespread.

Localized areas of tissue hypoxia do not, however, have significant effects on the total cardiovascular response to spinal anesthesia. Release of an arterial tourniquet applied for 2 hours to a lower extremity during spinal anesthesia has no significant effect on arterial blood pressure, pulmonary arterial pressure, TPR, CVP, pulmonary wedge pressure, CO, HR, or ventricular work (Samii, *et al.*, 1979).

That cellular environment plays a key role in vasomotor activity is well known, and in addition to the effects of anoxia, hypercarbia, and local metabolites on microvasculature, other factors have been described recently that also modify vascular changes induced by sympathectomy. The vascular endothelial layers of cells represent another mechanism involved in modulation of vascular reactivity (Furchgott, 1983). Among other substances (Vane, *et al.*, 1990; Ignarro, 1989), these endothelial cells contain the angiotensin-converting enzyme (ACE) responsible for the synthesis of the potent vasoconstrictor angiotensin II. ACE is also responsible for the inactivation of the potent vasodilator bradykinin. Endothelial cells also produce significant amounts of prostacyclin (Eldor, *et al.*, 1981; Moncada, *et al.*, 1977; Voelkel, *et al.*, 1981) in response to hydrodynamic disturbances (van Grondelle, *et al.*, 1984; Higgs, *et al.*, 1979). Studies of these endothelial layers of cells led to the finding (Furchgott and Zawadski, 1980) that vasodilation induced by acetylcholine was dependent on the presence of an intact endothelial layer. Furthermore, vascular endothelial cells produce a short-lived peptide (Peach, *et al.*, 1985 a), endothelium-derived relaxing factor (EDRF), a potent vascular smooth muscle relaxant. Sudden increases in blood flow or the introduction of pulsatile flow in experimental vasculature induce the release of EDRF (Rubanyi, *et al.*, 1986), while hypoxia produces an endothelium-dependent vasoconstriction based on inhibition of EDRF (Peach, *et al.*, 1985 b). In vitro, local anesthetics can inhibit the endothelium-dependent vasodilation by interfering with the cytoplasmic calcium influx necessary for EDRF production and release (Johns, 1989). Of the local anesthetics studied, bupivacaine has proven to be more potent in its inhibition of vascular relaxation than lidocaine, etidocaine, or 2-chloroprocaine (Johns, 1989). In 1987, the identity of EDRF was elucidated as nitric oxide (NO) (Vane, *et al.*, 1990; Ignarro, *et al.*, 1987; Palmer, *et al.*, 1987; Khan and Furchgott, 1987).

In 1988, Yanagisawa, *et al.* discovered yet another of several vascular smooth muscle vasoconstricting factors released by the endothelium, endothelin (Yanagisawa, *et al.*, 1988). Although there are three structurally and pharmacologically separate endothelin isopeptides, only endothelin-1 (also called porcine or human endothelin) is released by the endothelial cells, and it may be involved in hypertensive or vasospastic disorders (Cernacek and Stewart, 1989; Miyauchi, *et al.*, 1989). Endothelin is the most potent vasoconstrictor substance known (Vanhoutte, 1987), approximately 10 times more potent than angiotensin II (Vane, *et al.*, 1990; Weinheimer, *et al.*, 1990). Recent reports which suggest that endothelin induces enhanced vasoconstriction in senescent rats (Weinheimer, *et al.*, 1990) may help to elucidate the etiology of hypertension in the elderly. Interestingly, the actions of endothelin are more potent on veins than on arteries, inducing constriction of veins at lower concentrations than those required for arterial constriction (Cocks, *et al.*, 1989; Miller, *et al.*, 1989). Because of this selectivity, it remains to be seen whether endothelin will prove of therapeutic benefit for treatment of hypotension induced by spinal anesthesia.

Although much has been learned about the many factors synthesized and released by the endothelial layer of cells, studies that investigated the effects of sympathetic denervation induced by spinal anesthesia on these factors have not yet been performed. Nor is it known how these factors may in turn modulate the vascular responses to spinal anesthesia. Both are subjects that merit investigation.

From the foregoing outline of the physiology of the postarteriolar circulation, the hemodynamics of this all-important area of the vascular system can now be considered from the point of view of the changes produced by spinal anesthesia. One of the first problems encountered in considering this complex subject is the definition of terms. The literature contains many discussions as to whether spinal anesthesia increases or decreases "peripheral blood flow." The term "peripheral blood flow" is vague and might well be abandoned, for it actually includes two distinct factors: velocity of blood flow and volume of tissue blood. The rate of blood flow may be measured either as the time required for an erythrocyte to travel a given distance (i.e., velocity) or as the number of cubic milliliters of blood passing through 100 g of tissue/min. "Peripheral blood flow" is not directly related to tissue blood volume, which is commonly measured as the number of cubic milliliters of blood in 100 grams of tissue at any given time. The volume of blood in a tissue may be increased after spinal anesthesia, but this may be associated with either a concurrent increase or decrease in the rate of blood flow through the tissue. As currently used, the term "increased peripheral blood flow" usually implies either increased volume or increased velocity, or both, although each one of these should be evaluated separately. It therefore becomes expedient to study the physiology of the postarteriolar circulation during spinal anesthesia with respect to the following individual, although closely interrelated, factors: (a) volume changes, (b) route of peripheral blood flow, (c) changes in postarteriolar hydrostatic pressure, and (d) changes in velocity of postarteriolar blood flow.

Volume Changes

Following sympathetic blockade the normal contractile activity of the precapillary sphincters and the metarteriolar muscle fibers ceases. Intrinsic vasomotion is suppressed, and with it, the mechanism of selective opening and closing of the entrances to the capillaries is lost. With relaxation of the muscular elements in the vessels of the postarteriolar bed, blood can now flow into all capillaries instead of into just some of them. As a result, the volume of blood present in the postarteriolar area is increased. However, the increased quantity of blood in the capillary units that is characteristic of spinal anesthesia is not entirely due to the greater number of patent vascular channels. There is also an increase in capacity of each component of the postarteriolar circulation (Foate, et al., 1985). Thus, a metarteriole can contain more blood when its wall is relaxed, and the volume of blood in each patent capillary is also augmented.

These two factors combine to produce a tissue hyperemia which is one of the conspicuous effects of spinal anesthesia on the postarteriolar circulation. The hyperemia occurring in such circumstances indicates that a greater than normal percentage of the total circulating blood volume is in the periphery. Most evident in skin and subcutaneous tissues, hyperemia is not necessarily associated with an increased rate of blood flow and may even be associated with hyperemic stagnation to the point where cutaneous oxygen tension decreases (Davis and Greene, 1959). The increase in skin temperature in denervated areas during spinal anesthesia is not necessarily associated with an increase in cutaneous oxygenation. Postarteriolar vascular volume also increases, though to a somewhat lesser degree, in skeletal muscles following sympathetic denervation (Warren, et al., 1942; Barcroft and Edholm, 1946; Halligan, et al., 1956; Eriksson and Lisander, 1972). Part of the difference between responses of cutaneous and skeletal muscle postarteriolar circulations following sympathetic denervation may be related to the absence of morphologically distinct precapillary sphincters in skeletal muscles (Eriksson and Lisander, 1972). Thus, capillary blood volume in sympathetically denervated skeletal muscle is influenced not by abolition of precapillary sphincter tone, but rather by changes in intraluminal pressures in endarterioles.

Changes in skin temperature following sympathectomy of spinal anesthesia are not only conspicuous but also are frequently of diagnostic value. Under normal conditions the surface of the skin is cooler than the underlying tissues. The range of this temperature gradient varies considerably according to many factors, but is usually about 10°C. Following sympathectomy of spinal anesthesia there is an increased volume of blood present in the skin. The skin becomes warmer and its temperature approximates more closely that of the body (Green, et al., 1944; Davis and Greene, 1959). An increased rate of blood flow through the skin, which may coincide with an increased volume of blood in the skin, is only of secondary importance in determining the increase in temperature. The relative increase is greatest in the distal portions of the limbs, where the temperature is normally lowest.

Without hyperemia a slight elevation of cutaneous temperature may follow sympathetic block as a result of sudomotor paralysis and absence of sweating (Barcroft and Swan, 1953). Bengtsson, et al. (1983) studied the effect of sympathetic blockade produced by spinal anesthesia on skin blood flow and temperature, and the correlation between induced changes in blood flow and skin temperature. The study was performed using a laser Doppler flowmetry. During spinal anesthesia with bupivacaine or tetracaine to a mean dermatomal level of T_8, a significant reduction in skin blood flow occurred (and was interpreted as evidence of vasoconstriction) in the chest and upper extremity, while an increase in skin blood flow was observed in the lower part of the body (interpreted as vasodilation). However, there was no correlation between changes in skin blood flow and changes in skin temperature during spinal anesthesia. The authors concluded that estimation of skin blood flow by laser Doppler flowmetry was of greater value in estimating the extent of sympathetic blockade produced by spinal anesthesia than recordings of temperature changes (Chapter 1).

Cutaneous hyperemia does not invariably occur after sympathetic denervation even though all vessels are anatomically patent, a situation especially likely to occur in patients with carcinomatosis (Morton and Scott, 1930). Nevertheless, vasodilation with consequent hyperemia and elevation of skin temperature is a consistent enough effect of spinal anesthesia (Brill and Lawrence, 1930; Foregger, 1943; Felder, et al., 1951) to serve as a valuable diagnostic, prognostic, and therapeutic procedure in the study of peripheral vascular disease. When spinal anesthesia is used for diagnostic purposes in a room where the temperature is kept constant at 20°C, normal digits with an initial temperature of about 21–22°C, as well as those with arterial insufficiency due to vasospasm and registering about 19°C, show an increase in skin temperature to approximately 33.5°C after high spinal anesthesia. Failure to effect an increase to this level indicates either that sympathetic block is not complete, or that organic obliterative disease is present in the arteries or arterioles. In evaluating the skin temperature response to spinal anesthesia, the main emphasis is on whether the temperature rises to a "normal vasodilation level" of 33.5°C (Morton and Scott, 1930), rather than upon the number of degrees increase in temperature. Even with organic arterial occlusion there may be a certain increase in temperature of the skin following spinal anesthesia due to vasodilation of collateral channels, but the increase will not be to a normal level of 33.5°C and therefore should not be regarded as indicative of normal arterial vessels.

The physiologically important feature of spinal anesthesia as a diagnostic and therapeutic measure in peripheral vascular disease is, of course, the concomitant block of sympathetic fibers. This specific effect may be, and sometimes should be, obtained by anesthetizing the sympathetic nerves by differential spinal block (Sarnoff and Arrowood, 1946, 1947; Sarnoff, et al., 1948), by epidural (including caudal) block (Hingson and Southworth, 1947; Curbello, 1949; Thistlewaite, et al., 1953), or by anesthetizing the paravertebral chains or ganglia (White, 1930; Freeman and Montgomery, 1942; Eichna, 1943; Ruben, 1950). Sympathetic block by subarachnoid injection has the advantages of technical ease and invariable predictability (Smith and Rees, 1948), although in trained hands diagnostic epidural anesthesia may prove of equal reliability. Paravertebral block of the sympathetic chain is technically more difficult and lacks the certainty of spinal or epidural anesthesia. If the skin temperature of the foot does not rise after paravertebral injection, the failure could be due either to organic vascular occlusion or to the fact that the sympathetic chain has not in actual fact been blocked. With spinal anesthesia such technical difficulties and doubt are avoided; if sensory anesthesia extends to the tenth thoracic segment, all sympathetic fibers to the lower extremity must be anesthetized. Stellate ganglion block remains, of course, the most satisfactory technic for evaluation of upper extremity circulatory adequacy, but for the lower extremities diagnostic spinal anesthesia remains unexcelled for ease of performance and reliability of results.

Route of Peripheral Blood Flow

The channels via which blood passes through the postarteriolar bed are altered by spinal anesthesia. The sympathetic block produced by the anesthesia causes precapillary sphincters to relax. This leads to an increase in the number of patent capillaries, and a greater percentage of the blood entering the postarteriolar bed passes through capillaries instead of flowing directly to the venules by way of the arteriovenous thoroughfare channels (Lee and Holze, 1950). Thus a greater percentage of the blood entering the postarteriolar circulation is exposed to capillary endothelial surfaces, where gas and electrolyte exchanges take place (Ericksson and Lisander, 1972). This was aptly demonstrated by Bridenbaugh, *et al.* (1971) who measured capillary oxygen tension (PO_2) before and after sympathetic blockade of the upper and lower extremities. The authors found that sympathetic blockade of the lower extremity resulted in a mean increase in capillary PO_2 of 11.59 ± 9.85 mmHg, while the upper extremity capillary PO_2 mean increase was 6.48 ± 7.44 mmHg. This increase in capillary oxygenation was attributed to maximal skin vessel dilation "when the sympathetic constrictor influence on them is eliminated." The increase in capillary blood flow following sympathectomy results in more arterial (oxygenated) blood being exposed to areas where gas exchange with tissues takes place. Tissue uptake of oxygen is thereby facilitated, and the arterio-mixed venous oxygen difference would be expected to increase. This is a consequence of redistribution of postarteriolar blood flow in sympathetically denervated areas, since arterial oxygen saturation *per se* is unaffected by spinal anesthesia.

Such an increase in arterio-mixed venous oxygen difference during spinal anesthesia has been demonstrated in experimental animals (Co Tui, 1936; Shaw, *et al.*, 1937; Nowak and Downing, 1938) and in man (Schuberth, 1936; Sancetta, *et al.*, 1952, 1953; Lynn, *et al.*, 1952; Cain and Hamilton, 1966; Stevens, *et al.*, 1968; Bergenwald, *et al.*, 1972). If mixed venous blood is used in determining the arteriovenous (A-V) oxygen difference, the degree of change is found to vary with the amount of postarteriolar dilation (i.e., with the height of the sympathetic denervation). With a very low spinal block, the region of postarteriolar dilation and the blood volume passing through it are so small that there is relatively little change in the oxygen content of mixed venous blood. On the other hand, during high spinal anesthesia with total or near-total sympathetic block, the postarteriolar dilation is extensive, and mixed venous blood shows a much greater decrease in oxygen content. Sancetta, et al., have aptly demonstrated this (1952). In five of their patients, the brachial artery-pulmonary artery oxygen difference before anesthesia averaged 3.81 volumes percent. Thirty minutes after low spinal block the average difference was 3.95 volumes percent, or a 3.5 percent increase. Five other patients with an average brachial artery-pulmonary artery oxygen difference of 3.91 volumes percent before induction showed a 5.05 volumes percent difference during high spinal block, an increase of 22.6 percent. Cain and Hamilton (1966) also observed an increase in the normal A-V oxygen difference. At a time when arterial oxygen saturation remained unaltered during high spinal anesthesia, they found that mixed venous oxygen saturation decreased an average of 5.5 percent in 13 of 17 patients studied. Similarly, Stevens, et al. (1968) found right atrial oxygen saturation to have decreased more (5.3 percent) during high spinal than during low spinal anesthesia (4.1 percent) in humans. Johnson (1951) failed to find changes in A-V oxygen differences in six patients undergoing spinal anesthesia to the level of the fourth thoracic segment. This, however, is not surprising in view of the fact that ephedrine was given to each patient prior to the subarachnoid block. Similarly, mean mixed venous oxygen tension increased minimally from 35 to 37 mmHg during T_4 sensory spinal anesthesia in sheep whose blood pressure was kept in the normal range by infusion of 0.9% saline (Runciman, et al., 1984 b).

On the basis of the above reports on changes in oxygen content of mixed venous blood during spinal anesthesia, one would expect comparable results from analysis of peripheral venous blood that has come from a denervated area. The study by Kety, et al. (1950) investigated regional venous blood oxygenation during sympathectomy. In 17 patients with total or nearly total sympathetic denervation produced by differential spinal block, it was found that the average oxygen content of blood from the internal jugular vein showed a significant decrease from 10.6 volumes percent before the block to 8.9 volumes percent during the block. Similarly, Kleinerman, et al. (1958) observed a slight decrease in internal jugular oxygen content from 9.4 to 8.7 volumes percent in nine normotensive patients during high spinal anesthesia.

On the other hand, Weiss, et al. (1933) studied the content of femoral venous blood in four patients during high spinal anesthesia and found increases in venous oxygen content. The protocol does not state whether these patients received vasopressors at the time the venous samples were obtained, a fact that would have altered the results. The absence of hypotension despite high levels of anesthesia and use of the lateral decubitus position suggest that vasopressors were employed in this study. Cain and Hamilton (1966) and Stevens, *et al.* (1968), however, did not administer vasopressors to their patients prior to obtaining venous blood samples from the lower extremity during spinal anesthesia. They found that venous oxygen saturation increased during both high and low levels of anesthesia. Cerilli and Engell (1966) also found that during spinal anesthesia femoral vein oxygen tension increased and the arterial-femoral vein oxygen difference decreased in normal patients as well as in patients with obliterative arterial disease of the lower extremities. The increase in venous oxygen tension observed by Cerilli and Engell was modest, averaging approximately 6 mmHg, and it is interesting that this degree of change in oxygen tension produced the increase in oxygen saturation that was detected by Cain and Hamilton and by Stevens, *et al.* These investigators also observed that during spinal anesthesia oxygen saturation of venous blood obtained from the upper extremity decreased unless the level of anesthesia was high enough to produce sympathetic denervation of the arms. When the upper extremities were denervated, venous oxygen saturation increased.

The findings of Cain and Hamilton, Stevens, *et al.*, and Cerilli and Engell are at variance with those reported by Antonin (1930), but represent data obtained under more controlled conditions. Stevens, *et al.*, and Cain and Hamilton found an increase in arterial-mixed venous oxygen difference at a time when femoral venous oxygen saturation was increased and arterial-femoral venous oxygen difference was decreased. This finding can be explained by the fact that blood returning to the right side of the heart from areas other than the lower extremities (i.e., trunk and upper extremities) was relatively more desaturated than normal during spinal anesthesia, even though lower extremity venous blood was more saturated than normal. During low levels of spinal anesthesia, a portion of the blood that was more desaturated than normal came from the upper extremities. During high levels of spinal anesthesia the increase in upper extremity venous oxygen saturation and the continued decrease in mixed venous oxygen saturation mean that blood coming from areas other than the upper extremities was abnormally desaturated to the point that this desaturation was not compensated for by elevated oxygenation of blood draining from the upper extremities; thus, mixed venous oxygenation decreased. The source(s) of the desaturated blood causing an increase in arterial-mixed venous oxygen difference during high spinal anesthesia is not defined. It most likely represents a decrease in cardiac output. Venous oxygen saturation depends not only on the route of postarteriolar blood flow in denervated areas, but also depends on the amount of blood flowing through denervated areas (measured as ml/100 gm tissue/min).

The difference in response of venous blood oxygen levels in different parts of the body illustrates the lack of uniformity of various organs to sympathetic denervation. Results of an increase in venous PO_2 were reported by Bridenbaugh, *et al.* (1971), who found a 20.4 ± 13.4 mmHg increase in the arm venous PO_2 following sympathetic blockade (by brachial plexus block), and a 14.8 ± 7.6 mmHg increase in the foot venous PO_2 (following sympathectomy by femoral-sciatic block). The arterial PO_2 measured in the radial and femoral arteries simultaneously with venous and capillary PO_2 failed to show a significant change following sympathectomy.

The increase in venous oxygenation and the decrease in arteriovenous oxygen difference in blood draining from the extremities during spinal anesthesia are best explained on the basis that sympathetic denervation of the postarteriolar bed of skeletal muscle results in a situation in which a greater than normal amount of the blood entering the postarteriolar circulation passes through A-V thoroughfare channels directly from metarterioles to collecting venules. It is also possible that true anatomic A-V shunts open up. The blood therefore bypasses the capillaries where the gas exchange occurs. The majority of flow in the femoral vein is derived from skeletal muscle, and it is unlikely that changes in cutaneous flow induced by spinal anesthesia contribute to the increase in femoral venous oxygen content. In fact, despite cutaneous hyperemia and elevation of skin temperature indicative of increased blood flow to the skin during spinal anesthesia, there is a decrease in oxygen tension within the denervated skin of the lower extremity (Davis and Greene, 1959), probably a result of postarteriolar stagnation. In any case, there is a redistribution of postarteriolar blood flow during spinal anesthesia. In skeletal muscle, redistribution results in an increase in the amount of arterial blood going directly into the venous system and, presumably, a decrease in the amount of blood flowing through muscle capillaries. This in turn results in less oxygen extraction by muscle. In other organs (e.g., skin), rerouting or redistribution of postarteriolar blood flow brings a great volume of arterial blood into contact with cell interfaces because of opening of more capillary channels. The resulting increase in capillary flow is associated with a greater uptake of oxygen from blood, and so, with a decrease in venous oxygen content and saturation. In either instance, changes in A-V oxygen differences caused by spinal anesthesia cannot by themselves be taken as proof of postarteriolar stagnation or of anoxia at the capillary level. Changes in venous oxygen content are an indication of the redistribution of blood flow that is occurring in the postarteriolar bed.

Changes in the velocity of capillary blood flow during spinal anesthesia may also contribute to alterations of the A-V oxygen difference, but rerouting of postarteriolar blood can by itself explain changes in venous oxygen content independently of changes in rate of flow. Metabolic evidences of cellular hypoxia are not associated with changes in venous oxygenation (Chapter 7).

In summary, changes in the amount of oxygen extracted by different organs are reflected by changes in local venous blood oxygen content, by mixed venous blood oxygen content, or by A-V oxygen content difference. These changes can be multifactorial in origin and may involve redistribution of blood flow (i.e., increase in capillary blood flow or increase in A-V shunting), or a change in the velocity of blood flow through tissue. Furthermore, other factors (such as reversible ischemia) can affect local tissue metabolism and can thus have profound effects on regional perfusion and oxygen delivery. Burton and Johnson (1972), for example, studied red cell velocity profiles in individual capillaries in cat measured by dual-slit photometry following a 60-sec period of arterial occlusion; they concluded that the primary source of reactive hyperemia that followed tourniquet release reflected augmentation of flow in previously open capillaries, and not opening of new ones.

Postarteriolar Hydrostatic Pressure

Under normal conditions, the largest decrease in the arterial pressure gradient occurs at the arteriolar level (Figs. 2.4 and 2.6, and Gore, 1974).

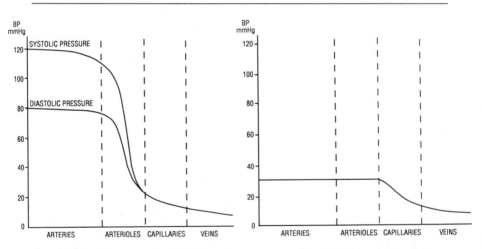

Figure 2.6. Diagrams of arterial blood pressure gradients. Left, normal gradient; right, following total sympathetic blockade. (Redrawn with permission from Griffiths, H. W. C., and Gillies, J.: Thoracolumbar splanchnicectomy and sympathectomy: anaesthetic procedure. Anaesthesia 3: 134, 1948.)

This corresponds to the fact that arteriolar tone accounts for 60 percent of the total peripheral vascular resistance. When dilated, however, the arterioles offer less resistance to the flow of blood through them, and the postarteriolar bed then becomes the site where peripheral vascular resistance is determined. In such a vasodilated area, the greatest decrease in arterial pressure occurs distal to the arterioles, rather than at the arteries. As a result, pressures in the postarteriolar bed are no longer independent of systemic arterial pressure as under normal conditions, but instead, they become directly related to arterial pressure. Thus, during vasodilation for example, increases in arterial pressure result in proportionate (though not equal) increases in postareriolar pressures in most (Landis, 1934; Eichna and Bordley, 1942) though not in all (Bohlen and Gore, 1977) areas. In normal digital vessels which have undergone vasodilation, the pressure in the arteriolar end of capillaries increases from normal levels of about 30 mmHg to levels as high as 43 mmHg (Landis, 1930; Eichna and Wilkins, 1942; Eichna, 1943; Eichna and Bordley, 1942; Gaskell and Krisman, 1958). In abnormally constricted vessels, dilation produces even more marked changes. In Raynaud's disease intracapillary pressures have been found to be 7.0–12.5 mmHg prior to sympathetic denervation, and 28–35 mmHg following denervation (Eichna and Wilkin, 1942). However, intracapillary pressures do not exceed approximately 45 mmHg no matter how complete vasodilation may be. There are two reasons for this. One is that there will always remain some gradient of pressure between arteries and capillaries because of the resistance to flow offered by friction alone. The other is that during vasodilation the pressure in the arterioles becomes dissipated over an increased number of open capillaries so that the pressure in any one capillary is increased only slightly, if at all (Gore, 1974; Bohlen and Gore, 1977). While vasodilation reduces the pressure gradient between arteries and capillaries, it does not eliminate it. During spinal anesthesia, therefore, intracapillary pressure may be expected to increase in denervated areas in the majority of patients. It would not increase in patients in whom organic vascular disease prevents vasodilation, and in patients in whom arterial pressure has decreased to such an extent that, even though vasodilation is present, arterial pressure is no longer adequate to maintain normal capillary pressure. In areas that have not been sympathetically denervated during spinal anesthesia, on the other hand, capillary pressures may actually decrease if there is compensatory vasoconstriction.

Intracapillary pressure determines both the volume of blood in capillaries and, most importantly, the rate of blood flow through the capillaries. Because capillary pressures are more directly related to arterial pressure during vasodilation than under normal conditions, sympathetic denervation results in maximal rate and volume of capillary blood flow at any given arterial pressure. Arterial hypotension with vasodilation may actually result in greater capillary blood flows than in situations in which arterial blood pressure is normal but vasoconstriction is present. This, of course, forms the rationale for deliberate induction of arterial hypotension by high spinal anesthesia or by ganglionic blocking agents to decrease surgical blood loss. It is also the basis of the theoretically sound but clinically hazardous practice of treating hemorrhagic shock by producing vasodilation.

Velocity of Postarteriolar Blood Flow

The rate at which blood flows through a capillary is determined by the difference in pressure at the arteriolar and venular ends of the capillary (Lee and Holze, 1950; Zweifach and Intaglietta, 1966). This difference is normally about 20 mmHg. It can be increased either by elevation of pressure at the arteriolar end of the capillary or by reduction of pressure at the venular end (Landis, 1934). Spinal anesthesia affects the pressure gradient in two ways. By producing arteriolar, metarteriolar, and capillary sphincter dilation, it tends to increase the hydrostatic pressure in the arteriolar limb of the capillary. By decreasing venous backpressure, it tends to lower resistance to outflow of blood at the venular end of the capillary. The pressure difference across the two ends of the capillary is therefore increased and the rate of capillary flow increases proportionately. Spinal anesthesia increases not only the volume of blood in the postarteriolar circulation and in each capillary, but also the rate at which this blood passes through the capillaries, as long as the arterial pressure is not decreased. The rate of postarteriolar blood flow will not, of course, change greatly in those areas of the vascular system in which vessels retain a high degree of intrinsic tone after sympathetic denervation (e.g., cerebral and renal circulations), but the rate of blood flow does increase in areas such as skin and skeletal muscle, where sympathetic denervation produces vasodilation. Following high spinal anesthesia, Sancetta, et al. (1952) found, using the finger occlusion plethysmograph, that following induction of anesthesia, blood flow to skin rose from an average resting level of 0.32 ml, to 1.11 ml of blood/10 ml of tissue/min. Similar increases have been shown to occur in skin after nerve block (Warren, et al., 1942; Marx and Schoop, 1956). Although not as marked as in skin, changes in blood flow through skeletal muscle following sympathetic denervation do take place (Prinzmetal and Wilson, 1936; Warren, et al., 1942; Barcroft, et al., 1943; Ederstrom, et al., 1956). There are, however, circumstances in which rate of blood flow may be decreased during spinal anesthesia both in those areas in which vasodilation takes place, as well as those in which vascular tone persists following sympathetic denervation. An example of this is seen when MAP decreases below about 35 mmHg. When this happens, there is reduction of pressure in the arteriolar end of the capillary to below 25 mmHg regardless of the degree of vasodilation. As soon as the pressure at the arteriolar end of the capillary decreases below 25 mmHg, the pressure gradient of 20 mmHg normally present between the two ends of the capillary can no longer be maintained. When this pressure gradient is reduced below 20 mmHg, a slower rate of capillary flow results. The same end result is, of course, obtained by elevation of the venous pressure: in the steep head-down position, it is likely that venous pressure may be so increased that, in the presence of arterial hypotension, the rate of blood flow through cerebral capillaries is decreased.

It can be seen from the preceding discussion that even in the normal cardiovascular system, factors regulating peripheral flow are so complex that categorical statements cannot be made to include all the effects of spinal anesthesia on the postarteriolar circulation. When only a few segments of the sympathetic outflow are interrupted, as during low spinal anesthesia, the arterial pressure is changed but little, and in these circumstances the relatively high perfusing pressure in the dilated peripheral vascular bed causes an increase in intracapillary pressure and in velocity of flow. At the same time that a low spinal block is producing an increased rate of capillary flow in denervated areas, there will be reflex vasoconstriction in certain of the unanesthetized portions of the body; in these areas the volume and rate of capillary flow will be simultaneously decreased. This has been well demonstrated by Berenyi, *et al.* (1964), who found that during spinal anesthesia with sensory denervation to T_{3-8} (i.e., subtotal sympathetic denervation), there was a 70 percent decrease in vascular resistance and a 160 percent increase in blood flow in skeletal muscle in the anesthetized area. There was a simultaneous 20 percent increase in vascular resistance and an 18 percent decrease in blood flow in the unanesthetized upper extremities. With high levels of anesthesia, arterial hypotension may develop and further alter the dynamics of postarteriolar circulation by decreasing the rate of capillary flow even though the capillary blood volume remains elevated. Therefore, one of the main determinants of the effects of spinal anesthesia on the postarteriolar circulation is the change in the arterial blood pressure, if any, produced by anesthesia. The question then arises as to the extent to which the arterial pressure can decrease before capillary circulation is impaired.

The following discussion does not apply to spinal anesthesia when sympathomimetic drugs are used to maintain normal arterial blood pressure. The vasoconstriction caused by such agents removes the direct relationship which exists between capillary and arterial pressures during spinal blockade.

Before attempting to define the minimal safe level of arterial blood pressure during vasodilation, it is necessary to consider in further detail how the factors of hydrostatic pressure, volume of flow, and rate of flow affect cellular metabolism and respiration. The importance of hydrostatic pressure (Hyman, 1944; Zweifach and Intaglietta, 1966) is based upon the fact that "the rate of net fluid movement across the capillary wall (is) simply proportional to the differences between hydrostatic osmotic forces acting across the capillary membranes" (Pappenheimer, et al., 1951). Blood pressure in the arteriolar limbs of capillaries must always exceed the osmotic pressure of the plasma in order to ensure transfer of liquids across capillary membranes. In humans, osmotic pressure averages about 25 mmHg (Landis, 1934; Fisch, et al., 1950). In the normally innervated postarteriolar bed, pressures in the arteriolar ends of the capillaries range from 21 to 48 mmHg, averaging about 32 mmHg. There is, therefore, a 7 mmHg mean difference between hydrostatic and colloid osmotic pressures which provides for fluid exchange between the vascular and extravascular compartments. However, hydrostatic pressure has little direct effect on gas exchange at the capillary level. The rate at which oxygen and carbon dioxide are transferred is determined by the differences in partial pressures of the gases on either side of the capillary membrane. These differences in partial pressures are (from the vascular point of view) primarily a function of the volume of capillary blood and the rate at which this blood flows through the capillary. Hydrostatic pressure has some influence on capillary blood volume in that increases in intraluminal pressure result in increases in diameter of denervated capillaries (Folkow, 1949; Bohlen and Gore, 1977). However, hydrostatic pressure has no direct effect on rate of capillary blood flow which, as stated above, is determined by the difference in hydrostatic pressures existing at the two ends of the capillary, rather than by the hydrostatic pressure itself. Rate of flow may actually be decreased in the presence of increased hydrostatic pressure as from obstruction to the venous outflow. Under normal conditions the arterial circulation brings to the capillaries blood with an oxygen tension greater than that found in the tissues. Oxygen therefore diffuses out of the capillary into the cells. Contrariwise, the tension of carbon dioxide in the arterial blood is less than that in the tissues, and so this gas diffuses out of the tissues into the capillaries. If, however, either the volume of arterial blood delivered to the capillaries or the rate at which capillary blood is replaced by fresh arterial blood decreases beyond a certain point, a situation will arise in which the tension of gases in tissues becomes the same as in capillary blood. Oxygen no longer diffuses out of the blood and carbon dioxide does not diffuse into it. Cellular anoxia supervenes and cell death occurs very rapidly. It should be noted, however, that at the present time there are no data that define the precise level at which tissue oxygen tension is no longer able to support aerobic tissue metabolism in vivo in normal humans. The critical level of tissue oxygen tension undoubtedly varies from organ to organ. It has been found that in the resting skeletal muscle of dogs, a 30 percent decrease in tissue oxygen tension during sympathetic paralysis and vasodilation is unaccompanied by metabolic evidence of anaerobiosis (Willenkin and Greene, 1963). In humans, however, comparable decreases in cellular oxygen tensions may result in impaired metabolism, particularly within the central nervous system (CNS).

The level of arterial pressure that is theoretically adequate to maintain normal cellular respiration and metabolism during vasodilation therefore becomes that pressure that will maintain normal rate and volume of flow as well as normal capillary hydrostatic pressures. The osmotic pressure is normally 25 mmHg and MAP has to be at least of this magnitude. A pressure of 25 mmHg at the arteriolar end of the capillary could also provide the 20 mmHg pressure gradient across the capillary that is required for normal rates of blood flow. But to ensure a pressure of 25 mmHg within the arteriolar end of the capillary would necessitate a mean pressure of at least 30–35 mmHg in the arteries to compensate for the 5–10 mmHg decrease in pressure that will exist between arteries and arterioles even in the presence of vasodilation. On a purely theoretical basis it can be said that during spinal anesthesia a MAP of at least 30–35 mmHg is necessary to provide adequate tissue oxygenation and metabolism in normal patients. This figure agrees with the work of Lynn, et al. (1952), who found that if the MAP decreased to below 30 mmHg during spinal anesthesia, the rate of blood flow in the hands and feet decreased.

In quoting the figure of 35 mmHg, however, several points should be emphasized. In the first place, the ability of such an arterial pressure to provide adequate tissue blood flow is dependent on the presence of vasodilation; during vasoconstriction, such a pressure will be grossly inadequate. Second, the figure represents MAP, not systolic pressure. Third, it represents the true intra-arterial pressure as determined by intra-arterial manometry. Pressures in this range cannot be determined reliably by sphygmomanometry. Fourth, the level of 30–35 mmHg MAP must never be used as a justification for viewing inadvertent hypotension with equanimity during clinical spinal anesthesia. At best, this theoretical figure applies only in cases in which the blood vessels are able to dilate fully and have no arteriosclerotic plaques or other obstructions. And finally, a level of 35 mmHg MAP, even in the presence of vasodilation, may not prove adequate for maintenance of normal function of many organs (e.g., kidney, brain). Such a pressure should, however, be consistent with tissue perfusion of blood that is adequate for the maintenance of cellular respiration (even though function may be depressed) at levels such that irreversible changes do not take place. Normal function can resume following restoration of normal blood pressure.

Certain clinical signs are useful in determining when spinal anesthesia is causing derangement of postarteriolar circulation to the extent that capillary blood flow is inadequate. One of the best of these signs is the capillary filling time. A clinical estimate can be made of the rate of capillary blood flow by applying pressure sufficient to cause blanching of the forehead, ears, or fingernail beds, and then noting the time required for return of normal color. If the filling time is longer than normal, immediate steps must be taken to elevate the arterial pressure. Sudden and extreme bradycardia developing after the establishment of spinal block often indicates a failing circulation. The onset of abnormal respiratory rates or rhythms also indicates the same thing. If tissue anoxia develops during spinal anesthesia, there may be an abrupt further decrease in blood pressure, to the extent that no arterial pulse is palpable. This is a result of further vasodilation secondary to anoxia and to the accumulation of metabolites during the period of inadequate capillary blood flow. These metabolites are then responsible for removal of the residual intrinsic vascular tone that remains following sympathetic denervation. Greater pooling of blood in the periphery then occurs, with still further reduction in venous return to the heart and in CO. Peripheral blood flow becomes increasingly inadequate, and the heart stops unless the vicious circle is promptly broken by immediate restoration of CO and blood pressure. The usual premonitory signs of anoxia and respiratory acidosis do not develop during high spinal anesthesia because of the sympathetic block produced by the anesthesia itself. Patients under high spinal anesthesia must be observed constantly and vigilantly for signs of impending circulatory inadequacy.

In the foregoing discussion of the effects of spinal anesthesia on the postarteriolar circulation, no account has been taken of the possible effects of sympathetic denervation on capillary permeability. Sympathetic denervation does alter the rate at which liquids and dyes pass through the capillary wall, but it has not yet been proven that this is due to any specific effect of the sympathectomy (Engel, 1940; Balourdas, 1955). Any alteration in capillary permeability accompanying sympathetic denervation is probably secondary to concomitant changes in intracapillary pressure and flow (McMaster, et al., 1932; Landis, 1934; Chambers and Zweifach, 1947; Pappenheimer, et al., 1951; Zweifach and Intaglietta, 1966; Mason and Bartter, 1968). Despite some opinions to the contrary (Turai, et al., 1956), changes in capillary permeability that take place during the sympathetic block of spinal anesthesia are of little if any significance, with the possible exception of renal electrolyte excretion (Chapter 5).

Before leaving the subject of the peripheral vascular system during spinal anesthesia, mention should be made of the effects of this technique on the blood itself. Although alterations in sympathetic tone produce well documented delayed changes in blood volume over a period of time (Mason and Bartter, 1968), total blood volume is not altered significantly by the acute sympathetic denervation of spinal blockade. Using the dye T-1824, Guest, *et al.* (1949) found that before spinal anesthesia the average blood volume of 25 normal patients was 5236 ml and the average plasma volume was 2652 ml. During anesthesia, the corresponding values were 5686 ml and 2750 ml. Both changes were within the range of error of the method employed. Using brilliant vital red dye, Goldfarb, *et al.* (1939) likewise found no significant changes in blood volume induced by spinal anesthesia. Using simultaneously injected chromium-tagged red blood cells and radioiodinated human serum albumin in one of the most carefully controlled studies reported, Armstrong and Finlayson (1967) found in 19 adult males that spinal anesthesia was unaccompanied by changes in red cell volume, plasma volume, or whole blood volume. However, these findings are at variance with those of Mann and Guest (1950), who found that there was a slight, but consistent and statistically significant increase in blood volume during spinal anesthesia. In their 25-patient study, Mann and Guest found that blood volume averaged 5236 ml before anesthesia, 5686 ml 10 min after spinal anesthesia was induced, and 6012 ml 1 hr later. Corresponding figures for plasma volume were 2652, 2750, and 2904 ml. The reasons for these observed increases are unclear but are probably related to details of technic, such as limitations inherent in blood volume determinations by T-1824 dye injections, as well as preanesthetic control measurements which were made several days prior to induction of anesthesia. Lorhan and Devine (1952), on the other hand, reported frequent and severe decreases in blood volume: 34 of 49 patients showed decreases in blood volume ranging from 1 percent to 15 percent following the induction of spinal anesthesia, while 9 patients had decreases of 16 percent to 30 percent. Only six of their patients failed to show any decrease in blood volume associated with spinal anesthesia. Sircar (1952) reported comparable decreases in blood volume during spinal anesthesia in patients, while Nakayama, *et al.* (1956) found similar changes in dogs. The reason for these reported decreases in blood volume is not clear, but is probably a matter of technic such as not allowing enough time for complete mixing of the test material in the vascular system. Although changes in circulating blood volume may and do occur with spinal anesthesia (Nylin and Pannier, 1947), there is no reason to believe that the anesthetic itself causes any significant changes in total blood volume.

A slight but constant hemodilution has, however, often been observed during spinal anesthesia. Sancetta, *et al.* (1952, 1953) found a consistent decrease in HCT levels, which averaged about 3.3 percent in 10 operative cases. Schuberth (1936) likewise found a decrease in HCT, although to a somewhat larger degree (17 percent). Nakayama, *et al.* (1956) as well as Tardieu, *et al.* (1957) also reported a decrease in hematocrit. Armstrong and Finlayson (1967), on the other hand, were unable to find any changes in whole body HCT, large-vessel HCT, or the ratio between the two. The only report indicating an increase in HCT due to spinal anesthesia is that by Turai, et al. (1956), but in their cases, operative and postoperative dehydration may well have been present. Some, but not all, of the reported hemodilution may be due to intravenous fluids used in the course of the experimental studies. In addition, some trapping of erythrocytes in the periphery may also occur during anesthesia. Such trapping is most likely to occur in the spleen which undergoes considerable enlargement following its sympathetic denervation (Barcoft and Elliott, 1936). Incidentally, the splenomegaly associated with spinal anesthesia is another reason why this type of anesthesia may be contraindicated for surgical treatment of a ruptured spleen: an enlargement of a ruptured spleen may be associated with renewed or more vigorous bleeding.

Effects on Coagulation

Although regional anesthesia does not influence the coagulation or fibrinolytic systems, thrombocyte aggregation may be influenced favorably (Kehlet, 1987). Lahnborg and Bergstrom (1975) were among the first to report the interesting, although anecdotal, finding that regional anesthesia administered following general anesthesia was associated with a lower incidence of thromboembolic events. Although their study investigated epidural anesthesia, it nevertheless prompted interest in assessing the effects of spinal anesthesia on the fibrinolytic system. Thus, Covert and Fox (1989) reviewed the incidence of complications related to thromboembolic phenomena in elderly patients having hip surgery under spinal or general anesthesia, and found that spinal anesthesia reduced the incidence of deep venous thrombosis (DVT) and pulmonary embolism (PE). The same benefits were reported by Davis, et al. (1989 b) who studied prospectively the incidence of DVT in 140 patients who received either a hypobaric tetracaine spinal or general anesthesia for total hip replacement. Deep vein thrombosis was diagnosed using impedance plethysmography and ^{125}I fibrinogen uptake test, combined with contrast venography. The overall incidence of DVT was 20 percent; 19 (27 percent) of patients having general anesthesia developed deep vein thrombosis, but only 9 (13 percent) of patients having spinal anesthesia had this complication postoperatively. The same group of investigators (Davis, et al., 1989 a), studied the incidence of DVT by fibrinogen scanning, impedance plethysmography, or ascending contrast venography. Of the 122 patients undergoing hip surgery, 65 had spinal anesthesia, and 57 had general anesthesia. Although the overall rate of DVT was 23 percent, only 14 percent of patients having spinal anesthesia had documented DVT, while in the general anesthesia group, the incidence of DVT was 33 percent. The beneficial effects of spinal anesthesia in reducing the incidence of deep venous thrombosis (and pulmonary embolization) have also been reported by Sharnoff, *et al.* (1976); Davis and Laurenson (1981); Davis, *et al.* (1987 b); Foate, *et al.* (1985); McKenzie, *et al.* (1985); Orr, *et al.* (1986); and Thorburn, *et al.* (1980).

Spinal anesthesia may offer another important advantage over general anesthesia: it has been shown that spinal anesthesia is associated with decreased intraoperative blood loss (460 ml vs. 792 ml) as compared to general anesthesia for intratrochanteric hip fractures (Covert and Fox, 1989). Similar decreases in intraoperative blood loss associated with spinal anesthesia (527 vs. 671 ml) were reported by Davis, *et al.* (1987 b), who studied hemostasis during total hip replacement in 101 patients. In their study, the lower intraoperative blood loss in patients receiving spinal anesthesia was associated with a 4% incidence of transfusion, while patients undergoing general anesthesia had a 12 percent incidence of transfusion. The decreased intraoperative blood loss associated with spinal anesthesia when compared to general anesthesia was also reported by Cook, *et al.* (1986); Davis, *et al.* (1987 b); Davis and Laurenson (1981); McGowan and Smith (1980); Sculco and Ranawat (1975); Thorburn, *et al.* (1980); and Valentin, *et al.* (1986).

The factors responsible for the beneficial effects of spinal anesthesia when compared to general anesthesia may be multifactorial and include the following. First, decreased blood loss associated with spinal anesthesia requires less intraoperative fluid replacement. The decreased requirement for fluid administration may in turn decrease the hypercoagulability induced by crystalloid administration (Janvrin, *et al.*, 1980). Second, the vasodilation induced by the sympathetic denervation increases the mean leg blood flow, thereby decreasing the likelihood of thrombosis (Foate, *et al.*, 1985). Third, sympathetic denervation decreases the capacity for activation of factor VIII, thereby improving the fibrinolytic function (Modig, *et al.*, 1983 a, b). Fourth, local anesthetics decrease the adhesiveness and migration of leukocytes and platelets, decrease the aggregation of erythrocytes, and alter plasma proteins to decrease the incidence of thrombosis following absorption of local anesthetics into the blood stream (Modig, 1988). This beneficial effect of local anesthetics also has been investigated by Orr, *et al.* (1986) who studied the effects of an intramuscular injection of 75 mg of lidocaine. Peak plasma lidocaine concentrations of 0.8 $\mu g \cdot ml^{-1}$ were obtained 30 min following injection. The concentrations obtained were similar to those reported by Giasi, *et al.* (1979) following subarachnoid administration of 75 mg of lidocaine (0.32 $\mu g \cdot ml^{-1}$). Although HCT and red cell deformability remained unchanged in the study by Orr, lidocaine caused a small but significant decrease in plasma and whole blood viscosity, both at high and low shear rates. The reductions in viscosity were considered to result from decreased red cell aggregation. Fifth, improved postoperative pain relief and comfort (Harrison and Allen, 1986) associated with spinal anesthesia may result in earlier ambulation and lower likelihood of thromboembolism.

Venous Circulation (Preload)

Preload is a measure of end-diastolic volume of the left ventricle, LVEDV (i.e., venous return to the left ventricle). However, the end-diastolic volume is not linearly related to the end-diastolic pressure of the left ventricle (LVEDP). LVEDP is determined by blood volume, ventricular compliance, ventricular afterload (i.e., pressure generated during systole), venous tone, and myocardial contractility. Traditionally, LVEDP has nevertheless been used as the standard to define pump function of the left ventricle, although this measurement is exceedingly difficult to obtain routinely. This difficulty may be overcome in part by measurement of pulmonary artery occlusion pressure (pulmonary capillary wedge pressure (PCWP)), which assumes normal left ventricular compliance, normal mitral valve function, and normal airway pressures. An even less accurate approximation of preload (i.e., LVEDV), may be obtained relatively easily in the clinical setting by measurement of right atrial or superior vena caval pressures. Either of these pressures, although not identical, has been referred to as central venous pressure (CVP). Measurement of CVP as an indicator of preload (i.e., LVEDV) assumes normal right ventricular compliance and tricuspid valve function, normal pulmonary vascular resistance, normal airway pressure and mitral valve function, and normal left ventricular compliance. Despite these multiple assumptions, it is nevertheless common in the clinical setting to monitor CVP as an indicator of preload.

Sympathetic denervation dilates not only the arterial and postarteriolar circulation (afterload), but also the larger veins and venules (Lewis and Landis, 1929–1931; Capps, 1936; Folkow and Mellander, 1964; Webb-Peploe and Shepherd, 1968). As innervation of the venous circulation is similar to that of corresponding vessels on the arterial side (Pereira, 1946; McDowall, *et al.*, 1956), areas in which venodilation occurs during spinal anesthesia are the same as those in which the arteries and arterioles are denervated. There is, however, an important difference in the vasodilation that occurs on the arterial side and that occurring in the veins. Because the walls of veins and venules contain fewer muscle fibers and other supporting structures than their arterial counterparts, they do not retain any demonstrable residual intrinsic tone following sympathetic denervation. In contrast, on the arterial side vasodilation is not maximal; denervated arteries and arterioles retain residual smooth muscle tone.

Shimosato and Etsten (1969) assessed the effect of spinal anesthesia on veins by measuring vascular distensibility of calf vessels, a function primarily of venous tone, in 15 nonpremedicated, nonoperative subjects before and after induction of spinal anesthesia with sensory levels to T_{4-7}. They studied five subjects before and after equal sensory levels of epidural anesthesia (without epinephrine). Results were similar after both forms of anesthesia and were consequently pooled. Mean vascular distensibility prior to anesthesia was 3.0 ± 0.2 (SEM) units. During anesthesia, it was 3.5 ± 0.3 units, and the 17 percent increase induced by anesthesia was statistically significant. Simultaneous vascular distensibility values in the forearm were 5.6 ± 0.5 and 5.1 ± 0.4, respectively, a change that was not statistically significant. Distensibility of lower extremity veins, therefore, increased with spinal anesthesia, while distensibility of the veins in the upper, sympathetically intact, extremity was not affected. Other authors have reported similar findings (Blake, et al., 1988). In their study, 50 patients underwent spinal anesthesia with cinchocaine (dibucaine), while the forearm blood flow was measured by a strain gauge plethysmograph. Spinal anesthesia was associated with a lowering of the systolic and diastolic blood pressures by 18 and 9 mmHg, respectively. This decrease in blood pressure was associated with a 32% decrease in mean forearm blood flow (secondary to reflex vasoconstriction). Foate, et al. (1985) studied the changes in lower limb blood flow during transurethral resection of the prostate in patients undergoing either spinal anesthesia with amethocaine (tetracaine) or general anesthesia. They found that under spinal anesthesia the mean leg blood flow doubled from controlled values, and remained elevated for 2 hr postoperatively. General anesthesia, on the other hand, was associated with only a 36 percent increase in mean leg blood flow, which, importantly, was found to decrease postoperatively to 28 percent of control value.

Because veins retain no residual tone following sympathetic blockade, the degree of their dilation is mainly intraluminal hydrostatic pressure. The latter, in turn, is determined principally by gravity. Normally, blood entering venules from the postarteriolar bed exerts a hydrostatic pressure sufficient to push blood through the venules into the veins and, ultimately, to the right side of the heart. With venodilation, however, hydrostatic pressure becomes disipated by the greatly increased capacitance of the venous bed, and it may no longer be adequate to force blood back to the heart. Pooling of an abnormally large volume of blood in the veins and venules then occurs, and gravity becomes the chief factor regulating venous return to the heart. Thus, positioning of the body so that its sympathectomized region is dependent causes peripheral venous pooling, whereas elevation of such an area causes drainage of blood from the periphery toward the heart. The additional volume of blood in the peripheral veins and venules during spinal anesthesia therefore has the effect of reducing the circulating blood volume and modifying not only venous return to the heart, but also CO and systemic arterial blood pressure. The percentage of the patient's total blood volume that is retained in the periphery depends both on the extent of sympathetic block and the position of the patient. During a total sympathetic block with the patient in the head-up or Fowler position, the effective circulating blood volume may be decreased by 50 percent or more.

Because of peripheral pooling in veins and venules during spinal anesthesia, a decrease in velocity of venous blood flow is to be expected. Theoretically this slowing would be greatest in the smaller venules, but the technical difficulties of measuring this are such that it has never been done in humans. In reports of measurements of venous circulation time during spinal anesthesia, the site for injection of the test substance has always been the large veins of the arm (Webb, et al., 1936; Goldfarb, et al., 1939; Doud and Rovenstine, 1940). It generally has been observed that there is no change in circulation time when the sensory level of the block is below the sixth thoracic segment. With a level of anesthesia above T_6, circulation time is prolonged by about 50 percent. It is only at higher levels of sensory blockade that significant numbers of sympathetic fibers to the upper extremity are denervated. Using a vein of the lower extremity as the site of injection, measurements of venous circulation time during low spinal anesthesia would probably show similar or even greater delay, especially if the limb were in the dependent position. Unfortunately, such studies have not been reported. During clinical spinal anesthesia there is no reason to expect slowing of the venous circulation outside the regions directly affected by the blockade. The rate of venous flow will remain normal except where veins and tributary venules have become dilated from sympathetic denervation. If slowing of the venous return to the heart were to occur outside the area functionally sympathectomized by the anesthesia, this would indicate a severe decrease in CO, and circulatory collapse would be imminent.

When measured in the arm, changes in venous circulation time cannot be correlated with alterations in arterial blood pressure during spinal anesthesia. Nor do changes in venous circulation time bear any relation to concurrent paralysis of intercostal muscles and a hypothetical reduction in intrathoracic negative pressure. Absence of the normal negative intrathoracic pressure during inspiration can modify venous filling of the right side of the heart and consequently the peripheral venous circulation. However, because of compensatory diaphragmatic action, negative intrathoracic pressure remains normal during inspiration even with spinal anesthesia high enough to block the intercostal nerves (Chapter 3).

Changes in peripheral venous pressure produced by spinal anesthesia closely parallel those in venous circulation time (Seevers and Waters,

1932 a; Schuberth, 1936; Goldfarb, *et al.*, 1939; Adriani and Rovenstine, 1940; Gregory and Levin, 1948). The venodilation of sympathetic denervation reduces both the intravenous pressure and the rate of blood flow through the veins. As in measurements of venous circulation time, reported studies of peripheral venous pressure during spinal anesthesia in humans have invariably employed the veins of the upper extremities. With low spinal anesthesia there is no significant change in the pressure in these veins. It is not until the sensory block is at or above the midthoracic dermatomes (i.e., when sympathetic denervation of the arms has occurred) that the venous pressure shows a fairly consistent decrease, amounting to 1.5–2.0 cm H_2O. The fact that the decrease in venous pressure in the arms coincides with prolongation of venous circulation times provides that the latter is not due to obstruction to venous blood because of a reduction in negative intrathoracic pressure during inspiration. If obstruction were present, the prolongation of venous circulation time would be associated with an increase in venous pressure and not a decrease. As with changes in circulation time, changes in venous pressure cannot be directly correlated with alterations in arterial pressure during spinal anesthesia. When the changes in venous pressure and arterial pressure coincide, the occurrence is fortuitous rather than mathematically predictable.

Reports of measurements of venous pressure in the superior vena cava during spinal anesthesia yield results too erratic to be informative (Graves and Klein, 1968). Right atrial pressure, on the other hand, is a somewhat more consistent indicator of changes taking place in the peripheral venous circulation during spinal anesthesia, and, indeed, right atrial pressure can be roughly correlated with the level of anesthesia. In five patients with sensory block to below the fourth thoracic segment, Sancetta, *et al.* (1952) found that right atrial pressure decreased from a preanesthetic mean of 5.98 mmHg (one patient showed an abnormally high pressure of 19.0 mmHg) to a mean of 3.81 mmHg, a decrease of 36 percent, during anesthesia. In five patients with high spinal anesthesia, the mean pressure was 3.93 mmHg before, and 1.84 mmHg during anesthesia, a decrease of 53 percent. Cain and Hamilton (1966) and Bergenwald, *et al.* (1972) found comparable decreases in right atrial pressure during spinal anesthesia with sensory levels of T_4 and above, the average decrease being 3.4 mmHg. Kennedy, *et al.* (1968, 1970 a, b) also found that right atrial pressure decreased following induction of high spinal anesthesia, though the magnitude of the decrease was less, averaging about 8 percent. On the other hand, low (T_{10}) sensory levels of spinal anesthesia are not associated with changes in right atrial pressure (Samii, *et al.*, 1979). The decrease in right atrial pressure parallels the decrease in cardiac output, although it is not always proportional to it. The reduction in the right atrial pressure is a reflection of decreased venous return to the right heart. Because of the decrease in venous return to the heart that it causes, spinal anesthesia has been advocated as a therapeutic measure in the treatment of pulmonary edema (Tuohy, 1952). While such a "bloodless phlebotomy" has proven successful (Sarnoff and Farr, 1944), the dangers of the procedure in clinical practice outweigh its possible advantages: not only is the duration of the block relatively brief, but also the dangers of arterial hypotension are considerable in such severely ill patients. Vasopressors cannot be used to maintain the arterial pressure during spinal anesthesia induced for this therapeutic purpose without eliminating the desired venodilation and decrease in preload. Furthermore, spinal anesthesia must be induced in an orthopneic patient in the worst possible position as far as CO and systemic pressure are concerned, namely, in Fowler's position. However, the effect of spinal anesthesia on venous return does suggest an advantage in patients who may be in, or bordering on, congestive heart failure and who are undergoing operations suitable for mid- or high-thoracic levels of spinal anesthesia.

Cardiac Function

Before discussing the specific effects of spinal anesthesia on cardiac function, it must be emphasized that most knowledge currently available regarding the effects of sympathetic denervation on the cardiovascular system is derived from older studies. There is currently an unfortunate paucity of data concerning changes in myocardial function, for instance, during the sympathetic denervation of spinal anesthesia. The advent of newer, noninvasive techniques of assessing myocardial function should provide the impetus for studying such changes during spinal anesthesia.

Pulse Rate

Spinal anesthesia is characteristically associated with slowing of the pulse rate. The degree of bradycardia, as well as the frequency with which it occurs, can be roughly correlated with the extent of sympathetic denervation. This is, however, by no means a precise relationship under clinical conditions. Changes in pulse rate during spinal anesthesia are also influenced by age (Dohi, et al., 1979), by the amount and type of drugs used for premedication, and most important, by position of the patient on the operating table. In some patients the pulse rate may decrease during spinal anesthesia to 60 beats/min or less. This is especially likely to occur in the head-up position or when for other reasons venous return to the heart is diminished. Pronounced bradycardia is observed most frequently when cardiac output and arterial blood pressure have decreased significantly during anesthesia. In other patients, the pulse rate may change little, if at all (Runciman, *et al.*, 1984 b; Baron, *et al.*, 1987) while in still others pulse rate may increase slightly (by 8–10 beats/min) following induction of spinal anesthesia. When pulse rate increases during spinal anesthesia in the absence of the administration of positive chronotropic drugs, there is usually an increase in venous return, most often because of use of the head-down position, and arterial blood pressure decreases little, if at all. The tendency, however, is for pulse rate to decrease during spinal anesthesia. Tachycardia of 20 beats/min above preanesthetic control levels does not occur during spinal anesthesia in the absence of drugs with positive chronotropic effects.

The extent to which pulse rate decreases in normal patients during total preganglionic sympathetic denervation produced by spinal anesthesia has been quantitated under controlled conditions in two studies. In one, 12 unpremedicated patients aged 18–40 years were given high spinal anesthetics (T_3 and above) (O'Rourke and Greene, 1970). In the supine horizontal position mean HR decreased to 90.3 ± 2.3 (SEM) percent of preanesthetic baseline levels and mean arterial blood pressure decreased to 80.3 ± 1.9 percent of baseline. Both changes were statistically significant. After the chronotropic response to total sympathetic block was established, vagal blockade was then produced by intravenous administration of atropine, 0.04 mg·kg^{-1}. Mean HR increased to 148.6 ± 8.1 percent of baseline, significantly above both baseline and postsympathetic block levels. After atropine, MAP was 105.2 ± 4.2 percent of control values, significantly above postsympathetic block levels but not significantly different from baseline levels. The object of the study was to identify components of the neurogenic control of resting heart rate in humans. These authors concluded that both sympathetic and parasympathetic nervous systems regulate resting HR, but that in normal individuals the latter predominates, a conclusion also reached by Glick and Braunwald (1965), based on data obtained in experimental animals. In the second study (Greene and Bachand, 1971), six patients were given high spinal anesthetics and, after steady pulse rates were established, some of the patients were given the same amount of intravenous atropine prior to administration of intravenous methoxamine 0.5 mg, while the others were given methoxamine without prior atropine. The object of this study was to determine whether the bradycardia associated with elevation of mean aortic pressure was due to an increase in vagal tone or to a decrease in sympathetic activity. Mean HR in these patients following total preganglionic sympathetic denervation was 84.7 percent of baseline values, while mean arterial blood pressure was 82.4 percent of baseline. The difference in response of HR to methoxamine with and without prior administration of atropine indicated that the increase in vagal tone contributes more to the decrease in HR when arterial pressure increases than does diminution of sympathetic tone. The data from these two studies also demonstrate that in normal unpremedicated patients HR decreases relatively moderately, only about 10 percent to 15 percent, during total sympathetic block produced by spinal anesthesia. These are, however, average responses. Severe bradycardia can and does develop, even to the point of cardiac arrest, in otherwise normal subjects during otherwise uneventful spinal anesthesia (Gerbershagen and Kennedy, 1971; Wetstone and Wong, 1974; Gregoretti, 1985). Recently, asystole during spinal anesthesia was reported in a marathon runner, and its occurrence was attributed to the "athletic heart syndrome" (Kreutz and Mazuzan, 1990).

An extreme manifestation of cardiovascular changes that may occur in response to changes in position has been described even in the absence of sympathetic denervation (Milstein, et al., 1989) in six patients with histories of recurrent syncope associated with hypotension and bradycardia. All six patients developed syncope and cardiovascular collapse during a tilt provocation test, illustrating the fact that certain individuals are prone to development of asystole and cardiovascular collapse on a neurally mediated basis (Bezold-Jarisch reflex) (p. 133, 164). The mechanism proposed for this scenario is that during periods of reduced venous return (i.e., during resumption of upright position from supine), cardiac mechanoreceptors promote reflex sympathetic stimulation (Almquist, et al., 1989; Abboud, 1989). The cardiac mechanoreflex originates in the heart from nerve endings that are located in the ventricles. These nerve endings may be activated mechanically either by cardiac distention or by vigorous systolic contraction. Stimulation of mechanoreceptors may occur during severe hemorrhage that is accompanied by excessive neurohumoral stimulation (Abboud, 1989; Oberg and Thoren, 1972). In susceptible individuals, the loss of central volume (as during massive hemorrhage) in conjunction with the excitatory effects of the catecholamine surge (even in the absence of sympathetic denervation), may lead to increased afferent neural traffic relayed to the vasomotor center by vagal fibers, resulting in paradoxical simultaneous bradycardia and vasodilation (Mark, 1983).

Other etiologies of heart rate changes during spinal anesthesia have been investigated. Anton, et al. (1977) studied the interrelationship between electroshock therapy (EST)-induced convulsions, autonomic function, plasma catecholamines levels, and cardiovascular homeostasis in dogs. They found that high spinal anesthesia was most effective in preventing the hypertension associated with EST. The prevention of hypertension was due to attenuation of the increase in circulating catecholamines. The authors also concluded that the source of the EST-induced increase in circulating catacholamines was the adrenal medulla. Furthermore, the asystole induced by EST in sympathectomized dogs supports the hypothesis that EST-induced activation of the autonomic nervous system in the presence of a sympathetic block can lead to a vagally induced protracted asystole. The above-mentioned studies may provide some insight as to why extreme decreases in HR (or even asystole) developed in normal patients during spinal anesthesia. Administration of drugs having parasympathomimetic effects can also produce extreme, if pharmacologically more explicable, bradycardia during spinal anesthesia (Hilgenberg and Johantgen, 1980). The prudent anesthesiologist monitors HR continuously throughout even the most "routine" spinal anesthetic.

Bradycardia during high spinal anesthesia is due to two causes: paralysis of preganglionic cardiac accelerator fibers and diminished venous return to the right side of the heart because of the increased peripheral venous capacitance. The relative effect of each may vary considerably from patient to patient. Since cardiac accelerator fibers arise from the first four thoracic spinal segments, blockade of these fibers with subsequent control of cardiac pacemakers by inhibitory vagal fibers occurs most commonly when sensory levels of anesthesia extend to at least the fourth thoracic level. Because such levels of anesthesia are also usually associated with decreases in venous return, it is often difficult to determine the effect of removal of cardiac accelerator tone alone. This problem has been solved partially by studies in which segmental peganglionic denervation has been employed to block cardiac accelerator fibers without affecting the remainder of the sympathetic nervous system or altering peripheral vascular hemodynamics.

Because of the importance of defining the role of cardiac accelerator nerves in determining physiologic responses to spinal anesthesia, it is appropriate to consider briefly the effect these nerves have not only on pulse rate but also on other functions of the heart. To date, such effects have been studied only during epidural anesthesia. It should be noted, however, that while studies employing segmental epidural blockade provide invaluable information not readily obtained by other means in humans, they are nevertheless based on three uncertain assumptions: first, the technics are assumed to be so accurate that sympathetic denervation does not extend below the level of T_{1-4}. Second, these studies assume that the entire cardiovascular response to blockade of sympathetic fibers from T_1 through T_4 is solely the result of blockade of cardiac accelerator fibers, and that sympathetic fibers at this level have no other function in cardiovascular regulation, including no effects on intrathoracic, upper extremity, and intracranial veins and arteries. Finally, since segmental cardiac accelerator blockade in humans has been performed only during epidural anesthesia, and not during spinal anesthesia, these studies also assume that the local anesthetic agents used to produce epidural anesthesia have no direct effect of their own on cardiac function following their absorption into the vascular system from the epidural space.

To differentiate the effects of sympathetic denervation on cardiac accelerator fibers from the effects of denervation on major portions of the peripheral vascular bed, three studies have been performed to date: in the first, segmental epidural anesthesia only blocked cardiac accelerator fibers (T_{1-4}), leaving peripheral vascular resistance intact (Otton and Wilson, 1966). The authors studied six normal subjects with epidural catheters inserted at the $C_7 - T_1$ level. Baseline measurements were made, after which, while the subjects remained in the supine, level position, 1 mg·kg^{-1} of mepivacaine (without epinephrine) was injected through the catheter. The resulting area of sensory anesthesia extended from cervical dermatomes to T_4 and was associated with evidence of sympathetic denervation of the head and upper extremities. Their results are described in Table 2.2.

The authors concluded that cardiac accelerator denervation interfered with cardiac function by slowing HR and by decreasing myocardial response to filling pressure. This conclusion may, however, be questioned. Cardiac output decreased, possibly due to a decrease in venous return brought about by venous sympathetic denervation. If venous return did decrease, this alone could explain the decrease in mean HRs (see below). On the other hand, CVP increased. This is not characteristic of a decrease in venous return. The increase in CVP with a decrease in cardiac index does indeed suggest, as the authors hypothesize, depression of myocardial contractility. But a decrease in mean pulse rates from 81.5 to 68 beats/ min should not decrease the force of ventricular contraction in normal subjects. In fact, it would be more likely to increase contractility by increasing ventricular end-diastolic filling volumes. The apparent decrease

Table 2.2.
Hemodynamic Parameters Following Segmental Cervical Epidural Block

Parameter	Baseline Values	Values After Cervical Epidural Block
Cardiac index (L·min^{-1}·m^{-2})	3.23 ± 0.28	2.70 ± 0.21
Central venous pressure (cm H$_2$O)	4.2 ± 0.4	6.1 ± 0.6
Heart rate (beats·min^{-1})	81.5 ± 8	68 ± 4
Stroke volume index (ml·stroke^{-1}·m^{-2})	41	41
Mean arterial pressure (mmHg)	96.2 ± 2.0	88.9 ± 2.8
Left ventricular work index (kg·min^{-1}·m^{-2})	4.19 ± 0.37	3.23 ± 0.39
Total peripheral resistance (dynes·sec·cm^{-5})	1405 ± 92	1513 ± 93

Adapted from Otton, P. E., and Wilson, E. J. The cardiovascular effects of upper thoracic analgesia. Can. Anaesth. Soc. J. *13*: 541, 1966.

in contractility in the patients reported by Otton and Wilson may have been associated with interruption of the sympathetic innervation of the ventricles. It may be equally likely that the decrease in contractility reflected the presence of enough pharmacologic concentrations of local anesthetic in the blood to produce a direct negative inotropic effect.

In the second of the three studies that attempted to dissociate the cardiac effects of sympathetic denervation from effects on peripheral vascular bed, McLean, et al. (1967) measured the same indices of cardiovascular function as did Otton and Wilson, but did so in subjects who had total sympathetic denervation induced by epidural anesthesia. Their results and conclusions were the same as those of Otton and Wilson, namely, that sympathetic denervation of cardiac accelerator fibers produced bradycardia and that the decrease in HR decreased CO. The same reservations apply to these conclusions as to those of Otton and Wilson.

More recently, a third study by Baron, et al. (1987) evaluated the effects of lumbar epidural anesthesia on left ventricular function during sensory levels so low that cardiac sympathetic denervation was not produced. The patients studied had mild, stable, effort-related angina pectoris, and their myocardial function (CO, left ventricular ejection fraction, end-systolic, and end-diastolic volumes) were measured prior to, as well as during, moderate intravascular volume loading with 500 ml lactated Ringer's solution. Using radionuclide angiography, the authors were able to demonstrate the following changes associated with lumbar epidural blockade: (a) HR remained unchanged between control and epidural groups, and volume loading had no effect. (b) Arterial pressures (systolic, diastolic, and mean), cardiac index, and end-systolic ventricular volume decreased significantly during epidural block, but returned to control values following volume loading. (c) Left ventricular ejection fraction increased statistically significantly (from 54 percent to 59 percent) during epidural blockade, but returned to baseline values after volume loading.

While these investigations demonstrate that blockade of sympathetic fibers to the heart may contribute to the cardiovascular response to spinal anesthesia, they do not prove that all the effects of clinical spinal anesthesia on the vascular system, including its effect on pulse rate, are mediated solely through sympathetic denervation of cardiac accelerator fibers. A considerable body of experimental evidence indicates that while sympathetic stimulation increases pulse rate and force of myocardial contraction, in resting human beings under basal conditions, the activity of the sympathetic nervous system exerts only a modest "tonic" effect. Evidence of this lies in the fact that in resting, normal humans beta-adrenergic receptor blockade does not lower HR, nor does it decrease CO or myocardial contractility significantly (Mason, 1968). In addition, a considerable amount of evidence, some of which has been discussed above, indicates that although paralysis of cardiac sympathetic fibers undoubtedly plays a role in the production of bradycardia, it is an over-simplification to say that this is the sole factor involved in slowing of the pulse. For example, close study reveals that bradycardia during spinal anesthesia is related more to the development of arterial hypotension than to the extent of anesthesia. The degree of arterial hypotension is also generally related to the extent of sensory blockade (Brull and Greene, 1989; Bigler, et al., 1986; Taivainen, et al., 1990; Roberts, et al., 1989), but this again is not an exact relationship.

The relation between the extent of denervation and the degree of hypotension is no more precise than that between extent of spinal anesthesia and degree of bradycardia. In a large series of patients, all with total sympathetic block due to spinal anesthesia, individual changes in pulse rate and blood pressure are widely variable, even though the degree of sympathetic denervation is complete in all. The cephalad extent of spinal anesthesia does not correlate in such instances with either changes in pulse or changes in blood pressure. A direct and almost precise relation does exist, however, between the changes in arterial pressure and in pulse rate. With equal levels of anesthesia, pulse slows in proportion to the decrease in arterial pressure. As emphasized by Assali and Prystowsky (1950 a), slowing of the pulse occurs only in patients who have a vasodepressor response to spinal anesthesia. This observation was confirmed by Pugh and Wyndham (1950) who noted that bradycardia developed only when the arterial pressure decreased 25 percent or more, regardless of the sensory level. If the slowing of the pulse were due entirely to block of cardiac accelerator fibers, one would expect not only that it could be correlated exactly with the level of anesthesia but also that the pulse rate would remain fixed at its lower rate as long as the block persisted. Neither of these situations is correct. The bradycardia is not immutable but may be influenced by procedures (excluding use of vasopressors) that alter arterial pressure. Thus, in a patient who is hypotensive and bradycardic during high spinal anesthesia, raising of the legs or placing the patient in the head-down position elevates both blood pressure and pulse rate. If bradycardia were due simply to neurogenic block, such postural changes would not increase HR. The relation between pulse rate and arterial pressure is demonstrated most dramatically under clinical conditions during deliberate induction of arterial hypotension by the "hypotensive spinal" technique. Here the pulse rate invariably decreases when the blood pressure decreases. If the latter does not decrease, the pulse changes little if at all.

During spinal anesthesia there is one factor which influences pulse rate and arterial blood pressure simultaneously: venous return to the right side of the heart. A decrease in venous return results in a reduction in CO, and, as discussed below, CO is one of the main determinants of the level of arterial blood pressure during spinal anesthesia. Venous return to the heart also determines the hydrostatic pressure which exists in the right side of the heart. The volume of venous return to the right ventricle determines right ventricular end-diastolic volume (RVEDV), which in turn, influences the amount of ventricular fiber stretch. Decreased venous return to the heart may induce bradycardia by one of three mechanisms.

First, hydrostatic pressure in the right heart may affect HR through intrinsic chronotropic stretch receptors (Pathak, 1966, 1973) located within the wall of the right ventricle and particularly in the right atrium. These baroreceptors, independent of neural connections to the CNS, form an intracardiac reflex in which heart rate is proportional to pacemaker stretch. They adjust HR to meet changes in venous return and consequent changes in pressure even in a denervated heart.

Second, elevation of pressure in the great veins or in the right atrium produces tachycardia reflexly via stretch receptors (Kappagoda, et al., 1972). Lowering this pressure results in bradycardia. In other words, HR is adjusted to the quantity of blood entering its chambers.

Third, within the walls of the ventricles there are nerve endings which may be activated mechanically either by ventricular distension and stretching, or by vigorous and rapid systolic contractions. The reflex, also called the Bezold-Jarisch reflex, arises from mechanoreceptors and chemoreceptors found primarily in the inferoposterior wall of the left ventricle. Activation of this reflex results in increased parasympathetic activity and inhibition of sympathetic activity (i.e., bradycardia, hypotension, and vasodilation) (Mark, 1983).

Because both pulse rate and CO (and so systemic pressure also) vary according to the pressure existing in the great veins and the right atrium, the relationship between systemic pressure and pulse rate during spinal anesthesia becomes understandably more exact than the relationship between height of spinal anesthesia and pulse rate. The theory that blockade of preganglionic cardiac accelerator fibers alone causes bradycardia cannot explain the slow pulse rate that may accompany spinal anesthesia so low that sympathetic block does not extend above the seventh thoracic segment. Nor does it explain the variation in pulse rate effected by change of posture alone. But these phenomena can be explained on the assumption that venous return and pressure in the right side of the heart are the most important determinants of pulse rate during spinal anesthesia. Failure to appreciate this etiology of bradycardia leads to the error of attempting to estimate the level of subarachnoid sympathetic block by pulse rate alone. In turn, this leads to several erroneous hypotheses, including one stating that preganglionic cardiac accelerator fibers are more sensitive to local anesthetic agents than preganglionic vasoconstrictor fibers because, following a selective subarachnoid total sympathetic block, vasoconstrictor tone returns in the hands before the pulse rate increases (Sarnoff and Arrowood, 1946; Greene, 1955). Different types of preganglionic sympathetic fibers may differ in their sensitivities to local anesthetics, but this particular phenomenon cannot be explained on this basis alone, inasmuch as the regulation of pulse rate during spinal anesthesia depends upon both pressure in the right heart and denervation of cardiac accelerator fibers.

Theoretically, the hypotension of spinal anesthesia should cause tachycardia mediated reflexly through the baroreceptors of the carotid sinus and aortic arch. That this does not happen during high spinal anesthesia is only partly because the efferent arc of these reflexes arising from the first four thoracic segments may be blocked by the anesthesia (the afferent arc is parasympathetic in origin and so remains unaffected). The main reason is that responses activated by baroreceptors in the great veins and the right side of the heart are dominant over those from aortic and carotid baroreceptors.

Cardiac Output

Reduced CO during spinal anesthesia and sympathetic blockade has been reported by almost all investigators in this field (Burch, et al., 1930; Polano, 1933; Schuberth, 1936; Goldfarb, et al., 1939; Smith, et al., 1939; Rovenstine, et al., 1942; Eckenhoff, et al., 1948; Eather, et al., 1949; May, et al., 1949; Pugh and Wyndham, 1950; Assali and Prystowsky, 1950 a; Johnson, 1951; Lynn, et al., 1952; Sancetta, et al., 1953; Quilligan, et al., 1957; Tardieu, et al., 1957; Duner, et al., 1960; Li, et al., 1963, 1965; Bonica, et al., 1966; Ward, et al., 1965, 1966 a; Kennedy, et al., 1968; Bergenwald, et al., 1972, Nolte, 1978; Pearl, et al., 1988).

There are, however, reports of slight increases in CO during spinal anesthesia. One of these (Sobin, 1949) can perhaps be discounted since ballistocardiography, a technique with recognized limitations in measurements of cardiac function, was used to measure output. In another study, De Angelis, et al., (1982) found that the cardiac index remained relatively constant before (2.6 $\pm$ 0.6) and after (2.8 $\pm$ 0.8) induction of spinal anesthesia with tetracaine in nine patients undergoing urological procedures. The maintenance of cardiac index (as well as the increase in CVP and pulmonary artery wedge pressure) noted in this study, however, may well be attributed to the relatively large quantities of bladder irrigant solution absorbed during surgery, which may amount to a mean of 1000 ml (12–4500 ml range) (Oster and Madsen, 1969).

Other studies which have found increases in CO during spinal anesthesia, however, cannot be questioned on methodologic grounds. Kennedy, et al. (1970 b), for example, found that CO increased 14.5 percent immediately after induction of spinal anesthesia to T_5 in 20 unpremedicated, nonoperative, healthy volunteers. Fifteen minutes following induction of anesthesia CO remained only 3.7 percent above preanesthetic control levels. Thereafter cardiac output decreased below preanesthetic levels. This is one of the few reports that combines determination of CO immediately after induction of spinal anesthesia with repeated measurements at frequent intervals thereafter. Perhaps a transient increase in CO preceding subsequent reduction in output is characteristic of spinal anesthesia. If so, the increase might be due to a decrease in left ventricular afterload (brought about by peripheral arteriolar vasodilation), and an increase in CO, both of which preceded any decrease in preload due to peripheral venodilation and reduction in venous return to the heart.

The predominant response of CO to spinal anesthesia is, nonetheless, one of depression. The extent to which the output of the heart is diminished by spinal anesthesia varies considerably, however, from case to case; in some there may be no change (Runciman, et al., 1984 b, 1985, 1986); in others a decrease to 40 percent of basal levels may occur (Lynn, et al., 1952). As with pulse rate, there is a general relationship between the cephalad extent of spinal anesthesia and the percent decrease in CO; with low spinal anesthesia there is little or no change in output, while with high anesthesia, decreases in CO are frequent. The relationship between levels of sensory anesthesia and decreases in CO is, again, not an exact one. In studies in sheep (Runciman, et al., 1984 a, c) designed to identify interactions between regional blood flow and disposition of different drugs, general anesthesia (1.5% end-tidal halothane) was associated with a 30% decrease in CO. In contrast, spinal anesthesia to T_4 was not associated with a significant change in CO, because of, in all probability, the intravenous infusion of "adequate volumes of saline at the time of blockade" (Runciman, et al., 1984 b).

Changes in CO during spinal anesthesia follow changes in venous return to the heart. These in turn are determined by the extent of the sympathetic denervation and peripheral vasodilation and, equally important, by the position of the patient. During low spinal anesthesia, the sympathetic innervation of most peripheral vessels remains intact. There is little peripheral pooling of blood, and venous return to the heart is affected little, if at all. In these circumstances CO remains essentially unaltered, regardless of the position of the patient. During high spinal anesthesia most, if not all, of the preganglionic sympathetic fibers are blocked. Generalized vasodilation takes place and a large proportion of the total blood volume is pooled in the periphery. Venous return to the heart is diminished, and CO is correspondingly decreased. The extent to which this occurs varies mainly with the position of the denervated area and, particularly on whether or not it is dependent. Even under normal conditions, position plays an important role in maintenance of venous return (Brigden, et al., 1950), and in the presence of a sympathetic block, it assumes still greater significance. By placing the patient in a slight head-down position during high spinal anesthesia, the decrease in venous return to the heart and in CO can be minimized. A head-up tilt during high spinal anesthesia may, on the other hand, diminish venous return and CO to such a degree that severe bradycardia and even cardiac arrest may occur. This has been demonstrated by Pugh and Wyndham (1950) who studied CO in 13 patients undergoing spinal anesthesia with sensory levels of T_6 to T_3, both in the supine horizontal position and in the 30° to 40° head-up position. While the patients remained in the horizontal position, the average decrease in cardiac output following induction of anesthesia was 21.1 percent; in the head-up position, the average decrease was 36.2 percent. In one patient there was a 17.7 percent decrease in output in the supine position, followed by a 48.2 percent decrease in the head-up position. In another, CO decreased 5.4 percent below the preanesthetic baseline level after induction of spinal anesthesia while still in the supine horizontal position, to 30.1 percent below preanesthetic levels in the head-up position.

The primary effect of spinal anesthesia on CO is mediated by changes in venous return and thus end-diastolic ventricular filling volumes. The effects of preload changes on cardiac output are opposite to the effects on CO produced by simultaneous changes in TPR (i.e., left ventricular afterload) produced by spinal anesthesia. If all other factors affecting CO are kept constant, a decrease in afterload results in an increase in CO. The decrease in CO brought about by a decrease in preload during spinal anesthesia should, therefore, be less than the decrease in CO associated with the same decrease in venous return if afterload were also decreased simultaneously. This theoretical point may be of relatively minor significance in most clinical situations. It might however, as mentioned above, explain some of the instances in which CO has been shown to increase slightly or transiently during high spinal anesthesia (Mather, *et al.*, 1986). It might also explain instances in which CO fails to decrease even in the presence of documented slight decreases in venous return. For example, the unexpected lack of change in CO reported by Shimosato and Etsten (1969) during spinal anesthesia in patients with sensory levels of T_{4-7} despite evidence of decreased venous return, may be attributed to the occurrence of a decrease in TPR. The decrease in left ventricular afterload associated with a decrease in TPR may not be due entirely to a decrease in total peripheral *vascular* resistance brought about by arteriolar vasodilation. Simultaneous changes in shear rate and viscosity may also contribute to observed reductions in TPR. Alternatively, other factors that can modulate cardiovascular responses during spinal anesthesia also must be taken into account. One of these factors may be the autonomically mediated increase in CO, arterial pressure, and tone of capacitance vessels induced by absorption of local anesthetics into the bloodstream (Blair, 1975).

A partial explanation for the increase in systemic resistance produced by local anesthetics is shunting of blood from certain vascular areas to the central compartment by increasing the tone of the capacitance vessels. Myocardial depression produced by subconvulsive doses of local anesthetics is seen only in the presence of depressant drugs such as barbiturates, other CNS depressants, or during sympathetic blockade.

The effect of spinal anesthesia on CO is as important as its effect on the distribution of CO. If CO remained unchanged at a time when peripheral vascular changes resulted in hyperperfusion of certain organs and hypoperfusion of other organs, a potentially inimical situation would arise. This might occur if important organs, such as the brain, were affected adversely by the redistribution of peripheral blood flow. The portion of CO perfusing the lower extremities has been reported to increase by as much as 77 percent during T_{4-7} sensory levels of spinal anesthesia (Shimosato and Etsten, 1969). What organs are hypoperfused to permit such hyperperfusion of the lower limbs? This has been evaluated most extensively by Sivarajan, et al. (1975) using radioactive microsphere injection techniques in Rhesus monkeys given either low (T_{10}) or high (T_1) spinal anesthetics (Tables 2.3 and 2.4). With low levels of anesthesia, no significant changes occurred in either distribution of CO, or in absolute levels of blood flow in various tissues and organs (Table 2.3). Regional vascular resistance in the right leg (arterial cannulation of the left leg precluded its use for flow and resistance studies) decreased significantly (Table 2.5), but elsewhere, regional vascular resistance remained unaffected. Why the decrease in leg vascular resistance was not associated with a statistically significant increase in flow (Table 2.3) remains unclear. Perhaps an increase in venous pressure in the denervated extremity took place and precluded an increase in total flow despite a decrease in resistance to flow on the arterial side of the postarteriolar bed. During T_{10} levels of anesthesia, MAP decreased significantly 10 and 20 min following the onset of spinal anesthesia, while CO and TPR remained unaltered. Only with T_1 levels of anesthesia did the proportion of CO perfusing the right leg increase at 10 min (Table 2.4); even then, there was no statistically significant increase in total blood flow to the extremity. With the exception of blood flow to the lungs, to the carcass, and to miscellaneous organs, T_1 levels of anesthesia were not accompanied by significant alterations in the distribution of CO to peripheral organs. Total blood flow to the kidneys, liver, carcass, and miscellaneous organs decreased, however. The carcass included all skin, muscles, bones (except in the lower extremities), and the spinal cord. Miscellaneous organs included reproductive organs (all monkeys were male),

Table 2.3.
Regional Blood Flow during T10 Spinal Anesthesia in Five Monkeys (Mean ± SEM)[a]

	Control	10 min	20 min	40 min	80 min
Heart					
Percent CO	4.9 ± 0.4	4.9 ± 0.4	54 ± 0.5	5 ± 0.5	4 ± 0.5
Flow/100 g/min	297 ± 54.4	312 ± 77.9	309 ± 29.3	302 ± 48.2	256 ± 57.6
Brain					
Percent CO	3.6 ± 0.22	3.5 ± 0.23	3.4 ± 0.27	3.6 ± 0.23	3.3 ± 0.36
Flow/100 g/min	61 ± 9.9	64 ± 15	59 ± 11.9	65 ± 14.9	60 ± 8.9
Kidneys					
Percent CO	13.9 ± 1.23	12.4 ± 1.03[b]	12 ± 1.11	11.9 ± 1.25	11.1 ± 0.98
Flow/100 g/min	687 ± 98.2	632 ± 99.1	574 ± 46.5	596 ± 84.7	558 ± 24
Liver (hepatic artery and portal vein)					
Percent CO	22 ± 3.3	20.2 ± 3.9	20.3 ± 4	21 ± 3.8	22.4 ± 4.5
Flow/100 g/min	200 ± 34.4	203 ± 56	193 ± 49.6	212 ± 59	221 ± 61.1
Lungs					
Percent CO	0.6 ± 0.07	1.61 ± 0.27[b]	1.32 ± 0.38	1.13 ± 0.29	0.55 ± 0.15
Flow/100 g/min	24 ± 2.9	64 ± 3.9[b]	47 ± 10.6	40 ± 6.8	21 ± 3.3
Right leg					
Percent CO	4.7 ± 0.71	6.9 ± 1.9	6.9 ± 1.68	6.3 ± 1.48	5.4 ± 1.26
Flow/100 g/min	8 ± 0.7	10 ± 0.7	11 ± 1.6	10 ± 1.4	10 ± 0.6
Carcass					
Percent CO	34 ± 2.76	34.1 ± 2.88	35.1 ± 1.78	34.6 ± 2.57	37.9 ± 2.15
Flow/100 g/min	15 ± 1.9	16 ± 2.1	16 ± 2.6	16 ± 2.5	18 ± 1.8
Miscellaneous					
Percent CO	11.8 ± 0.95	11.4 ± 1.5	10.6 ± 1.2	11.8 ± 1.4	10.4 ± 1.0
Flow/100 g/min	38 ± 4.9	39 ± 8.2	34 ± 4.6	40 ± 7.2	35 ± 6.4

[a] Reproduced with permission from Sivarajan M., Amory, D. W., Lindbloom, L. E., and Schwettman, R.S.: Systemic and regional blood-flow changes during spinal anesthesia in the Rhesus monkey. Anesthesiology 43: 78, 1975.
[b] $P < 0.005$.

bladder, thyroid, salivary glands, adrenals, trachea, and esophagus. Liver blood flow included circulation to the gastrointestinal tract, mesentery, pancreas, and spleen. The authors ascribed the increased concentration of microspheres in the lungs to peripheral arteriovenous shunting of blood which resulted in less trapping of microspheres in peripheral tissues. Although this appears reasonable, if such extensive arteriovenous shunting occurred in peripheral tissues, then the adequacy of the microsphere injection to detect changes in capillary circulation of peripheral tissues becomes problematic. Nevertheless, if applicable to humans under clinical conditions, these data suggest that redistribution of CO is probably not a significant problem during clinical spinal anesthesia. This is all the more striking since arterial blood pressure and CO (at 20 min) decreased significantly during T_1 levels of anesthesia in the animals studied (Sivarajan, et al., 1975).

Although a full discussion of the etiology of arterial hypotension is not necessary at this point, the close relationship between CO and systemic arterial pressure during spinal anesthesia deserves amplification. Once

Table 2.4.
Regional Blood Flow during T1 Spinal Anesthesia in Five Monkeys (Mean ± SEM)[a]

	Control	10 min	20 min	40 min	80 min
Heart					
Percent CO	5.1 ± 0.63	4.9 ± 0.67	5.8 ± 0.65	5.2 ± 0.51	5.3 ± 0.72
Flow/100 g/min	384 ± 48.7	346 ± 49.5	348 ± 56.4	310 ± 51.2	318 ± 38.9
Brain					
Percent CO	3.7 ± 0.57	3.2 ± 0.39	4.1 ± 0.57	3.9 ± 0.65	3.8 ± 0.73
Flow/100 g/min	71 ± 11.9	58 ± 5.4	63 ± 6.1	58 ± 7.2	57 ± 8.0
Kidneys					
Percent CO	15.5 ± 1.36	16.0 ± 2.46	14.6 ± 1.12	13.0 ± 1.38	12.3 ± 1.03[b]
Flow/100 g/min	960 ± 73.3	896 ± 64.7	717 ± 53[b]	614 ± 19.9[c]	611 ± 21.2[c]
Liver (hepatic artery and portal vein)					
Percent CO	19.7 ± 1.41	18.5 ± 1.38	20 ± 1.39	19.9 ± 1.89	19.5 ± 1.94
Flow/100 g/min	207 ± 20.6	180 ± 16.9	166 ± 18.7[b]	160 ± 16.3[b]	162 ± 12.7
Lungs					
Percent CO	0.5 ± 0.15	1.7 ± 0.33[c]	2.9 ± 0.96[b]	1.9 ± 0.54[b]	2.3 ± 1.22
Flow/100 g/min	21 ± 58	64 ± 9.6[c]	89 ± 23[b]	62 ± 13.3*	78 ± 39.2
Right leg					
Percent CO	5.31 ± 0.8	8.4 ± 0.99[b]	8.8 ± 0.8[b]	8.1 ± 0.66[b]	7.43 ± 0.91
Flow/100 g/min	11 ± 1.6	18 ± 3.9	16 ± 2.6	14 ± 2.1	13 ± 1.8
Carcass					
Percent CO	37.1 ± 1.3	34.1 ± 2.8	31.7 ± 0.85[b]	36 ± 2.7	35.6 ± 3.4
Flow/100 g/min	21 ± 2.2	17 ± 2.4	14 ± 1.7[c]	16 ± 2.1[b]	16 ± 1.6
Miscellaneous					
Percent CO	10.7 ± 1.2	6.3 ± 0.6[b]	5.8 ± 0.8[b]	5.3 ± 0.6[b]	7.6 ± 0.4[b]
Flow/100 g/min	57 ± 12.1	35 ± 12.8[b]	27 ± 7.7[b]	22 ± 4.2[b]	35 ± 8.4[c]

[a] Reproduced with permission from Sivarajan, M., Amory, D. W., Lindbloom, L. E., and Schwettman, R.S.: Systemic and regional blood-flow changes during spinal anesthesia in the Rhesus monkey. Anesthesiology 43: 78, 1975.
[b] $P < 0.05$.
[c] $P < 0.01$.

the peripheral resistance has been reduced as a result of spinal anesthesia and vasodilation, it tends to remain relatively constant. In the presence of a constant peripheral resistance, any increase in CO is followed by an increase in arterial pressure; a decrease in output lowers the pressure (Eather, et al., 1949; Rashkind, et al., 1953). Any further decrease in blood pressure after the first 20 min of spinal anesthesia is usually due primarily to a change in CO. This can best be treated by specific correction of the particular factor that is causing the decrease in output rather than by increasing peripheral resistance. Such decreases in CO are usually the result of diminution of venous return secondary either to additional peripheral pooling of blood, in which case proper positioning of the patient is effective, or to operative blood loss, which must be treated by infusion of crystalloid or colloid solutions, or blood and blood products.

The negative intrathoracic pressure that normally exists during the

Table 2.5.
Regional Vascular Resistance during T10 and T1 Spinal Anesthesia[a,b]

	Control	10 min	20 min	40 min	80 min
Heart					
T10	0.4 ± 0.08	0.36 ± 0.08	0.31 ± 0.02	0.37 ± 0.04	0.47 ± 0.12
T1	0.31 ± 0.07	0.26 ± 0.03	0.24 ± 0.03	0.28 ± 0.03	0.49 ± 0.18
Brain					
T10	2.0 ± 0.46	1.88 ± 0.51	1.96 ± 0.4	1.87 ± 0.41	1.86 ± 0.31
T1	1.66 ± 0.23	1.49 ± 0.15	1.36 ± 0.21	1.48 ± 0.18	1.76 ± 0.25
Kidneys					
T10	0.16 ± 0.03	0.15 ± 0.03	0.16 ± 0.01	0.17 ± 0.02	0.18 ± 0.01
T1	0.11 ± 0.01	0.09 ± 0.01[c]	0.11 ± 0.01	0.13 ± 0.01	0.15 ± 0.01
Liver					
T10	0.59 ± 0.11	0.63 ± 0.19	0.61 ± 0.12	0.61 ± 0.14	0.56 ± 0.11
T1	0.54 ± 0.07	0.47 ± 0.05	0.5 ± 0.05	0.51 ± 0.04	0.59 ± 0.06
Right leg					
T10	13.6 ± 0.42	9.13 ± 1.15[c]	9.05 ± 0.89[c]	10.65 ± 1.72	11.07 ± 0.9
T1	10.58 ± 1.64	5.25 ± 0.56[c]	5.59 ± 0.59[c]	6.26 ± 0.52	8.16 ± 1.77

[a] Reproduced with permission from Sivarajan, M., Amory, D. W., Lindbloom, L. E., and Schwettman, R. S.: Systemic and regional blood-flow changes during spinal anesthesia in the Rhesus monkey. Anesthesiology 43: 78, 1975.
[b] Data represent means ± SEM from five monkeys for each level of anesthesia. Peripheral vascular resistance is expressed as mmHg/ml/100 g of tissue/min.
[c] $P < 0.05$.

inspiratory phase of respiration aids the flow of blood in the great veins and the filling of the right atrium. This negative pressure, normally maintained even during high spinal anesthesia, assumes special importance in the maintenance of venous return to the heart if the CO is already low. The elimination of the negative intrathoracic pressure by intermittent positive pressure applied to the airway during mechanical ventilation can further impair an already embarrassed cardiovascular system. If respiratory inadequacy develops during spinal anesthesia, pulmonary ventilation must be either assisted or controlled. If this is accomplished by intermittent positive-pressure ventilation, it must be realized that unless steps are taken to increase venous return by positioning and by the use of venoconstrictor drugs, positive-pressure ventilation may further decrease an already reduced cardiac output to a dangerous level. Guyton, *et al.* (1958) have demonstrated that increases in right atrial pressure must be pronounced before venous return to the heart is altered significantly. Sarnoff, *et al.* (1950), however, have shown, in animals in whom respiratory arrest was produced by spinal anesthesia, that intermittent positive-pressure ventilation may further reduce an already low CO. Electrophrenic artificial respiration, on the other hand, does not have this deleterious effect, because it maintains normal cycles of negative intrathoracic pressures. Under clinical conditions, the use of manual pressure on a rebreathing bag (i.e., assisted ventilation) is necessary in the majority of cases of respiratory inadequacy during spinal anesthesia. Theoretically, use of either electrophrenic or mechanical respirators capable of providing a negative as well as a positive phase during the respiratory cycle is best. Such equipment, however, may not be immediately available and in an emergency, oxygenation should be attained as rapidly as possible with the equipment on hand, bearing in mind that venous return will have to be increased artificially if positive-pressure ventilation is used.

The maintenance of adequate CO becomes the *sine qua non* of safe spinal anesthesia. Cardiac output determines not only the amount of oxygen in arterial blood, but also the rate at which the oxygenated blood is delivered to the tissues. If CO falls below the level necessary for normal tissue metabolism, the life of the patient is immediately endangered. It is imperative that the anesthesiologist performing a spinal anesthetic should devote all attention, skill, and knowledge to maintaining an adequate level of CO, peripheral blood flow, and oxygenation. This can best be accomplished by aiding the venous return to the heart through correct positioning of the patient and by providing increased inspired oxygen concentration by supplemental oxygen via nasal cannulae or face masks. Sole reliance on vasopressors for maintenance of normotension is to be condemned, as is sole reliance on the administration of large volumes of intravenous fluids in the absence of hypovolemia.

Myocardial Work

The amount of work performed by ventricular muscle per unit of time decreases during spinal anesthesia. Johnson (1951), in a report dealing with right ventricular work in humans, showed this to be true of the right side of the heart. In five patients not undergoing supplemental (barbiturate) anesthesia, the calculated mean work rate of the right ventricle was 1.28 kg·min^{-1} before high spinal anesthesia and 0.94 kg·min^{-1} during spinal anesthesia. Quantitatively, Johnson's data cannot be regarded as accurate because all patients were given ephedrine preanesthetically. Qualitatively, however, the data agree both with the results of left ventricular work studies obtained without the concurrent administration of vasopressors, as well as with studies of right ventricular work done in animals before and after sympathetic blockade (Brewster, *et al.*, 1956). Sensory levels of spinal anesthesia to T_{10} have been reported in humans as unassociated with changes in right ventricular stroke work index (Samii, *et al.*, 1979). This is not surprising in view of the absence of changes in cardiac index or venous return associated with T_{10} levels of anesthesia.

Eckenhoff and his associates (1948) were the first to study the effects of total sympathetic block on left ventricular work. They observed in six dogs that high spinal anesthesia reduced the work of the left ventricle, from an average baseline value of 4.72 kg·min^{-1} to 1.62 kg·min^{-1} during anesthesia, a statistically significant 66 percent decrease. Coincident with this reduction in work, CO decreased 42 percent, from an average of 2791 ml/min to 1618 ml/min. Oxygen consumption of the left ventricle also was reduced, although not proportionately. Similar findings have been reported in dogs by Brewster, et al. (1956) and in humans by Johnson (1951), Sancetta, et al. (1952), Lynn, et al. (1952), Li, et al. (1963), and Li, et al. (1965). Among the nonoperative cases reported by Sancetta's group (1952), those with sensory levels below T_4 showed an average decrease of 30 percent in left ventricular work; patients with higher levels had an average decrease of 62 percent. Working in the same laboratory but in a clinical study of operative patients with sensory levels of approximately the same extent as those obtained by Sancetta's group, Lynn, et al. (1952) found that left ventricular work decreased by 85 percent, a striking example of how laboratory and clinical results may differ.

Left ventricular work decreases during high spinal anesthesia for three reasons. One is the decrease in frequency of myocardial contraction, that is, slowing of the heart rate, seen in most patients with high levels of spinal anesthesia. The second reason for the decrease in left ventricular work is the reduction in peripheral resistance and the pressure against which the ventricle must force blood during systole, that is, reduction in afterload. The third reason is a decrease in SV, that is, reduction in preload, reported by most investigators (Schuberth, 1936; Johnson, 1951; Lynn, et al., 1952; Sancetta, et al., 1952, 1953; Duner, et al., 1960; Li, et al., 1963, 1965; Ward, et al., 1965; Bergenwald, et al., 1972). The diminution of SV during spinal anesthesia is a manifestation of decreased ventricular filling during diastole as a result of decreased venous return. For this reason, the extent to which ventricular SV decreases during spinal anesthesia can be correlated with the extent of sympathetic nerve block and the position of the patient. Sancetta's (1952) nonoperative cases showed little or no changes in stroke volume during low spinal blockade, but with high level of blockade, there were decreases averaging 23 percent. Before induction of anesthesia, the average left ventricular SV was 57.0 ml, while during anesthesia it was 43.5 ml. Similarly, Li, et al. (1965) found in seven unpremedicated, nonoperative subjects with sensory levels of T_{3-10} a decrease in stroke volume index from preanesthetic control levels of 36.6 to 33.0 ml/beat/m^2 during anesthesia. This decrease of approximately 10 percent was of greater magnitude than that found in the same laboratory in a separate group of patients (Li, et al., 1963).

Stroke volume is, however, determined not only by venous return, but also by pulse rate. If pulse rate decreases to the same extent as venous return, SV remains unaltered. Thus, Kennedy, et al. (1968, 1970 b) found SV to increase slightly during high spinal anesthesia. This most likely occurred because in their subjects pulse rate decreased proportionately more than venous return.

During surgery, changes in SV may be even more pronounced. In their study of operative cases undergoing spinal anesthesia, Lynn, *et al.* (1952) found the average left ventricular SV to be 57.3 ml before, and 28.3 ml during anesthesia, a decrease of 51 percent. The reduction in left ventricular SV that accompanies high spinal anesthesia and which is usually associated with low systemic arterial pressure is quantitatively less than that which occurs when an equal degree of hypotension follows blood loss and peripheral vasoconstriction. In each case the diminution of venous return to the heart is approximately the same, but in the former case this is associated with bradycardia, while in the latter it is associated with tachycardia. Since diastole is shortened during tachycardia, the volume of blood in the ventricle at the start of systole (i.e., the potential stroke volume) will therefore be less during tachycardia than during bradycardia.

All of the studies cited previously reported various degrees of left ventricular work decreases associated with the sympathectomy of spinal anesthesia. However, studies have also reported increases in myocardial work in the presence of sympathetic blockade (achieved by ganglionic blockade) (Frye and Braunwald, 1960) during spinal anesthesia in healthy parturients (Palmer, *et al.*, 1990), or during epidural anesthesia in nonpregnant (Nishimura, *et al.*, 1985) or pregnant patients (Elstein and Marx, 1990). These studies, however, found such increases in myocardial work during sympathetic blockade most likely as a result of the hypervolemia induced by infusion of 1600–2000 ml of intravenous crystalloid solutions.

Ventricular stroke work index measures the amount of work performed per ventricular contraction per square meter of body surface area. Stroke work index thus differs from the above-mentioned measurements of ventricular work expressed not per contraction, but rather per unit of time. Ventricular stroke work index is determined by the same factors that determine stroke volume (i.e., venous return and pulse rate), plus afterload. Left ventricular stroke work index thus would be expected to vary during spinal anesthesia in parallel with changes in stroke volume and peripheral resistance. The only report of left ventricular stroke work index in humans during spinal anesthesia is that by Samii, *et al.* (1979) who found no change in stroke work index during T_{10} levels of sensory anesthesia. More recently, Malmqvist, *et al.* (1987) investigated the changes in the hemodynamic parameters that occur during spinal anesthesia. They found that in 25 of their 30 patients, only minor alterations in CO, heart rate, stroke volume, MAP, and SVR were seen when the sensory level was T_{4-5}. In the patients in whom anesthesia reached T_{3-4}, MAP decreased more than 30%, although CO was well preserved. In this study, however, CO was measured by thoracic impedance cardiography, and the results obtained differed from those obtained using dye dilution technique by "roughly 24%." Nevertheless, their results indicate that hemodynamic parameters (including left ventricular SV) tend to be maintained during spinal anesthesia to sensory levels of T_4. Ventricular stroke work index is not as useful as ventricular work per unit of time when attempting to determine the ratio between myocardial oxygen demand (work) and myocardial oxygen supply (coronary blood flow). Myocardial oxygen supply is measured per unit of time (minutes), not per stroke.

In addition to the changes in cardiac physiology already mentioned, some decrease in the strength of ventricular muscle contraction during spinal anesthesia probably occurs. This could result from one or a combination of three factors. First, the decreased force of contraction could be the result of decreased ventricular filling. It has already been shown that ventricular SV is decreased during spinal anesthesia, and according to Starling's law, reduced end-diastolic ventricular volume is associated with a diminution in force of myocardial contraction. This in itself could explain much of the decreased myocardial contractility during sympathetic blockade. Second, sympathetic denervation might also result in lowered blood levels of circulating catecholamines, contributing to a decreased force of myocardial contraction (Bigler, et al., 1986; Halter and Pflug, 1980). Blood levels of both epinephrine and norepinephrine in humans are essentially unchanged, however, during low spinal anesthesia and in the resting state (Shimosato and Etsten, 1969; Roizen, et al., 1981). Third, blockade of cardiac accelerator fibers during high spinal anesthesia may reduce contractile force independently of other concurrent changes in the cardiovascular system.

The effect of spinal anesthesia on myocardial irritability is a matter that has not been completely determined. It seems unlikely that spinal anesthesia increases irritability of cardiac tissue, but whether it decreases it or not, has not been studied. Clinical impression suggests that, aside from sinus bradycardia, spinal anesthesia is not associated with a greater increase of intraoperative tachyarrhythmias than is general anesthesia and may actually be associated with a lower incidence. Isolated reports of occurrence of asystole and sick sinus syndrome following spinal anesthesia do exist, however (Underwood and Glynn, 1988). In a case report, Cohen concluded that while sinus bradycardia with normal blood pressure was generally beneficial because of its reduction in myocardial oxygen demand, progressive sinus bradycardia "in the setting of sick sinus syndrome and spinal anesthesia warrants heightened awareness and possibly, earlier intervention" (Cohen, 1988). Patients with heart blocks appear, however, to do well during and after spinal anesthesia (Berg and Kotler, 1971; Kunstadt, et al., 1973; Venkataraman, et al., 1975; Pastore, et al., 1978), despite these reports of asystole in patients with sick sinus syndrome. Clinical impression further suggests that the development of arrhythmias other than sinus bradycardia during spinal anesthesia is more often precipitated by drugs, including vasopressors, hypnotics, and analgesics, by general anesthetics, or by upper airway obstruction, rather than by spinal anesthesia itself. In addition, development of arrhythmias may be precipitated by withdrawal of chronic beta-receptor blockade prior to induction of spinal anesthesia (Ponten, et al., 1982). Safe administration of a spinal anesthetic has been reported in a patient with a prolonged QT interval syndrome (Palkar and Crawford, 1986).

The effect of spinal anesthesia on left atrial pressure as determined by pulmonary capillary wedge pressures has only been reported once as of the time of writing. Left atrial pressure was unchanged in this report (Samii, et al., 1979). This is not surprising, since the patients studied had T_{10} sensory levels of anesthesia; such levels are not expected to affect atrial or left ventricular pressures or hemodynamics. Furthermore, all patients in their study underwent intravascular volume expansion with transfusion of 650–1050 ml of blood.

The effects of spinal anesthesia on pulmonary arterial pressures are reviewed in Chapter 3.

Coronary Blood Flow

Rate and volume of coronary blood flow depend mainly on perfusion pressure and coronary vascular resistance. An increase in mean aortic pressure increases the difference between the pressures at the arterial and venous ends of the coronary arteries and so augments both volume and rate of coronary blood flow. A decrease in mean aortic pressure has the opposite effect. But while the coronary circulation is influenced passively by changes in aortic pressure, it also possesses an inherent ability to autoregulate by vasoconstriction or dilation. Vasodilation occurs when myocardial metabolic requirements increase. An increase in myocardial work and a demand for more oxygen result in greater coronary flow. Reduction in work has the opposite effect. But coronary vascular resistance also depends on factors other than the degree of vasodilation or vasoconstriction of coronary vessels. Most notable are the effects on coronary flow exerted by pressure generated by ventricular muscles during systole. An increase in either the frequency or the state of contractility of ventricular muscles will generate increased intramural pressures. These increases may be to such a degree that the only compressible part of the ventricular walls, the coronary vessels, may be constricted to the point that coronary flow decreases markedly or even ceases. An increase in myocardial work often is associated with an increase in frequency of force of ventricular contraction. Thus, the increase in coronary flow resulting from coronary vasodilation that is mediated by increased metabolic demands may be partially or even totally offset by the increased resistance offered by compressive forces generated outside the coronary vasculature.

Spinal anesthesia may affect aortic pressure and may thus influence coronary blood flow. Simultaneously, spinal anesthesia may also affect myocardial work and thereby further affect coronary blood flow. And, finally, spinal anesthesia may alter the inotropic state of the ventricles and thus influence coronary flow. The effects of spinal anesthesia on coronary blood flow are therefore complex.

In 1948, Eckenhoff, et al. first reported on the effect of spinal anesthesia on coronary blood flow. In six dogs made hypotensive by high spinal anesthesia, they found an average decrease in MAP of 47 mmHg (37 percent). At the same time there was an average decrease in coronary blood flow of 26 ml/100 g of tissue per minute (29 percent). Although the decrease in coronary blood flow was coincident with the decrease in arterial pressure, the decrease in flow was, on a percentage basis, less than the reduction in arterial pressure. Equally important was the demonstration that when arterial pressure and coronary flow were diminished, there was also a 65 percent decrease in left ventricular work. During anesthesia, ventricular work decreased to an average of 4.72 kg·min^{-1} mainly because of decreased peripheral resistance and slowing of the pulse. Although in these experiments oxygen supply to the myocardium (as measured from coronary blood flow) decreased by 29 percent during spinal anesthesia, myocardial oxygen requirements (as measured from work performed), were reduced by 65 percent. In other words, even though spinal anesthesia decreased blood supply to the myocardium, the oxygen requirement of the myocardium was decreased to an even greater extent. Similar results also were obtained in the study performed on coronary blood flow in humans during spinal anesthesia (Hackel, et al., 1956). In six patients given high spinal anesthesia, MAP decreased from average levels of 119.5 ± 9.9 mmHg to 62.0 ± 8.2 mmHg. At the same time, the coronary blood flow decreased from 153.2 ± 21.7 to 73.6 ± 12.3 ml/100 g of tissue/min. There also was a concurrent decrease in myocardial work, and oxygen utilization decreased from 16.1 ± 1.8 to 7.5 ± 0.9 ml of oxygen/100 g of tissue/min. Thus, although coronary flow decreased, so did oxygen requirements and consequently myocardial hypoxia did not ensure (coronary sinus oxygen saturation and the percentage of oxygen extracted from blood by the myocardium did not change). Similar results were also observed by Sivarajan, et al. (1975) in monkeys during T_1 sensory levels of spinal anesthesia. Coronary flow was 25, 29, 35, and 32 percent below control levels 10, 20, 40, and 80 min after induction of anesthesia, a decrease due not to changes in vascular resistance of the coronary circulation (Table 2.5), but rather to a decrease in perfusion pressure. At the time coronary flow had decreased, cardiac work decreased, however, to 29 percent, 39 percent, 43 percent, and 25 percent below control levels at the corresponding time intervals.

The above data suggest that while decreasing coronary blood flow, spinal anesthesia also produces a decrease in myocardial metabolic requirements of at least equal magnitude. The above data also illustrate the similarities between spinal anesthesia and the effects of pharmacologic agents such as organic nitrates on coronary flow and myocardial oxygen requirements (Williams, et al., 1965; Mason, et al., 1971; Majid, et al., 1980). Widely used in management of angina pectoris and other conditions associated with myocardial ischemia, nitrates are effective because, like spinal anesthesia, they increase venous capacitance, reduce diastolic filling by diminishing venous return, and, by decreasing myocardial work, have a salutary effect on the balance between myocardial oxygen supply and myocardial oxygen requirements. This may suggest that spinal anesthesia might be appropriate in the anesthetic management of patients with coronary insufficiency. Indeed, Urmey and Lambert (1986) provided a case report in which induction of spinal anesthesia with isobaric tetracaine in a patient with ongoing myocardial ischemia (3 mm ST segment depression) was associated with improvement of ischemic changes when pinprick anesthetic levels reached T_{10} dermatome, and with complete resolution of ischemia with T_7 dermatomal level of anesthesia. Similar beneficial effects of sympathetic blockade have been reported in patients with coronary artery disease following induction of thoracic epidural anesthesia (Kock, et al., 1990; Blomberg, et al., 1990; Blomberg, et al., 1989) or following lumbar epidural anesthesia (Baron, et al., 1987). The analogy between nitrates and spinal anesthesia, however, cannot always be extrapolated to patients with preexisting coronary artery disease; injudiciously high levels of spinal anesthesia may induce significant hypotension, thus decreasing myocardial oxygen supply and worsening ischemia.

The preceding data do not indicate the location of coronary blood flow distribution during spinal anesthesia. Distribution of coronary flow is as important as its volume. Coronary blood flow could be distributed during spinal anesthesia in such a manner that regional areas of ischemia might develop even if total coronary blood flow matched total myocardial oxygen demand. Although distribution of coronary flow has not been studied during spinal anesthesia, it has been studied during epidural anesthesia. Using a multiple-microsphere technique, Klassen, et al. (1980) found in normal dogs that cervicothoracic epidural anesthesia (without epinephrine) was associated with no change in the ratio of endocardial to epicardial blood flow. When coronary blood flow was artificially decreased by 50 percent prior to induction of anesthesia, subsequent epidural anesthesia resulted in an 18 percent increase in the ratio of endocardial to epicardial blood flow. When myocardial infarctions were produced prior to initiation of epidural anesthesia, the ratio of endocardial to epicardial flow increased by 43 percent during anesthesia when coronary flow was unrestricted. When myocardial infarction was combined with a 50 percent reduction in coronary flow, subsequent induction of epidural anesthesia increased the endocardial to epicardial flow ratio by 76 percent. These changes were associated both with anesthetically induced decreases in MAP, as well as with increases in coronary vascular resistance that accompanied decreases in myocardial work. The authors concluded that in the presence of decreased coronary flow, sympathetic blockade produced by epidural anesthesia affects distribution of coronary blood flow favorably by increasing endocardial flow more than epicardial flow. These important data, while encouraging, should be applied only with caution to clinical situations (Klocke, et al., 1980). Furthermore, whether or not these data apply to spinal anesthesia is uncertain in the absence of data on how blood levels of local anesthetics associated with epidural anesthesia may have affected myocardial oxygen consumption and distribution of coronary blood flow in the study by Klassen, et al.. Were their results due solely to sympathetic denervation produced by the anesthesia? Or were they related, at least in part, to high circulating concentrations of local anesthetic? If the latter be the case, the effects of spinal anesthesia may prove different than the effects of epidural anesthesia. On the other hand, the beneficial effects of thoracic epidural anesthesia are clearly not the result of high plasma concentrations of local anesthetics, as only approximately 20 mg of bupivacaine (3.8–4.3 ml of 0.5% bupivacaine) were used in the studies by Blomberg, et al. Nevertheless, results obtained during thoracic epidural anesthesia may not necessarily be used to infer similar beneficial effects of spinal anesthesia, as the total sympathetic denervation of spinal anesthesia and its concurrent vascular resistance changes are not produced by thoracic epidural anesthesia. With or without anesthesia, much still remains to be determined about local oxygen supply and demand in various areas of the heart, particularly those with ventricular hypertrophy.

Similar caveats can be applied to indices designed to evaluate the balance between myocardial oxygen delivery and myocardial oxygen consumption in humans under clinical conditions. Four such indices have been proposed (Braunwald, 1971; Bland and Lowenstein, 1976; Wilkinson, et al., 1980; Barash and Kopriva, 1980) based on the products of (a) HR and pulse pressure, (b) HR and mean aortic pressure, (c) systolic ejection period and mean systolic pressure, and (d) HR and peak systolic pressure. The last index mentioned, rate pressure product (RPP), has received particular attention. It has been suggested that RPP values in excess of 11,000 units may indicate potential for development of myocardial ischemia, that is, myocardial oxygen consumption that exceeds myocardial oxygen supply. If applied to spinal anesthesia, RPP would in most instances be below 11,000 units, since pulse rate and peak systolic pressure usually decrease in tandem. As Barash and Kopriva (1980) point out, however, RPP may be misleading, especially if increases in HR are such that the interval available for diastolic coronary flow becomes too abbreviated to allow sufficient flow, regardless of the systolic arterial pressure. At the present time, RPP cannot be recommended with confidence as a means for assuring a proper balance between myocardial oxygen consumption and myocardial oxygen supply during spinal anesthesia. Much the same caution seems appropriate, at least at the present time, with regard to the other proposed indices of myocardial oxygen consumption. While they may be used in certain situations, their applicability in all situations, including local myocardial oxygenation in patients with myocardial heart disease, remains to be proven. Thus, their value is as yet limited in estimating the adequacy of coronary blood flow during spinal anesthesia in humans.

Hypotension

Etiology

Arterial hypotension is the most common immediate complication of spinal anesthesia. Over the years many theories have been offered as to its etiology. Some older theories have been proven untenable, but they are of sufficient interest to warrant brief review, as much for their historical value, as to emphasize the factors which indeed are NOT responsible for development of arterial hypotension during spinal anesthesia. For example, Klapp (1905) and Nowak (1933) proposed the theory of "hematogenous intoxication" in which it was postulated that, following its vascular absorption from the subarachnoid space, the agent used to produce spinal anesthesia was carried by the bloodstream to the CNS where it depressed the vasomotor center directly. Bower, et al. (1932) refuted this idea by showing that intra-arterial or intravenous injection of equivalent amounts of amylocaine (Stovaine) and procaine into dogs caused only minor and transient alterations in arterial blood pressure. Moreover, the inadequacy of this theory has been made obvious by the practice of intravenous local anesthesia (i.e., Bier block). This technique employs dosages of local anesthetics considerably in excess of those used for spinal anesthesia without the occurrence of severe cardiovascular depression after deflation of the arterial tourniquet.

Another theory (Perl, 1932; Hadenfeldt, 1932; Schotte, 1933; Philipowicz, 1933), which proposed that spinal anesthesia functionally denervates the adrenal glands and that the resulting "oligoadrenalemia" causes hypotension, has also been proven inaccurate. Arterial hypotension following total spinal anesthesia in normal dogs is essentially the same as that following total spinal anesthesia in bilaterally adrenalecto-mized dogs (Hilton, 1957); this indicates that denervation of the adrenals by anesthesia plays no significant role in the development of hypoten-sion. In addition, of course, hypotension of spinal anesthesia is profound and immediate. Hypotension following surgical adrenalectomy is usu-ally delayed for several hours and is usually less pronounced than that which follows spinal anesthesia. Similarly, decreases in circulating levels of renin (or angiotensin) during spinal anesthesia do not contribute to the development of hypotension. Plasma renin activity is unaffected by either spinal anesthesia itself or by surgery performed during spinal anesthesia (Oyama, et al., 1979; Robertson and Michelakis, 1972). How-ever, although plasma renin activity may not be lowered, regional anes-thesia attenuates or even inhibits the increase of the endocrine-metabolic (stress) response to surgery (Chapter 6).

In an attempt to explain hypotension associated with spinal anes-thesia, it also has been suggested that the nerve block reduces the tone of skeletal muscles to such a degree that the veins, deprived of their normal surrounding support, dilate, and thus allow peripheral pooling of blood (Smith, et al., 1939). Although dilation of the venous portion of the cardiovascular system does occur with spinal anesthesia and is of considerable importance in the etiology of systemic hypotension, there is no evidence that venodilation is caused by skeletal muscle paralysis. Actual measurements have shown that skeletal muscle tone is the same during rest as it is during the paralysis of spinal anesthesia (Milwidsky and De Vries, 1948). Furthermore, the vascular changes which accom-pany spinal anesthesia can be produced without any skeletal muscular paralysis by means of a differential sympathetic spinal block which leaves somatic motor nerves unimpaired (Sarnoff and Arrowood, 1946). Conversely, paralysis of skeletal muscles in the absence of sympathetic denervation produces no change in blood pressure: hypotension or other evidence of venous pooling of blood does not occur during the clinical use of muscle relaxants such as succinylcholine. If further proof be needed, it can be obtained from the demonstration that block of motor nerves in previously sympathectomized limbs does not produce venous pooling or changes in blood flow (Barcroft, et al., 1943; Barcroft and Edholm, 1946).

A popular early theory, still responsible for some anachronistic clinical practices today, claimed that local anesthetics injected into the lumbar subarachnoid space could ascend in the cerebrospinal fluid to the ventri-cles in concentrations sufficient to paralyze the vasomotor and respira-tory centers directly (Heineke and Laewen, 1906; Co Tui and Standard, 1932; Co Tui, 1934, 1936). Although the theory has been discussed in Chapter 1, it also deserves brief review here. It was based primarily on laboratory demonstration by Co Tui that 75 mg of procaine (2.5 ml of a 3 percent solution) injected intracisternally in dogs produced respiratory arrest and cardiovascular collapse. In this work, no provision was made to prevent downward diffusion of the procaine into the spinal subarachnoid space, where such a concentration could indeed produce preganglionic denervation. Instead, it was assumed that all the effects of the intracisternal injection were due to the direct action of the procaine on the brainstem. Local anesthetics can undoubtedly produce direct medullary depression if present in unusually high concentrations in the ventricular fluid. Such concentrations, however, are rarely if ever attained in clinical practice. The concentrations necessary to depress the brainstem are indicated in Co Tui's original work, in which he showed that the intracisternal injection of 40 mg of procaine did not produce the same effect as 75 mg. Johnston and Henderson (1932) injected 50 mg of procaine (1 ml of a 5 percent solution or 0.5 ml of a 10 percent solution) directly into the fourth ventricle (not into the cisternal magna) without any effect on the systemic blood pressure. Additionally, the direct application of pledgets (soaked in 2.5 percent Neocaine) to the medullae of dogs did not cause significant vascular changes, even though it produced general anesthesia (Koster and Kasman, 1929). These observations are supported by Haranath and Venkatakrishna-Bhatt (1968) and by Loeschke and Koepchen (1958). On the basis of similar studies, these investigators concluded that local anesthetics introduced into cerebrospinal fluid reach neither the respiratory nor the vasomotor center in pharmacologically active concentrations. Finally, during a clinical trial of intracisternal anesthesia, Vehrs (1931, 1934) found that 240 mg of procaine injected into the cisterna magna of humans did not result in vasomotor paralysis. In a series of cases reported by Koster, et al. (1938) the concentration of procaine in cisternal fluid during high spinal anesthesia was less than 0.002 percent in two thirds of their patients, and between 0.006 and 0.02 percent in one third. In view of the concentrations quoted as necessary to produce direct medullary paralysis, it is unlikely that the dilute solutions of local anesthetic actually found in cisternal fluid during high spinal anesthesia could produce paralysis of the medullary centers. If further proof is needed that the hypotension of spinal anesthesia is not due to direct paralysis of the vasomotor centers, it can be shown that all the cardiovascular effects of spinal blockade are produced if the local anesthetic agent is injected into the thoracic subarachnoid space after isolation of the latter by ligatures placed so that none of the anesthetic agent can ascend to the brainstem (Ferguson and North, 1932).

In 1912, Gray and Parsons put forward the theory that hypotension accompanying spinal anesthesia was secondary to concurrent respiratory insufficiency. Noting that the higher levels of anesthesia were associated both with intercostal muscular paralysis and more frequent and severe episodes of hypotension, they concluded that the latter were due to the intercostal paralysis. On the basis of carefully constructed but purely theoretical diagrams showing the mechanical factors involved in respiration, they stated, without actual measurements, that the diaphragm could not compensate for intercostal paralysis, and that with high spinal anesthesia, therefore, there was a decrease in intrathoracic negative pressure during inspiration. With loss of this "sucking action" of respiration, venous return to the heart was diminished and the consequent decrease in CO resulted in arterial hypotension. This theory attracted attention for a time (Bower, et al., 1926, 1932; Seevers and Waters, 1932 a, b), but it has since been discredited (Lewis and Palser, 1938). Intrathoracic negative pressure during inspiration does assist venous return and maintenance of CO. However, even with the assumption that this factor is modified by spinal anesthesia, the decrease in systemic pressure associated with high spinal anesthesia is greater than can be explained on this basis alone. Increasing the negative pressure in the great veins to the point beyond which any further increase collapses them, increases the systemic arterial pressure by 20 percent at most (Guyton and Harris, 1951). Since the decrease in blood pressure with high spinal anesthesia may exceed 20 percent of resting levels, loss of intrathoracic negative pressure cannot be the sole cause of hypotension. Actually, the diaphragm can and does compensate for intercostal muscle paralysis to the extent that tidal volume and effective alveolar ventilation are unaltered (Chapter 3). Neither tidal volume nor effective alveolar ventilation can be maintained at normal levels spontaneously without the continuance of normal inspiratory negative pressures. Further, increasing the negative pressure of inspiration by producing hyperpnea with carbon dioxide inhalation during spinal anesthesia not only fails to increase the blood pressure (Smith, et al., 1939) but also usually has the opposite effect (Seevers and Waters, 1932 a; Co Tui, 1936; Burstein, 1939) for reasons already mentioned (pp. 139–140). In addition, hypotension develops during differential spinal block even though the intercostal muscles are not paralyzed (Sarnoff and Arrowood, 1946).

As a corollary to the theory of Gray and Parsons, it was suggested that respiration is so impaired by spinal anesthesia, that the hypoxia that was said to develop is the cause of the arterial hypotension (Seevers and Waters, 1932 a, b). This explanation is invalidated by the fact that arterial oxygen saturation remains normal during spinal anesthesia even though the blood pressure may decrease (Chapter 3).

Hypotension following spinal anesthesia is primarily the result of paralysis of preganglionic sympathetic fibers that transmit motor impulses to the smooth muscle of the peripheral vasculature. The importance of sympathetic denervation in such circumstances was first demonstrated by Tuffier and Hallion in 1900, only 1 year after the introduction of spinal anesthesia by Bier (1899), and was later confirmed by the classic experiments of Smith and Porter in 1915. Using cats, Smith and Porter showed that both the incidence and severity of hypotension were related to the area of the subarachnoid space in which the anesthetic agent was deposited. Following injection of the anesthetic into the lumbar subarachnoid space, only 5 percent of the animals became hypotensive, the average decrease in blood pressure being 19 percent. The same amount of anesthetic injected into the thoracic subarachnoid space caused hypotension in 47 percent of the animals, with an average decrease in blood pressure of 43 percent. After cervical subarachnoid space injection, 38 percent of the animals became hypotensive, with an average decrease in blood pressure of 27 percent. These experiments did not exclude spread of the anesthetic agent from one part of the subarachnoid space to another, a factor that was controlled in later work by Schilf and Ziegner (1924) and Ferguson and North (1932). Isolating the injected section of the subarachnoid space by ligatures, Ferguson and North repeated and confirmed Smith and Porter's results. With additional information derived from serial sectioning of nerves, they concluded that the degree of blood pressure decrease during spinal anesthesia was proportional to the number of sympathetic fibers blocked. This observation was further substantiated by the fact that spinal anesthesia given to a totally sympathectomized animal produced no change in blood pressure (Wilson, et al., 1936; Bradshaw, 1936).

Clinically, arterial hypotension is related to the height of sensory anesthesia (Halter and Pflug, 1980; Roberts, et al., 1989; Taivainen, et al., 1990; Callesen, et al., 1991). For example, in one study involving normal subjects, the average decrease in systolic blood pressure ($\pm$SD) was 5.6 $\pm$ 1.2 percent when sensory levels were at the T_{10} level, 11.8 $\pm$ 2.4 percent when they were at T_8, 15.8 $\pm$ 3.0 percent at T_6, 20.9 $\pm$ 1.5 percent at T_4, and 23.1 $\pm$ 0.6 percent at T_3 (Defalque, 1962). As hypotension becomes especially marked with sensory levels above the mid-thoracic region, it was originally believed that sympathetic denervation of the area supplied by fibers from the lower and mid-thoracic segments was mainly, if not entirely, responsible for the hypotension, and that the most important single factor was blockade of the splanchnic nerves with consequent pooling of blood in the abdominal viscera (Smith and Porter, 1915; Schilf and Ziegner, 1924; Demel and Burke, 1930; Saklad, 1931; Roeder, 1931). Clinically, however, there is no visceral engorgement during spinal anesthesia to support this theory. It has been shown experimentally that the splanchnic vessels contribute to the circulatory changes of spinal anesthesia only in proportion to the percentage of the volume of blood which passes through the vasculature. Spinal anesthesia can still produce arterial hypotension, but proportionately less, after either ligation of the splanchnic arteries to prevent any excessive pooling of

blood in this area (Nowak, 1933) or after surgical division of the splanchnic nerves (Domenech-Alsina, 1932; Pannett, 1933). There is nothing
inherent in the splanchnic circulation that causes it to play a special
or specific role in the production of hypotension. Denervation of the
splanchnic vessels affects the arterial pressure no more than sympathetic
denervation of an equally large portion of the somatic circulation. There
is even some evidence to suggest that the splanchnic vessels in this
respect may actually be less important than the peripheral vessels. Mueller, *et al.* (1952) found no significant change in splanchnic vascular resistance during high spinal anesthesia at a time when total peripheral vascular resistance was decreased. Although measurement of vascular
resistance cannot indicate the amount of postarteriolar and venular pooling of blood that accompanies sympathetic denervation, the findings of
Mueller do suggest that the splanchnic arteries and arterioles are inher-
ently no more likely to dilate than are other peripheral vessels.

After it was generally agreed that the sympathectomy of spinal anesthesia was the primary cause of arterial hypotension, debate continued
for some time as to the exact mechanism whereby sympathetic blockade
lowered blood pressure. There were two schools of thought. One postulated that generalized arterial and arteriolar dilation caused a decrease
in peripheral vascular resistance great enough to account for the major
portion of the decrease in arterial pressure (Babcock, 1928; Burch and
Harrison, 1930; Ferguson and North, 1932; Neuman, *et al.*, 1945; Gregory
and Levin, 1948). The other postulated that the hypotension was secondary to a decrease in CO as a result of peripheral pooling and a diminution
in venous return to the heart (Smith, *et al.*, 1939; Rovenstine, *et al.*, 1942;
Pugh and Wyndham, 1950; Assali, *et al.*, 1951). While both theories are
correct, neither is by itself adequate to explain all the alterations in circulatory physiology caused by spinal anesthesia. In some circumstances
hypotension may be due predominantly to a decrease in CO; in others
it is primarily the result of decreased peripheral resistance; or it may
result from a combination of both factors. When CO and peripheral
resistance decrease during spinal anesthesia, the latter precedes the former (Eather, *et al.*, 1949), thus eliminating any theoretical possibility that
changes in peripheral resistance are secondary to changes in CO.

The relative importance of these two factors in the causation of hypotension varies from case to case. It has been estimated that in 80 percent
of operative patients, the decrease in arterial blood pressure is primarily
the result of decreased peripheral resistance. In the remaining 20 percent
it is due mainly to decreased CO (King and Dripps, 1950). The opposite
is true in most nonoperative cases studied under laboratory conditions,
and many errors have been made in the study of physiology of spinal
anesthesia when laboratory results were assumed to apply to clinical
conditions. If the position of the patient is such that venous return to

the heart is adequate to maintain CO, changes in arterial pressure are chiefly the result of alterations in peripheral resistance. If, when vasoconstrictors are administered to maintain the peripheral resistance, the blood pressure still decreases, then such changes must result from decreases in CO.

The extent to which blood pressure decreases is indicative of the relative role played by changes in peripheral resistance and by changes in CO. Analysis of published investigations shows that relatively minor degrees of arterial hypotension stem mainly from changes in peripheral vascular resistance, but if the pressure continues to decrease below a certain critical level, then such further degrees of hypotension are most frequently due to changes in cardiac output. The critical level below which changes in pressure are the result of changes in CO during spinal anesthesia is about 90 mmHg systolic in a normal patient. While the systemic arterial pressure may decrease to this level without any significant change in CO, any further decrease is frequently due to decreases in CO (May, et al., 1949). This can be demonstrated when spinal anesthesia high enough to produce a total subarachnoid sympathetic block is administered to a patient who has, for example, a normal preanesthetic systolic blood pressure of 120 mmHg. If such a patient is kept in the Trendelenburg position so that venous return to the heart, and therefore CO, are maintained at near-normal values, systolic pressure decreases to 90–100 mmHg and remains at this level. This is the result of decreased peripheral vascular resistance. If the position of the patient is then changed to head-up or even to horizontal, further decreases in arterial pressure occur secondary to gravitational pooling of blood. Cardiac output decreases abruptly and severe hypotension develops.

Although arterial pressure during spinal anesthesia is affected primarily by alterations in CO and by the extent of the sympathetic block, other factors also are involved. One of these is the amount of trauma and organ manipulation (i.e., surgery) to which the patient is subjected following induction of spinal anesthesia. This becomes apparent when a comparison is made between the blood pressure changes in response to equal levels of spinal anesthesia induced under clinical and laboratory conditions.

Only 25 percent of patients given spinal anesthesia for simple investigative procedures develop "moderately severe" hypotension. In contrast, approximately 40 percent of operative patients develop equal degrees of hypotension (Smith, et al., 1939; Papper, et al., 1943; Assali and Prystowsky, 1950 b; Lynn, et al., 1952). Frequently in investigative cases the anesthetic agent is either injected into the subarachnoid space through a spinal catheter while the patient remains in the supine position, or the patient is merely turned from the lateral to the supine position after induction of anesthesia, without further positional changes or surgery. Laboratory investigators studying the circulatory effects of high thoracic or even cervical sensory blocks often find that the degree of hypotension is small, while clinical anesthesiologists recognize that decreases in blood pressure are frequent and severe with equally high levels of spinal anesthesia.

In addition to external trauma, postural changes and organ manipulation, certain constitutional factors of the patient may affect the cardiovascular response to a given level of spinal anesthesia. If blood pressures are studied in a large series of patients undergoing spinal anesthesia to the same level and all are kept in the same position, a number will show relatively little decrease in pressure, while others will exhibit more pronounced hypotension. There are many reasons for this variability, the most frequent being conditions such as pregnancy (Chapter 8), preexisting hypertension, old age, coexisting cardiovascular disease, and abnormalities of blood volume. One of the most important factors in determining the degree of blood pressure change following the sympathectomy of spinal anesthesia is preoperative high blood pressure. In hypertensive patients, the decrease in blood pressure following induction of spinal anesthesia is proportionately greater than in normotensive patients. Frequently blood pressure may be reduced to a normal or subnormal level by a relatively low spinal block (Allen, et al., 1936; Taylor, et al., 1948 a; Pugh and Wyndham, 1950; Kety, et al., 1950). The magnitude of the difference in response between normotensive and hypertensive patients is illustrated by the studies of Kleinerman, et al. (1958). Two groups of patients, one hypertensive and the other normotensive, were studied under similar conditions of experimentally induced spinal anesthesia with levels of blockade which were high enough to produce sympathetic denervation of the upper extremities. In the hypertensive group (four subjects), MAP decreased from hypertensive control levels of 158 mmHg, to 79 mmHg during anesthesia, a decrease of 50 percent. In the normotensive patients (nine subjects), mean arterial pressure decreased from control levels of 92.5 mmHg, to 63.4 mmHg during anesthesia, a decrease of 31 percent. In other words, the percent decrease in mean blood pressure was greater in hypertensive patients than in normal subjects. However, arterial pressure remained at significantly higher levels in the hypertensive patients during spinal anesthesia than in the normotensive patients. The greater decrease in blood pressure in hypertensive patients was associated with greater decreases in peripheral vascular resistance. In the normotensive subjects, peripheral vascular resistance decreased an average of 28 percent, while in hypertensive patients the decrease in vascular resistance averaged 40 percent. The greater response of arterial pressure to spinal anesthesia in hypertensive patients is related more to the greater degree of arterial and arteriolar vasodilation such patients experience than to greater decreases in CO (or venous return).

Whether hypertension is "essential" or of renal origin does not influence the degree of hypotension, and although the use of spinal anesthesia has been advocated in the past to differentiate between the several types of hypertension, it has been found to be unsatisfactory for this purpose (Page, et al., 1944; Gregory and Levin, 1945; Taylor, et al., 1948 b; Soloff, et al., 1948). There also is no reliable correlation between the degree of hypotension produced by pharmacologic sympathetic block of spinal anesthesia and that produced surgically by equally extensive sympathectomy.

Along with postural changes, degree of external trauma and organ manipulation, and preoperative existence of hypertension, age also has been shown to influence the degree of cardiovascular changes induced by spinal anesthesia (see also pp. 176–177). Younger patients usually show less severe decreases in blood pressure than older ones under equal levels of spinal anesthesia. The data of Dohi, et al. (1979) provide a particularly striking (and unique) demonstration of this. They studied 65 children (aged 8 months to 15 years) and 17 adults. All patients had spinal anesthetics with sensory levels of T_{3-5}. There was no significant change in systolic blood pressure in patients 5 years of age and younger. Patients aged 6–10 years experienced highly variable changes in blood pressure. In some patients, blood pressure decreased to such an extent (30 to 50 percent) that vasopressors had to be administered; in others blood pressure remained unchanged. In patients above the age of 10 years, blood pressure changes paralleled those of the adults. Patients aged 15 and over were indistinguishable from adults in terms of their blood pressure responses to spinal anesthesia. Even among adults, age appears to be an important factor which influences the degree of hemodynamic response to spinal anesthesia. Economacos and Skountzos (1980) studied the hemodynamics and incidence of complications in 3012 patients undergoing spinal anesthesia with lidocaine or prilocaine to a level of T_{5-6}. They found that in patients 20–32 years old there were no significant changes in blood pressure following spinal anesthesia. In patients from 32 to 58 years old, blood pressure decreased by 10–20 mmHg, while older patients (58–82 years old) showed the highest reduction in blood pressure (30–40 mmHg). These authors' findings are similar to those of Graves and Klein (1968), who investigated CVP during routine spinal anesthesia, and found that the incidence of hypotension was higher in older patients. In patients over 50 years of age, 75% developed hypotension, compared to a 36% incidence in patients under 50 years of age. These age-dependent changes in blood pressure are probably related to the higher residual autonomous vascular tone that persists in the younger patients following sympathetic denervation, as well as to more active compensatory reflexes. Older patients not only show less active reflex vasoconstriction in unanesthetized areas of the body, but also they appear to have less residual vascular tone following sympathetic denervation. The fact that CO normally decreases with advancing years may also explain why there is a proportionately greater decrease in CO in elderly patients following a given degree of peripheral vasodilation.

The severity of concurrent medical disease as reflected by the American Society of Anesthesiologists (ASA) physical status classification also may determine the relative hemodynamic changes associated with spinal anesthesia. Thus, Hemmingsen, et al. (1989) found that in 48 patients distributed evenly to ASA groups I, II, and III, all patients in ASA class III who did not receive hydration (7 ml/kg) or ephedrine prophylaxis developed decreases in MAP exceeding 20 percent. In this group, MAP decreased from a baseline level of approximately 106 mmHg to 75 mmHg 40 min following induction of spinal anesthesia. In contrast, the mean blood pressure decreases from baseline in ASA I group (95 to 85 mmHg) and in ASA II group (103 to 90 mmHg) were less pronounced. Perhaps these differences among ASA groups reflect the higher incidence of hypertension in the ASA III group, which would therefore be expected to exhibit a greater blood pressure decrease following sympathectomy of spinal anesthesia.

Other less frequent factors influencing the hemodynamic responses to spinal anesthesia are the use of methylmethacrylate (MMA) for cementation in orthopedic surgery (Svartling, et al., 1986), and the preoperative existence of idiopathic hypertrophic subaortic stenosis (IHSS) (Loubser, et al., 1984). Both Svartling, et al. and Loubser, et al. reported the development of exaggerated hypotension in response to induction of spinal anesthesia in their patients.

Patients with low blood volumes also show disproportionately severe decreases in arterial pressure after induction of spinal anesthesia. In such patients, a given degree of peripheral vasodilation results in pooling in the periphery of a greater proportion of the circulating blood volume than in a normal individual. As a result, there is a disproportionately large reduction in venous return to the heart and in cardiac output. For example, in a patient with a normal total blood volume of 5 L, the volume of blood in one lower extremity during spinal blockade is approximately 800 ml, or 16 percent of the total blood volume. In a hypovolemic patient with an equal body weight but with a blood volume of only 3.5 L, the same area of vasodilation (i.e., a lower extremity) contains 23 percent of the circulating blood volume.

In addition to hemorrhage, one of the clinical conditions frequently associated with low blood volume is carcinomatosis (Berlin, et al., 1952).

Patients with abnormally low blood volumes may have normal or near-normal preanesthetic blood pressures, but although the blood pressure may be normal, even low levels of spinal anesthesia should be avoided.

Because of the dangers of decreased blood volume in the presence of sympathetic block, patients under high spinal anesthesia do not tolerate major blood loss during surgery (Burch, et al., 1930; Roome, et al., 1933; Schlossberg and Sawyer, 1933; Freeman, et al., 1938). The normal reflexive vasoconstrictor response to hemorrhage is absent, and a loss of 500 ml of blood (which might otherwise have little effect on the blood pressure of a patient undergoing general anesthesia) may cause severe hypotension in a patient whose peripheral vasculature is dilated by a high spinal anesthetic. In addition, in certain instances where low blood volume is due to active bleeding (e.g., bleeding from premature partial separation of the placenta), the induction of spinal anesthesia may accelerate the loss of blood by producing vasodilation in the bleeding area.

The dangers of spinal anesthesia in the presence of blood loss have been demonstrated graphically and quantitatively by Kennedy, et al. (1968). These investigators studied 15 unpremedicated, nonoperative normal subjects during spinal anesthesia before and after phlebotomy of 10 ml of blood/kg body weight over 11–35 min. Thirty minutes after induction of spinal anesthesia to T_5 in the absence of blood loss, MAP was 8.4 percent below baseline levels, cardiac output decreased 3.7 percent, SV increased 3.3 percent, and CVP decreased 8.3 percent. Thirty minutes after 10 ml/kg phlebotomy in the presence of spinal anesthesia, the same measurements revealed that MAP was 18.7 percent below baseline levels, CO decreased 14.1 percent, SV diminished by 12.6 percent, and CVP was 57.5 percent below baseline levels.

It has been suggested that vasodilation, including that associated with spinal anesthesia, may help to prevent hemorrhagic shock from becoming irreversible. It has been shown experimentally that animals obtain some degree of protection against otherwise lethal hemorrhage when given drugs which depress sympathetic activity, especially if the drugs are administered prior to onset of shock (Nickerson and Carter, 1959; Overton and DeBakey, 1956). This protection may be due to prevention of normal reflexive vasoconstriction following blood loss, since such vasoconstriction, occurring in the presence of a lowered arterial pressure, may lead to cellular hypoxia with consequent production of toxic metabolites (Nuwayhid, et al., 1978). In turn, the metabolites may accentuate the shock and contribute to making it irreversible. The pharmacologic agents employed to produce vasodilation in the shock state have included ganglionic as well as adrenolytic agents. The latter have included the administration of alpha-adrenergic blocking compounds (to inhibit arterial and arteriolar vasoconstriction) together with beta-adrenergic stimulating agents (to produce maximal peripheral vasodilation and to increase CO). It also has been suggested that because it produces vasodilation, spinal anesthesia is a desirable and effective means of protecting against shock, as well as a means of treating it. Whether or not the production of peripheral vasodilation is a safe and appropriate method of treating shock under clinical circumstances is doubtful, regardless of its demonstrated efficacy in experimental animals under controlled laboratory conditions. Certainly the production of vasodilation without the simultaneous administration of blood or plasma volume expanders during oligemic shock accentuates the metabolic evidence of cellular anoxia and leads to increased mortality (Danoff and Greene, 1964). But there are also significant physiologic differences between the response to spinal anesthesia and the response to many of the pharmacologic agents recommended. The former produces denervation of both alpha- and beta-adrenergic receptors and does not impair the ability of these receptors to respond to normal humoral or pharmacologic stimuli. The majority of adrenolytic compounds employed either block both alpha- and beta-adrenergic receptors simultaneously, in which case the result is the same as with spinal anesthesia except that the receptors no longer respond to normal stimuli, or they selectively block alpha-receptors alone, in which case inotropic and vasodilator beta-receptors remain unaffected. The differences in response can be critical in a condition as complex and potentially lethal as clinical shock. It is unlikely that spinal anesthesia represents a safe clinical method of treating established shock. There may be theoretical advantages in using spinal anesthesia in shock because of the vasodilation it produces, but these remain highly theoretical and include the assumption that while the blood vessels are dilating, the blood volume of the patient in shock can be increased simultaneously by transfusion of blood in amounts adequate to fill the enlarged capacity of the vascular bed. Unless this can be accomplished, peripheral vascular collapse will ensue and the patient will be in worse condition than before the vasodilation of spinal anesthesia.

Afferent stimuli have been proposed as etiologic factors in the pathogenesis of shock. Crile's theory of anoci-association, for example, suggested that noxious afferent stimuli arising from traumatized areas constitute a major factor in the development of shock (Crile and Lower, 1915; Phemister, et al., 1944). On the other hand, another popular school of thought holds that afferent stimuli are of no importance whatsoever. This theory is exemplified by the use of the lightest possible levels of general anesthesia during surgery, levels amounting to little more than analgesia (and, it is hoped, sufficient for amnesia), but which are combined with muscle relaxants in doses large enough to prevent somatic motor responses to painful stimuli. Probably neither concept is entirely correct. Afferent stimuli can affect the cardiovascular system. The response is usually characterized by vasopressor responses, but vasodepressor reactions are also possible in response to painful stimuli. It is unlikely, however, that shock, as currently defined, is due principally to noxious afferent stimuli. Certainly spinal anesthesia completely blocks all afferent stimuli from operative areas. However, aside from blocking certain specific reflexes such as those that arise during rectal or upper abdominal surgery, its role remains uncertain in the prevention of the so-called traumatic shock. Often it is not possible in certain clinical situations to determine whether the beneficial effects of spinal anesthesia are due to afferent blockade of the operative area or to avoidance of deep general anesthesia. For example, during and after rectal operations under spinal anesthesia, there is generally less physiologic derangement, especially of the cardiovascular system, than in cases performed under general anesthesia deep enough to provide similar operating conditions. But this result is probably attributable more to the adverse cardiovascular effects of deep general anesthesia than to blocking of painful surgical stimuli. On the other hand, during upper abdominal surgery, any theoretical benefits obtained from blocking of painful stimuli by spinal anesthesia are considerably offset by the cardiovascular effects of a high block. A well-administered general anesthetic, especially in conjunction with muscle relaxants, can provide the same desirable operating conditions in the upper abdomen as can spinal anesthesia, but without producing the profound physiologic alterations associated with the latter. Aside from the possible cardiovascular benefits of spinal anesthesia, however, there have been several reports of other types of long-term benefits. These include the decreased incidence of postoperative residual pain (Tverskoy, *et al.*, 1990; Brull, *et al.*, 1992) and the lower requirements for postoperative narcotics (Thomas, *et al.*, 1983; Owen, *et al.*, 1985; Patel, *et al.*, 1983; Lewis and Thompson, 1953; Levack, *et al.*, 1986; Sinclair, *et al.*, 1988).

It is apparent that the hypotension of spinal anesthesia is completely different from hypotension due to blood loss. The only feature common to both is low blood pressure. The two types of hypotension are quite distinct from each other etiologically, physiologically, and biochemically, making the clinical significance and management of each entirely different. The hypovolemic, hypotensive patient is cold, sweating, apprehensive, restless, and thirsty. His primary deficit is reduced blood volume. The homeostatic mechanism attempts to compensate for this by vasoconstriction, which may be so intense that blood flow is impaired and tissues become hypoxic. The biochemical changes in patients in hemorrhagic shock reflect these abnormalities of peripheral blood flow. Elevations of serum lactate and pyruvate levels take place as a result of anaerobic carbohydrate metabolism. Serum potassium levels increase following an increase in cell membrane permeability due to lack of oxygen. A patient equally hypotensive but with a normal blood volume during spinal anesthesia is warm and dry because of vasodilation. Despite lowered arterial pressure, such patients do not show evidence of cellular hypoxia or metabolic disturbances (Greene, et al., 1954). The treatment of hypotension caused by blood loss consists of restoration of normal blood volume by replacement of intravascular fluid. The treatment of hypotension of spinal anesthesia consists of maintenance of adequate CO by appropriate positioning of the patient and, if necessary, administration of a vasopressor.

When hypotension occurs during spinal anesthesia, it usually develops during the first 15–20 min; left untreated, the blood pressure reaches its lowest level 20 to 25 minutes following the subarachnoid injection. For this reason, the first half-hour of a spinal anesthetic is considered to be its most dangerous period, although the initial decrease in blood pressure may develop with alarming rapidity in certain individuals. This immediate hypotension develops particularly frequently in patients with low blood volume and in those who have been ineptly positioned on the operating table (pp. 163, 165–166). After the blood pressure has reached its lowest point, the systolic pressure often increases spontaneously 5–10 mmHg over the next 10–15 min, after which it levels off and remains relatively fixed until the effect of the anesthetic on the nerve roots has worn off. This small increase is a manifestation of compensatory circulatory activity mediated reflexly by those portions of the sympathetic outflow that have not been blocked and perhaps by a slight return of smooth muscle tone in the denervated portions of the peripheral vasculature. It is not due to increases in CO. This was well demonstrated by Kennedy, et al. (1968) in their study of 15 subjects who had serial determinations of cardiovascular function until spinal anesthesia had worn off. These investigators found, for example, that while MAP was 10.2 percent below baseline levels 15 min following administration of spinal anesthesia, it was 8.4 percent of baseline values 30 min after induction of anesthesia (and before the anesthetic had started to wear off). This modest return of arterial pressure toward preanesthetic levels was associated with a CO that was higher at 15 min than at 30 min, and with an increase in total peripheral vascular resistance from 13.2 percent below baseline levels at 15 min, to 3.2 percent below baseline at 30 min.

As already discussed, the initial lowering of arterial pressure during spinal anesthesia is usually mainly the result of reduced peripheral vascular resistance. A decrease in CO may accentuate the hypotension during this initial period, but any further decrease in pressure after 20 or 30 min is almost invariably the result of a further decrease in CO. At this stage the CO may decrease as a result of operative blood loss, but is most frequently affected by an alteration of the patient's position whereby an additional gravitational or obstructive factor is imposed on the venous return to the heart. Elevation of the trunk and head as in the reverse

Trendelenburg position, and angulation of the body as in the prone and lateral jackknife positions are likely to cause delay or obstruction of venous return, with abrupt and serious decreases in blood pressure. Such positions should be avoided in patients with high levels of spinal anesthesia.

Another obvious cause of hypotension after the first half-hour of spinal blockade is the wearing off of the effects of a vasopressor given prophylactically. This type of hypotension develops relatively slowly and is easily recognized.

Untreated arterial hypotension during spinal anesthesia will, in the absence of appreciable intraoperative blood loss, persist simply for the duration of sympathetic denervation, provided the patient's position is not altered (Kim, et al., 1977). In a patient with a sensory level of anesthesia at T_3 who is maintained in the horizontal or slight head-down position, blood pressure gradually returns toward normal as vascular absorption of local anesthetic causes a decrease in the anesthetic concentration within the subarachnoid space and thus brings about regression of anesthesia. When levels of local anesthetic within neural elements rostral to the level of L_2 have decreased below minimum effective concentrations, there is no longer any significant sympathetic blockade. At this time, the anesthetic no longer has any cardiovascular effects and the position of the patient may be altered with impunity. However, although sympathetic function may have returned at the L_2 levels, around the level of the cauda equina there may still be local anesthetic in sufficient concentration to cause continuing areas of hypesthesia, anesthesia or deranged motor function of the lower extremities or perineum. Ambulation may therefore prove hazardous even though assumption of the erect position has no cardiovascular effects (Pflug, et al., 1978). The length of time required for the sympathetic block to regress completely following spinal anesthesia depends upon the amount of local anesthetic injected per segment of anesthesia produced, the lipid solubility of the anesthetic, and whether or not a vasoconstrictor was injected into the subarachnoid space along with the local anesthetic.

The duration of sympathetic denervation associated with spinal anesthesia commonly exceeds the duration of surgery. The danger of arterial hypotension is thus frequently as great in the immediate postoperative period as it is intraoperatively. A patient who has been in the head-down position during surgery performed under spinal anesthesia must be kept in the same position when moved from the operating table to the stretcher, if hypotension is to be avoided.

Management of Hypotension

Arterial hypotension following induction of spinal anesthesia must not be ignored. The fact that the hypotension of spinal anesthesia is associated with a decrease in operative blood loss (Madsen and Madsen, 1967; Moir, 1968) and that in selected cases severe degrees of hypotension can be intentionally induced in order to decrease operative bleeding (Griffiths and Gillies, 1948; Gillies, 1949, 1950; Greene, 1952; Greene, et al., 1954; Moir, 1968) does not warrant the inference that inadvertent hypotension in unselected patients should be viewed with complacency. Deaths associated with spinal anesthesia have been and continue to be reported (Hingson and Hellman, 1951; Lorhan and Merriam, 1952; Hampton and Little, 1953 a, b; Beecher and Todd, 1954; Turk and Glenn, 1954; Wasserman, et al., 1955; Caplan, et al., 1988). The great majority of such fatalities are caused by a decrease in CO to the point where coronary and cerebral blood flows become inadequate, although other factors have been implicated as well, as shown by Caplan, et al. (1988) in their closed claims analysis of predisposing factors for the development of cardiac arrest during spinal anesthesia. Their review of 900 closed insurance claims revealed 14 cases of sudden cardiac arrest in healthy patients. Although all patients were resuscitated from the intraoperative cardiac arrest, six suffered neurologic injury that ultimately led to their death while still in the hospital. Only one of the eight survivors recovered sufficiently to allow independent self-care. Of the factors analyzed, two predisposing factors were identified: first was intraoperative oversedation in which cyanosis heralded the onset of cardiac arrest. The second predisposing factor was inadequate appreciation of the profound physiologic changes induced by spinal anesthesia and of the mechanisms of cardiopulmonary resuscitation in the setting of sympathetic denervation. The authors therefore suggested that "prompt augmentation of central venous filling through the use of a potent alpha agonist and positional change might have improved organ perfusion, shorten the duration of cardiac arrest, and lessen the degree of neurologic damage." Mackey, et al. (1989) reported three cases of bradycardia and asystole that occurred during spinal anesthesia. Prior to development of asystole, these patients were all hemodynamically stable, well oxygenated, and they were not heavily sedated. The authors proposed that the mechanism for the occurrence of the bradycardia and asystole in their cases may have involved sensory receptors located principally in the inferoposterior wall of the left ventricle. Stimulation of these inhibitory cardiac receptors by stretching of the myocardium (mechanoreceptors), or by chemical substances or drugs (chemoreceptors) increases parasympathetic activity and inhibits sympathetic activity, promoting reflex bradycardia, vasodilation, and hypotension. This reflex, first described in 1867, bears the names of two of its first proponents, Bezold and Jarisch. Normally, a decrease in left ventricular end-diastolic volume decreases the tonic receptor activity of the mechanoreceptors, thereby decreasing parasympathetic, and increasing sympathetic activity. This results in vasoconstriction and an increase in blood pressure. However, a rapid, sudden decrease in ventricular volume can actually stimulate the activity of these receptors, presumably due to vigorous ventricular contraction around an almost empty chamber. The paradoxic increased activity of the receptors leads to bradycardia and hypotension (Bezold-Jarisch reflex).

The important question concerns the degree of hypotension that should be regarded as dangerous and that therefore requires active corrective measures. It is impossible to give a categorical answer to this question because the different situations in which the hypotension can develop must be taken into account. There are situations in which hypotension of even mild degrees should be corrected as soon as detected. Even minor degrees of hypotension should probably not go untreated in patients with preanesthetic abnormalities of coronary or cerebral blood flow. Similarly, patients who develop even mild degrees of hypotension immediately after the induction of anesthesia should be treated promptly. If a patient's systolic pressure decreases 10 percent in the first 2 min after the spinal anesthetic has been injected, it should be assumed from the rapidity of this decrease that unless corrective measures are taken, the pressure will reach dangerously low levels within the next 10 min. On the other hand, if a young healthy adult experiences a gradual 20 percent decrease in systolic pressure over a period of 20 min, usually nothing need be done.

As a general rule, if a patient's normal systolic blood pressure decreases by more than 25 percent of the preanesthetic level, steps should be taken to correct it. A patient with a preanesthetic systolic pressure of 100 mmHg can usually tolerate a level of 75 mmHg in the absence of medical contraindications. Similarly, the blood pressure of a hypertensive patient with a systolic level of 200 mmHg can safely be lowered by spinal anesthesia to about 150 mmHg provided no organic vascular changes are present to make this decrease dangerous. Such lowering of the blood pressure can be tolerated, of course, only if it occurs as a result of sympathetic blockade; a similar degree of hypotension resulting from blood loss is more dangerous and must be corrected immediately.

When arterial hypotension develops during spinal anesthesia, treatment should be directed at the specific etiology. In cases in which hypotension is due to decreased CO or to decreased CO plus reduced TPR, the administration of vasoconstrictors that merely increase peripheral vascular resistance is not as effective as reliance on measures designed to increase CO. On the other hand, increasing CO alone cannot be expected to completely reverse the hypotension due to a markedly decreased peripheral vascular resistance. Since a severe decrease in arterial pressure during spinal anesthesia is usually the result of decreased CO and since the latter follows a diminution in venous return to the heart caused by faulty positioning of the patient, correct positioning of the patient during spinal anesthesia should be a primary concern of the anesthesiologist. It has been said that position is everything in life. This is particularly true during spinal anesthesia. Unless the position is so arranged that venous return to the heart and CO remain adequate, treatment of severe arterial hypotension is futile. Perhaps one of the more unfortunate pieces of advice about spinal anesthesia is that the patient's head should be kept elevated to prevent the ascent of local anesthetic agent to the brain stem. Certainly this should be done when a hyperbaric solution is used and a low level of anesthesia is required. But, if the drug inadvertently reaches a high level, or if severe hypotension develops, elevation of the head is dangerous, since CO may decrease to a point where cardiac arrest occurs (Caplan, *et al.*, 1988; Mackey, *et al.*, 1989; Nishikawa, *et al.*, 1988; Underwood and Glynn, 1988). The slight head-down position should always be used during severe degrees of hypotension associated with spinal anesthesia. Obviously, maintenance of a patent airway and its protection from aspiration of gastric contents should also be of primary importance to the anesthesiologist.

Recognition of the importance of the head-down position in maintaining an adequate venous return and CO is not new. It has been noted, by those who employed the somewhat debatable technique of total spinal anesthesia for head and neck surgery, that patients did well so long as they were kept in the Trendelenburg position (Payne, 1901; Jonnesco, 1909; Koster, 1928; Koster and Kasman, 1929; Labat, 1930; Wright, 1930–1931; Vehrs, 1931, 1934). The importance of the head-down position has long been emphasized and reemphasized by clinical and by experimental studies relating blood pressure to position during spinal anesthesia (Evans, 1928, 1929; Brigden, *et al.*, 1950; Cole, 1952; Caplan, *et al.*, 1988). Gordh (1945) showed that during spinal anesthesia blood pressure could be raised from 80/70 to 130/100 mmHg by position alone. Assali and Prystowsky (1950 a, b) found that elevation of the lower extremities alone is effective in increasing blood pressure, although less so than by taking advantage of the maximal effects of gravity with the use of slight head-down position. In experimental work in animals, Graham and Douglas (1949) increased CO and arterial blood pressure by 28 percent and 30 percent, respectively, during hypotension induced by high spinal anesthesia combined with bleeding. Their results were confirmed in humans by Johnson (1951) who found that during T_4 spinal anesthesia, movement of patients from the supine level position to the Trendelenburg position caused an average increase in cardiac output of 31 percent, along with an average elevation of the blood pressure from 96/67 to 117/80 mmHg. Sheskey, *et al.* (1983) likewise underscored the importance of maintenance of cardiac output and venous return by positioning (i.e., by use of lithotomy position), in their study in which patients with sensory blocks involving cervical dermatomes still exhibited no significant hypotension (9–17 percent decrease), or bradycardia (8–17 percent decrease), regardless of whether 10, 15, or 20 mg of subarachnoid bupivacaine was used. The dangers of the head-up position have been classically demonstrated by Pugh and Wyndham (1950); they recorded alarming decreases in CO and blood pressure, often associated with severe CNS symptoms in all patients placed in reverse Trendelenburg position during high spinal anesthesia. More recently, Nishikawa, *et al.* (1988) reported a case of asystole during spinal anesthesia following a change from the Trendelenburg to the horizontal position.

The foregoing discussion is not intended to imply either that the head-down position should be used routinely immediately after injection of a spinal anesthetic, or that unnecessarily high levels of anesthesia should be viewed with nonchalance. Every effort should be made to keep the level of anesthesia as low as compatible with the projected surgery, including the use of the head-up position; but if hypotension should develop, the head-down position must be adopted without hesitation. Once normal CO has been assured by proper positioning, vasopressors and other therapy, including oxygen, should then be employed as indicated.

Oxygen should be administered during high spinal anesthesia, especially if severe arterial hypotension develops or if there is a question regarding the adequacy of pulmonary function. The purpose of oxygen administration during hypotension is to increase arterial oxygen content so that although CO and peripheral blood flow are decreased, the rate of oxygen delivery to tissue is not decreased proportionately. It is debatable if oxygen should be routinely administered to all patients during spinal anesthesia since high concentrations of oxygen during spinal anesthesia have been shown to accentuate some of the deleterious physiologic responses its administration is meant to relieve. Ward, *et al.* (1966 a) found that during high spinal anesthesia (sensory levels of T_5), the administration of 100 percent oxygen to spontaneously ventilating patients decreased CO and increased peripheral vasoconstriction, as evidenced by an increase in peripheral vascular resistance. In other words, the slight increase in arterial oxygen content produced by breathing 100 percent oxygen instead of room air was achieved only at the cost of decreasing the rate at which the oxygen-enriched arterial blood was delivered to peripheral tissues. It is not known whether or not the increased arterial oxygen content compensates for the decrease in CO and the decrease in tissue perfusion under these conditions. These effects of high oxygen concentrations on CO and peripheral blood flow during spinal anesthesia also occur in unanesthetized subjects. It is interesting that the vascular effects of high oxygen concentration persist in the presence of sympathetic denervation, perhaps reflecting humoral factors involved, such as increase in the release of vasopressin (Peters, *et al.*, 1990).

In other settings, however, delivery of supplemental oxygen has salutary effects. Muravchick and Johnson (1986) studied the continuous transcutaneous oxygen of the anterior chest wall below the clavicle during spinal anesthesia, with and without supplemental inspired oxygen, in young and elderly patients. They found that, although anesthesia itself did not change the peripheral tissue oxygenation, peripheral oxygen tension increased statistically significantly during conventional nasal prong oxygen therapy in both young and elderly patients. Since spinal anesthesia may be associated with periods of hypotension and decreased peripheral oxygenation, the authors therefore recommended routine application of conservative oxygen therapy, such as oxygen delivered via nasal prongs, during clinical spinal anesthesia. In addition, other studies have demonstrated the value of supplemental oxygen in patients given intravenous sedation during spinal anesthesia. Manara, *et al.* (1989), for example, studied the effect of sedation with midazolam on arterial oxygen saturation during spinal anesthesia with and without delivery of supplementary oxygen. Oxygen saturation decreased significantly in 40% of the patients breathing room air and in none of the patients given supplemental oxygen. The need for supplemental oxygen when sedatives are given during spinal anesthesia was also demonstrated by Reinhart, *et al.* (1983) who found that midazolam, as well as diazepam, promethazine, and meperidine invariably decreased intraoperative arterial oxygen tension significantly when given in amounts adequate to induce sleep. The importance of delivery of supplemental oxygen during spinal anesthesia in elderly patients undergoing total hip replacement and cementing with methylmethacrylate (MMA), was underscored by Svartling, *et al.* (1985) and Modig, *et al.* (1975), who also found significant decreases in arterial oxygenation and blood pressure following cementation with MMA.

Alternatively, sympathetic denervation almost completely abolishes the normal cardiovascular responses to hypoxemia. Although not investigated during spinal anesthesia, this has been demonstrated by Peters, *et al.* (1990) during epidural anesthesia. In the absence of sympathetic denervation, hypoxemia evoked an increase in mean blood pressure of approximately 35%, while heart rate was increased by 50 beats/min. In the presence of sympathetic blockade, a similar degree of hypoxemia did not change blood pressure, and heart rate increased only 15 beats/min. In both sympathectomized and intact dogs in this study, hypoxia induced a similar degree of hypocarbia (partial pressure of carbon dioxide (PCO_2) = 25 mmHg). The authors concluded that the sympathetic denervation associated with high epidural anesthesia markedly blunted the normal cardiovascular responses (such as hypertension and tachycardia) to hypoxemia.

Vasopressors have a limited but definite role in the prevention and treatment of arterial hypotension during spinal anesthesia. They should not be employed as a substitute for maintenance of adequate CO by appropriate positioning of the patient. Vasopressors are useful, however, if employed when use of the head-down position alone has proven inadequate to restore blood pressure to acceptable levels.

Since hypotension profound enough to require pharmacologic treatment is due to decreases in CO rather than to decreases in TPR, the most rational vasopressors to use in correction of hypotension are those that restore CO, rather than those that primarily or solely increase peripheral resistance. Alpha-adrenergic agonists such as phenylephrine and methoxamine are best avoided during spinal anesthesia, as their administration makes little pharmacologic or physiologic sense. Their use may also prove deleterious (Li, *et al.*, 1965; Smith and Corbascio, 1970) by producing such marked increases in left ventricular afterload and left ventricular work, that CO may be decreased further, with adverse effects in the balance between myocardial oxygen requirements and myocardial oxygen supply.

Vasopressors that increase CO during spinal anesthesia are of two types: those that act solely and directly on the heart to increase its output, and those that increase CO by virtue of their ability to produce venoconstriction, thereby restoring venous return to the heart. The former type includes atropine which, in usual clinical doses during spinal anesthesia, has no effect on the peripheral vasculature on either the arterial or the venous side. Atropine also has no direct effect on myocardial contractility; it increases cardiac output during spinal anesthesia solely through its chronotropic effect. By increasing heart rate, atropine increases CO and thus elevates arterial blood pressure, since peripheral resistance remains unchanged. Atropine alone, however, is not always an effective vasopressor during spinal anesthesia. It may be relatively effective when given intravenously in large doses (0.04 mg·kg^{-1}) (O'Rourke and Greene, 1970; Greene and Bachand, 1971), but is less reliable when given in usual doses of 0.4–0.6 mg (Ward, *et al.*, 1966 b; Graves, *et al.*, 1968). Disadvantages of atropine also include unpleasant dryness of the mouth it produces in awake patients, as well as the more important disadvantage that tachycardia may be inadvisable in patients with certain types of heart disease. An increase in HR may be especially poorly tolerated in patients with mitral stenosis or other conditions in which diastolic ventricular filling may be shortened. An increase in HR also may be poorly tolerated in patients with myocardial ischemia secondary to coronary artery disease. The diastolic time interval during which coronary blood flow takes place is decreased during tachycardia. The increase in myocardial work and oxygen requirements produced by the tachycardia may thus aggravate preexisting myocardial ischemia because tachycardia may further impair an already marginal coronary blood flow.

Given the fact that severe hypotension during spinal anesthesia is due to venodilation with decrease in preload, the ideal vasopressor would be one that had no effect except production of venoconstriction. None of the clinically available vasopressors are pure venoconstrictors, however. All have at least some effects on both venous and arterial vessels as well as effects on the inotropic state of the myocardium. The relative effects on venous and arterial circulation vary considerably among the different sympathomimetic amines. These effects have been quantitated by Zimmerman, *et al.* (1963) using the formula:

$$\frac{\text{(Change in venous resistance)}}{\text{(Change in total vascular resistance)}} \times 100$$

Application of this formula to norepinephrine yields a figure of 13.8. With metaraminol, the figure is 7.2, with ephedrine 3.3, with mephentermine 1.9, with phenylephrine 1.8, and with methoxamine 1.4. On this basis, ephedrine, metaraminol, and norepinephrine would be more appropriate than mephentermine, phenylephrine, or methoxamine for treatment of hypotension during spinal anesthesia. These data, however, do not tell the full story. They fail to consider other equally important cardiovascular effects of these vasopressors, particularly effects on cardiac contractility and HR. Nor do they take into account clinically relevant factors such as rapidity of onset and duration of action, effect on the CNS, and the potential for development of tachyphylaxis. When these considerations are taken into account and added to experimental data on cardiovascular responses to vasopressors as diverse as phenylephrine (Butterworth, *et al.*, 1986); dobutamine (Butterworth, *et al.*, 1987); ephedrine (Stevens, *et al.*, 1968; Butterworth, *et al.*, 1986; Taivainen, 1991; Thorburn, 1985); methoxamine (Li, *et al.*, 1965; Stevens, *et al.*, 1968); mephentermine (Li, *et al.*, 1963; Cucchiara and Restall, 1973); dopamine (Cabalum, *et al.*, 1979; Rolbin, *et al.*, 1979; Butterworth, *et al.*, 1987; ergotamine (Klingenstrom, 1960; Castenfors, *et al.*, 1975; Hilke, *et al.*, 1978); etilefrine (Taivainen, 1991); and isoproterenol (Butterworth, *et al.*, 1986), it becomes apparent that clinically, certain vasopressors are not only more practical, but also more rational than others for the prevention and treatment of hypotension during spinal anesthesia.

In an elegant model, Butterworth, *et al.* (1986) demonstrated in anesthetized dogs undergoing cardiopulmonary bypass (CPB) that mixed adrenergic agonists (such as ephedrine) corrected the noncardiac circulatory sequelae of spinal anesthesia more effectively than either a pure alpha- or beta-adrenergic agonist. The model used in their study consisted of measuring the volume of blood in the venous reservoir and the MAP as indices of changes in venous capacitance and arterial resistance, respectively, produced by adrenergic agonists. CPB technique was chosen to prevent direct drug effects on the heart from influencing the results. This model also facilitated measurement of venous capacitance. The authors demonstrated that spinal anesthesia significantly increased venous capacitance and decreased mean arterial pressure relative to steady-state CPB values. Correction of hemodynamic alterations produced by spinal anesthesia was attempted using a pure alpha-agonist (phenylephrine), a beta-agonist (isoproterenol), and a mixed adrenergic agent (ephedrine). Phenylephrine induced arterial vasoconstriction and increased MAP, but had no effect on venous capacitance. Isoproterenol decreased capacitance (i.e., increased venous return) but also further decreased MAP. Ephedrine, however, was associated with an increase in MAP and a decrease in venous capacitance. These results provided further proof that a mixed adrenergic agonist such as ephedrine (or mephentermine) might well be the agents of choice for correcting the noncardiac circulatory sequelae of spinal anesthesia (i.e., decreased CO based on decreased venous return). The authors also hypothesized that a predominantly beta-adrenergic agent such as isoproterenol is able to cause venoconstriction (i.e., decreased capacitance) because beta-receptor stimulation increases venous return in much in the same way that cross-clamping the aorta at the diaphragm increases venous return (Butterworth, et al., 1986). Beta-adrenergic receptor stimulation redirected, in other words, blood flow from the slow transit system (i.e., splanchnic bed) to the fast transit system (heart, brain, and kidney). The net effect was an effective autotransfusion (or of generalized venoconstriction). The authors thus introduced the concept that redistribution of blood flow, rather than venoconstriction might be the mechanism by which adrenergic agonists increase venous return during the total sympathectomy produced by spinal anesthesia. Such a concept is also supported by the studies of Green (1977), Permutt and Caldini (1978), and Rutlen, et al. (1979).

Other vasoactive substances have also been investigated regarding their cardiovascular effects in the presence of sympathetic denervation produced by spinal or epidural anesthesia. Castenfors, et al. (1975) studied the effect of dihydroergotamine (DHE) on the peripheral circulation during epidurally induced sympathectomy in humans. They found that DHE induced a significant increase in blood flow if sympathetic innervation were left intact, and a significant decrease in blood flow in the sympathectomized calf. On the average, however, the arterial blood pressure increased. Cabalum, et al. (1979) investigated the effectiveness of dopamine in reversing the hypotension induced by spinal anesthesia. They found that autonomic blockade associated with spinal anesthesia in pregnant sheep induced a decrease in the systemic arterial pressure, HR, and uterine blood flow, while uterine vascular resistance increased. Intravenous dopamine corrected these circulatory changes. Taivainen (1991) compared ephedrine and etilefrine for treatment of arterial hypotension induced by spinal anesthesia in elderly patients. Both sympathomimetic drugs (alpha- and beta$_1$-receptor agonists) increased systolic blood pressure and HR in a similar fashion, and neither one was associated with the development of tachyphylaxis. Thorburn (1985) in a study performed in patients undergoing total hip replacement, confirmed that intravenous ephedrine was effective in maintaining normal blood pressures following induction of spinal anesthesia and had no effects on blood transfusion requirements or on postoperative hemoglobin concentrations.

From the above studies it is apparent that pure alpha- or beta-receptor agonists may not be effective in reversing the circulatory changes (hypotension and bradycardia) associated with high spinal anesthesia. Dihydroergotamine, although associated with increases in both capacitance and resistance vessels, does not have a consistent and predictable effect in the setting of sympathetic denervation. Dopamine, although effective in restoring spinal anesthesia-induced blood pressure, is used infrequently clinically because of the need for continuous infusion. On the other hand, mixed agents, such as ephedrine, mephentermine, and etilefrine are effective and practical in the clinical setting for restoring blood pressure and HR during spinal anesthesia.

Another method for treating arterial hypotension during clinical anesthesia consists of the rapid intravenous infusion of relatively large volumes of fluids, usually in the range of 1.0 to 1.5 L/70 kg body weight within 10 min or less (Venn, et al., 1989). Balanced electrolyte solutions are used most frequently, as they tend to remain in the vascular system longer than noncrystalloid solutions such as dextrose in water, while hypertonic solutions of dextrose often produce osmotic diuresis. Thus, while increasing blood volume transiently, hypertonic solutions may eventually decrease it. Use of intravenous solutions for the management of hypotension during spinal anesthesia is not, however, designed to treat preanesthetic hypovolemia or electrolyte deficits. Such abnormalities should be treated prior to induction of spinal anesthesia.

Coe and Revanäs (1990) studied whether crystalloid preloading would be useful for prevention of hemodynamic instability in elderly patients undergoing spinal anesthesia. The 60 patients in this study, aged 60 years or older, were separated randomly into two groups: they were either given no volume preload, or a rapid volume preload with Ringer's acetate solution (8 ml·kg^{-1} or 16 ml·kg^{-1}). Significant hypotension was defined as a 25% decrease in systolic arterial pressure, and bradycardia was defined as a HR under 50 beats/min. The overall incidence of hypotension was 27%, and did not differ significantly among treatment groups. Hypotension occurred in 60% of patients who experienced a loss of cold sensation to T$_7$, and in 100% of those patients in whom cold sensation was blocked to T_4 or above. The incidence of hypotension was not affected by crystalloid preloading. The authors therefore concluded that crystalloid preloading had no affect on the incidence of hypotension during spinal anesthesia, and that intravenous ephedrine should be given prophylactically to patients in whom it is anticipated that the level of anesthesia might extend more cephalad than T_7. Somewhat different conclusions were offered by Venn, *et al.* (1989) who studied the effects on systemic arterial pressure of fluid preloading with 1 L of crystalloid prior to induction of spinal anesthesia. They suggested that "a fluid preload may be of value in reducing the maximum decrease of arterial pressure, but only in patients with blocks extending above the T_6 dermatome." Furthermore, these authors found that vasopressors (ephedrine) were always effective in treating hypotension, even when 1 L of crystalloid was ineffective.

When rapid infusion of large volumes of balanced salt solutions is able to restore blood pressure during spinal anesthesia to normal levels, it does so simply by increasing venous return, an effect analogous to that produced by use of the head-down position (Sidi, *et al.*, 1984). Sheskey, *et al.* (1983) underscored the importance of maintenance of CO and venous return during spinal anesthesia by positioning (i.e., by use of the lithotomy position), in their study in which patients with cervical levels of anesthesia still exhibited no significant hypotension or bradycardia (the average maximal decrease in MAP was 9 percent to 17 percent).

Large volumes of intravenous fluids also produce hemodilution. By decreasing the hematocrit, fluids alter peripheral blood flow, as well. At any given perfusion pressure, the flow of blood through vessels with small diameters, such as those in the postarteriolar bed, increases as the HCT decreases (Crowell and Smith, 1967; Laks, *et al.*, 1973; Replogle, *et al.*, 1967; Gordon and Ravin, 1978). Flow increases because resistance decreases; resistance decreases because viscosity is decreased. The viscosity of blood is directly related to hematocrit. But viscosity of a nonnewtonian fluid such as blood is also inversely related to flow rate, that is, velocity gradient. Thus, if velocity gradient is constant at 106 sec^{-1}, the viscosity of blood at 37°C decreases from 4.4 centipoise (cp) at a HCT of 40 percent to a viscosity of 2.6 cp at a HCT of 20 percent, amounting to a decrease in viscosity of 40 percent. Similarly, if HCT is constant at 40 percent, viscosity is 4.4 cp at a velocity gradient of 106 sec^{-1}, but increases by 20 percent to 5.3 cp when the velocity gradient is increased to 42 sec^{-1} (Gordon and Ravin, 1978). But viscosity is but one of the two components of TPR, the other being vascular resistance. From the above it is apparent that TPR increases as CO decreases, even though the HCT remains unchanged, because viscosity is inversely related to velocity gradient. This is one of the reasons for the lack of linearity between TPR and the degree of sympathetic denervation (i.e., vasodilation) during spinal anesthesia. Spinal anesthesia may also decrease CO that, by decreasing transcapillary velocity gradients, may increase viscosity and thus resistance. For the same reason, TPR decreases during infusion of crystalloids and, if CO remains constant, blood pressure decreases. Intravenous crystalloid solutions increase blood pressure during spinal anesthesia despite the decrease in TPR produced by the hemodilution. This is so because such fluids increase venous return and CO more than they decrease TPR due to changes in blood viscosity. Thus, hemodilution resulting from the administration of large volumes of crystalloids increases peripheral perfusion through two mechanisms. By increasing CO (i.e., peripheral velocity gradients), resistance to flow of blood through the postarteriolar bed is decreased. By decreasing HCT, large volumes of crystalloids decrease the viscosity of blood at any given velocity gradient, thus increasing peripheral perfusion.

These salutary effects of the rapid infusion of large volumes of balanced salt solutions may in part be offset, however, insofar as tissue oxygenation is concerned, because large volumes of electrolyte solutions also decrease the oxygen carrying capacity of blood. By decreasing HCT through hemodilution and by increasing CO, blood flow through peripheral tissues increases. But the amount of oxygen being delivered per unit of blood flow decreases as the HCT decreases. This gives rise to the concept of optimal HCT, that is, the HCT at which total systemic transport of oxygen remains adequate, despite the conflicting effects of hemodilution on postarteriolar oxygenation: an increase in flow associated with hemodilution and a decrease in the amount of oxygen carried by blood. If systemic transport of oxygen is considered to be 100 percent at a HCT of 40 percent, a 25 percent decrease in HCT to 30 percent is associated with a decrease in systemic transport of oxygen of only about 2 percent. The decrease in oxygen transport is trivial at this level of HCT because the relationship between HCT and viscosity is exponential, not linear. Below a HCT of 30 percent, systemic oxygen transport falls off more rapidly. When the HCT is 15 percent, systemic oxygen transport is decreased to approximately 78 percent of what it was at a HCT of 40 percent (Crowell and Smith, 1967; Gordon and Ravin, 1978).

Crystalloid solutions are an useful adjunct to maintenance of cardiovascular function during spinal anesthesia when used in modest amounts. Used in excessive volumes they may do more harm than good. The anesthesiologist who uses rapid intravenous infusion of fluid for management of hypotension during spinal anesthesia should bear in mind the following.

1. In normovolemic patients arterial blood pressure cannot be maintained predictably merely by intravenous infusion of crystalloids (Graves, et al., 1968; Coe and Revanäs, 1990). Intravenous crystalloids

must be combined with the use of the head-down position and the judicious use of vasopressors. Sidi, *et al.* (1984) reported that despite crystalloid preloading to achieve a CVP between 5 and 10 cm H_2O in all 40 patients in their study, blood pressure decreased by more than 10% below baseline values in 80% of the cases, and more than 30% below baseline in 35% of the cases. In their study, the upper level of sensory denervation was T_{7-12}.

2. Intravenous crystalloids increase peripheral blood flow by decreasing the viscosity of blood and increasing CO, but do so at the expense of decreasing oxygen content of arterial blood. If hemodilution is carried too far, the decrease in oxygen content may exceed the beneficial effects of increased tissue flow.

3. Blood pressure is not an accurate index of systemic oxygen transport. An increase in blood pressure produced by alpha-adrenergic agonists has a well-recognized potential for decreasing systemic oxygen transport because of arterial and arteriolar vasoconstriction. An increase in blood pressure accomplished by volume hemodilution is also not associated with proportionate increase in systemic oxygen transport because of the associated decrease in the oxygen carrying capacity of arterial blood.

4. Large volumes of balanced salt solutions rapidly administered intravenously may be tolerated poorly by patients with diminished myocardial reserve or valvular heart disease.

5. Volumes of intravenous fluids in excess of those required to maintain normal fluid and electrolyte concentrations expose patients given spinal anesthesia to the risks associated with postoperative catheterization of the bladder. Urinary retention due to prolonged paralysis of parasympathetic motor nerves involved in micturition becomes more frequent when large volumes of intravenous fluids are administered to maintain normal blood pressure during spinal anesthesia.

6. Crystalloid administration may exert untoward effects on the hemostatic system. Janvrin, *et al.* (1980) in their study of the incidence of postoperative deep vein thrombosis found that patients given intravenous crystalloid infusions perioperatively had increased blood coagulability, and increased incidence of deep venous thrombosis (an incidence of 30 percent). In contrast, patients not given intravenous crystalloids perioperatively did not exhibit any change in coagulability, and had only a 7 percent incidence of deep venous thrombosis.

Finally, inflatable boots or cushions extending from toes to umbilicus have been suggested as a method for prevention or treatment of arterial hypotension during spinal anesthesia. The rationale is that such devices prevent peripheral pooling of the blood in the venous circulation. In practice, they have been found inadequate (James and Greiss, 1973), probably because the portion of the venous circulation they can affect significantly constitutes a relatively small part of the total area in which venous pooling may occur during spinal anesthesia.

Hemodynamic Effects of Spinal Anesthesia in Pediatrics

Pediatric regional anesthesia, and in particular, spinal, epidural and caudal anesthesia are established techniques of providing both intraoperative anesthesia, as well as postoperative analgesia (Eige and Bell, 1991). The use of regional anesthesia has increased dramatically in the last decade, as evidenced by the number of pediatric regional anesthesia textbooks published (Bell, et al., 1991; Dalens, 1990; Saint-Maurice, 1990).

Although reference has already been made to the effects of age on the hemodynamic responses to spinal anesthesia, a review of cardiovascular changes in the pediatric population deserves emphasis. Dohi, et al. (1979) studied the changes in hemodynamics and duration of motor block associated with spinal anesthesia in patients ranging in age from 8 months to adulthood. The authors induced spinal anesthesia with tetracaine plus phenylephrine in 65 children and 17 adults. Although all patients included in this study had similar levels of sensory anesthesia, ranging from T_3–T_5, children less than 5 years of age had little or no change in blood pressure or HR in response to the sympathectomy of spinal anesthesia. Children 5–8 years of age had variable changes in blood pressure in response to spinal anesthesia, while children 8–15 years of age had blood pressure and HR responses much more similar to the adults. The authors suggested that responsible factors for the differences between children and adults with respect to hemodynamic responses include: (a) immaturity of the sympathetic nervous system in young children; and (b) physical and physiologic differences, including the amount of cerebrospinal fluid and the surface area of the spinal cord.

The results reported by Dohi, et al. (1979) have been confirmed by other groups of investigators. Gallagher and Crean (1989) for example, studied the cardiovascular effects of spinal anesthesia with hyperbaric bupivacaine in infants born prematurely; they found that none of the 25 infants had any episodes of hemodynamic instability. This finding was also reported by Rice, et al. (1987) who studied hemodynamic responses to spinal anesthesia in infants under 1 year of age, and found that blood pressure and HR changes were less than 5% from preoperative values. Rice, et al. concluded that spinal anesthesia is a safe and effective alternative to general anesthesia. Similarly, Harnik, et al. (1986) reported on spinal anesthesia in 20 premature infants who were recovering from respiratory distress syndrome. Even in this group of high-risk infants, the authors found no hypotension or bradycardia. Similar cardiovascular stability during spinal anesthesia in high-risk infants was also reported by Abajian, *et al.* (1984). And finally, Mahe and Ecoffey (1988) found the duration of analgesia to be shorter in infants than in adults, and, despite the relatively high levels of cutaneous analgesia reached (T_3), maximal blood pressure decrease was only 24%.

It is not only the hemodynamic stability exhibited by infants undergoing spinal anesthesia which has prompted clinicians to recommend it as a safe alternative to general anesthesia. Several investigators have reported lack of respiratory side effects (Rice, *et al.*, 1987; Gallagher and Crean, 1989), while some have even concluded that spinal anesthesia with tetracaine may avoid the "increased incidence of postoperative respiratory complications associated with general anesthesia and reduce the requirement for postoperative mechanical ventilatory support" in premature infants (Harnik, *et al.*, 1986). It is encouraging to note that spinal anesthesia has become an accepted and safe technique of providing perioperative comfort and hemodynamic stability, even in high-risk, premature infants, with the caveat, however, that spinal anesthesia does not change the need for intensive monitoring and vigilance. Regional anesthesia, and in particular, spinal anesthesia, need to be investigated further in the pediatric population, especially with regard to long-term outcome.

Pharmacokinetics of Intravenous Drugs

In view of the many ways in which spinal anesthesia may affect cardiovascular function, the pharmacokinetics of drugs administered intravenously might be expected to be affected by high spinal anesthesia. Theoretically, the apparent volume of distribution might be altered. So, too, might elimination of drugs, insofar as the anesthesia might affect blood flow to the liver and kidneys. Unfortunately, few data exist on the effects of spinal anesthesia on the rate of onset, magnitude of peak response, or duration of peak response of intravenous drugs. One of the few studies of the effect of spinal anesthesia on drug disposition is that by Whelan, *et al.* (1989), in which the authors used propranolol as a model compound in dogs. The authors found that low sacral to mid-thoracic levels of spinal anesthesia had no significant effects on the clearance, the volume of distribution, or the elimination half-life of propranolol, and spinal anesthesia induced no decrease in hepatic plasma flow. These findings were in contrast to the inhalational anesthetics, fentanyl, and propofol, all of which had been found to inhibit hepatic drug metabolism. In another report, Adams, et al. (1989) studied the sympathoadrenergic response to intravenous administration of theophylline during general or spinal anesthesia by measuring the plasma levels of epinephrine and norepinephrine in response to an intraoperative injection of 4 mg·kg^{-1} body weight of theophylline. Both epinephrine and norepinephrine levels increased from baseline levels following administration of theophylline, with epinephrine concentrations increasing significantly more than those of norepinephrine. However, the increase in plasma catecholamines in response to theophylline injection showed no statistically significant difference among patients who received general or spinal anesthesia. The authors therefore concluded that the mechanism of action of theophylline is one of release of endogenous catecholamines and this mechanism is not blocked by spinal anesthesia. For this reason, patients with cardiovascular disease should be monitored closely with regard to possible cardiac arrhythmias associated with theophylline administration, even during spinal anesthesia.

Another group of investigators has studied the pharmacokinetics of intravenously administered drugs during spinal anesthesia (Runciman, et al., 1984 b, c; Runciman, et al., 1986; Runciman, et al., 1985; Mather, et al., 1986). These investigators, using a sheep preparation, found that spinal anesthesia, in contradistinction to general anesthesia, induced no significant changes in the hepatic extraction ratio or the clearance of meperidine, cefoxitin, or chlormethiazole. In addition, Ponten, et al. (1982) and Viegas, et al. (1983) have reported on the interaction between spinal anesthesia-induced sympathectomy and chronic beta-blockade therapy. Despite lack of data regarding the pharmacokinetics of betablockers during spinal anesthesia, these two studies deserve brief mentioning. In the first report, Ponten, et al. (1982) studied the effects of beta-receptor blockade during spinal anesthesia in two groups of patients receiving chronic beta-blocker therapy. One group underwent gradual beta-blocker withdrawal prior to induction of spinal anesthesia, while the other group continued the therapy. In the patients who underwent beta-receptor blockade withdrawal, a mean anesthetic level of T_6 induced an increase in HR, and was associated with a high incidence of arrhythmias, angina pectoris, and postoperative ST-T segment changes. In contrast, these effects were not seen in the patients who continued their beta-receptor blockade therapy. The study therefore suggested that patients on long term beta-receptor blockade should continue the therapy during and following spinal anesthesia.

In the second investigation, Viegas, et al. (1983) studied cardiovascular responses following spinal blockade in patients with and without chronic treatment with propranolol; they found that although there were no significant differences in blood pressure among patients regardless of propranolol administration, a significantly lower heart rate was seen in patients on chronic beta-blocker therapy. The authors concluded that induction of spinal anesthesia in patients receiving chronic beta-blockade may nevertheless be safe, as long as total sympathetic blockade is avoided.

Lastly, one other pharmacokinetic study, that by Kauto, *et al.* (1979), was performed during spinal anesthesia, but it was designed to evaluate the effects of age, and not the effects of the anesthetic, on the pharmacokinetics of intravenously administered diazepam. In this study it is impossible to dissociate the effects of age from the effects of anesthesia. It is hoped that this potentially fruitful area of investigation will be addressed in the future.

REFERENCES

ABAJIAN, J. C., MELLISH, R. W. P., BROWNE, A. F., PERKINS, F. M., LAMBERT, D. H., AND MAZUZAN, J. E., JR.: Spinal anesthesia for surgery in the high-risk infant. Anesth. Analg. *63:* 359, 1984.

ABBOUD, F. M.: Ventricular syncope. Is the heart a sensory organ? N. Engl. J. Med. *320:* 390, 1989.

ABRAMSON, D. I., AND FERRIS, E. B.: Responses of blood vessels in the resting hand and forearm to various stimuli. Am. Heart J. *19:* 541, 1940.

ABRAMSON, D. I., ZAZEELA, H., AND OPPENHEIMER, B. S.: Plethysmographic studies of peripheral blood flow in man: III. Effect of smoking on the vascular beds in the hand, forearm, and foot. Am. Heart J. *18:* 290, 1939.

ADAMS, H. A., WEIDACHER, A., BORGMANN, A., BOLDT, J., AND HEMPELMANN, G.: Sympathoadrenerge reaktionen nach theophyllin-applikation bei anwendung verschiedener anaesthesieverfahren. Anaesthesist *38:* 309, 1989.

ADRIANI, J., AND ROVENSTINE, E. A.: Effects of spinal anesthesia upon venous pressure in man. Proc. Soc. Exp. Biol. Med. *45:* 415, 1940.

ALLEN, E. V., LUNDY, J. S., AND ADSON, A. W.: Preoperative prediction of effects on blood pressure of neurosurgical treatment of hypertension. Proc. Staff Meet. Mayo Clin. *11:* 401, 1936.

ALMQUIST, A., GOLDENBERG, I. F., MILSTEIN, S., CHEN, M-E., CHEN, X., HANSEN, R., GORNICK, C. C., AND BENDITT, D.G.: Provocation of bradycardia and hypotension by isoproterenol and upright posture in patients with unexplained syncope. N. Engl. J. Med. *320:* 346, 1989.

ANDERSON, B. M.: A rational basis for the use of spinal anesthesia. Calif. Med. *105:* 307, 1966.

ANTON, A. H., UY, D. S., AND REDDERSON, C. L.: Autonomic blockade and the cardiovascular and catecholamine response to electroshock. Anesth. Analg. *56:* 46, 1977.

ANTONIN, V.: Einfluss der Lokal- und Lumbalanasthesie auf den acido-basischen Haushalt in der postoperative Zeit und die Bedeutung der Vorbereitung des Kranken auf diese Verhaltnisse. Acta Chir. Scand. *66:* 79, 1930.

ARMSTRONG, D. J., AND FINLAYSON, D. C.: The effect of spinal anaesthesia on blood volume in man. Can. Anaesth. Soc. J. *14:* 399, 1967.

ASSALI, N. S., AND PRYSTOWSKY, H.: Studies on autonomic blockade. I. Comparison between the effects of tetraethylammonium chloride (TEAC) and high selective spinal anesthesia on the blood pressure of normal and toxemic pregnancy. J. Clin. Invest. *29:* 1354, 1950 a.

ASSALI, N. S., AND PRYSTOWSKY, H.: Studies on autonomic blockade. II. Observations on the nature of blood pressure fall with high selective spinal anesthesia on pregnant women. J. Clin. Invest. 29: 1367, 1950 b.

ASSALI, N. S., KAPLAN, S. A., FOMON, S. J., DOUGLASS, R. A., AND TADA, Y.: The effect of high spinal anesthesia on the renal hemodynamics and the excretion of electrolytes during osmotic diuresis in the hydropenic normal pregnant woman. J. Clin. Invest. 30: 916, 1951.

BABCOCK, W. W.: Spinal anesthesia: an experience of 24 years. Am. J. Surg. 5: 571, 1928.

BALOURDAS, T. A.: Disassociation of sympathetic vascular tonus and permeability in the capillary blood vessels. Fed. Proc. 14: 7, 1955.

BARASH, P. G., AND KOPRIVA, C.: The rate-pressure product in clinical anesthesia: boon or bane? Anesth. Analg. 59: 229, 1980.

BARCROFT, H., AND ELLIOTT, R. H. E.: Some observations on the denervated spleen. J. Physiol. 87: 189, 1936.

BARCROFT, H., AND EDHOLM, O. G.: Sympathetic control of blood vessels of human skeletal muscle. Lancet 151: 513, 1946.

BARCROFT, H., AND SWAN, H. J. C.: Sympathetic Control of Human Blood Vessels. London: Edward Arnold & Co., 1953.

BARCROFT, H., BONNAR, W. M., EDHOLM, O. G., AND EFFRON, A. S.: On sympathetic vaso-constrictor tone in human skeletal muscle. J. Physiol. 102: 21, 1943.

BARON, J. F., CORIAT, P., MUNDLER, O., FAUCHET, M., BOUSSEAU, D., AND VIARS, P.: Left ventricular global and regional function during lumbar epidural anesthesia in patients with and without angina pectoris. Influence of volume loading. Anesthesiology 66: 621, 1987.

BAZETT, H. C.: Factors concerned in the control of capillary pressure as indicated in a circulation schema. Am. J. Physiol. 149: 389, 1947.

BEDDER, M. D., KOZODY, R., PALAHNIUK, R. J., CUMMING, M. O., AND PUCCI, W. R.: Clonidine prolongs canine tetracaine spinal anaesthesia. Can. Anaesth. Soc. J. 33: 591, 1986.

BEECHER, H. K.: The active control of all parts of the capillary wall by the sympathetic nervous system. Scand. Arch. Physiol. 73: 123, 1936.

BEECHER, H. K., AND TODD, D. P.: A study of deaths associated with anesthesia and surgery. Ann. Surg. 140: 2, 1954.

BELL, C., HUGHES, C. W., AND OH, T. H.: The Pediatric Anesthesia Handbook. St. Louis: Mosby-Year Book, Inc., 1991.

BENGTSSON, M., NILSSON, G. E., AND LOFSTROM, J. B.: The effect of spinal analgesia on skin blood flow, evaluated by laser Doppler flowmetry. Acta Anaesthesiol. Scand. 27: 206, 1983.

BERENYI, K. J., SHIMOSATO, S., AND ETSTEN, B. E.: Effect of mephentermine upon venous circulation during spinal anesthesia. Anesthesiology 25: 90, 1964.

BERG, G. R., AND KOTLER, M. N.: The significance of bilateral bundle branch block in the preoperative patient. A retrospective electrocardiographic and clinical study in 30 patients. Chest 59: 62, 1971.

BERGENWALD, L., EKLUND, B., KAIJSER, L., KLINGENSTROM, P., AND WESTERMARK, L.: Haemodynamic effects of dihydroergotamine during spinal anaesthesia in man. Acta Anaesthesiol. Scand. 16: 235, 1972.

BERLIN, N. I., HYDE, G. M., PARSONS, R. J., AND LAWRENCE, J. H.: The blood volume in various medical and surgical conditions. N. Engl. J. Med. 247: 675, 1952.

BIER, A.: Versuche uber Cocainisierung des Ruckenmarks. Dtsch. Ztschr. f. Chir. 51: 361, 1899.

BIGLER, D., HJORTSO, N. C., EDSTROM, H., CHRISTENSEN, N. J., AND KEHLET, H.: Comparative effects of intrathecal bupivacaine and tetracaine on analgesia, cardiovascular function and plasma catecholamines. Acta Anaesthesiol. Scand. 30: 199, 1986.

BLAIR, M. R.: Cardiovascular pharmacology of local anaesthetics. Br. J. Anaesth. 47: 247, 1975.

BLAKE, D. W., DONNAN, G., NOVELLA, J., AND HACKMAN, C.: Cardiovascular effects of sedative infusions of propofol and midazolam after spinal anaesthesia. Anaesth. Intens. Care 16: 292, 1988.

BLAND, J. H. L., AND LOWENSTEIN, E.: Halothane-induced decrease in experimental myocardial ischemia in the non-failing canine heart. Anesthesiology 45: 287, 1976.

BLOMBERG, S., EMANUELSSON, H., AND RICKSTEN, S.-E.: Thoracic epidural anesthesia and central hemodynamics in patients with unstable angina pectoris. Anesth. Analg. 69: 558, 1989.

BLOMBERG, S., EMANUELSSON, H., KVIST, H., LAMM, C., PONTEN, J., WAAGSTEIN, F., AND RICKSTEN, S.-E.: Effects of thoracic epidural anesthesia on coronary arteries and arterioles in patients with coronary artery disease. Anesthesiology 73: 840, 1990.

BOHLEN, H. G., AND GORE, R. W.: Comparison of microvascular pressures and diameters in the innervated and denervated rat intestine. Microvasc. Res. 74: 251, 1977.

BONICA, J. J., KENNEDY, W. F., JR., WARD, R. J., AND TOLAS, A. G.: A comparison of the effects of high subarachnoid and epidural anaesthesia. Acta Anaesthesiol. Scand. Suppl. 23: 429, 1966.

BONNET, F., DIALLO, A., SAADA, M., BELON, M., GUILBAUD, M., AND BOICO, O.: Prevention of tourniquet pain by spinal isobaric bupivacaine with clonidine. Br. J. Anaesth 63: 93, 1989.

BONNET, F., BRUN-BUISSON, V., SAADA, M., BOICO, O., ROSTAING, S., AND TOUBOUL, C.: Dose-related prolongation of hyperbaric tetracaine spinal anesthesia by clonidine in humans. Anesth. Analg. 68: 619, 1989.

BOWER, J. O., CLARK, J. H., WAGONER, G., AND BURNS, J. C.: Spinal anesthesia; a summary of clinical and experimental investigations with practical deductions. Surg. Gynecol. Obstet. 54: 882, 1932.

BOWER, J. O., WAGONER, G., AND CLARK, J. H.: Clinical and experimental investigation in spinal anesthesia. Anesth. Analg. 5: 95, 1926.

BRADSHAW, H. H.: The fall in blood pressure during spinal anesthesia. Ann. Surg. 104: 41, 1936.

BRAUNWALD, E.: Control of myocardial oxygen consumption: physiologic and clinical considerations. Am. J. Cardiol. 27: 416, 1971.

BREWSTER, W. R., JR., ISAACS, J. P., OSGOOD, P. F., AND KING, T. L.: The hemodynamic and metabolic interrelationships in the activity of epinephrine, norepinephrine and the thyroid hormones. Circulation 13: 1, 1956.

BRIDENBAUGH, P. O., MOORE, D. C., AND BRIDENBAUGH, L. D.: Capillary PO_2 as a measure of sympathetic blockade. Anesth. Analg. 50: 26, 1971.

BRIGDEN, W., HOWARTH, S., AND SHARPEY-SCHAFER, E. P.: Postural changes in the peripheral blood-flow of normal subjects with observations on vasovagal fainting reactions as a result of tilting, the lordotic posture, pregnancy, and spinal anesthesia. Clin. Sci. 9: 79, 1950.

BRILL, S., AND LAWRENCE, L. B.: Changes in temperature of the lower extremities following the induction of spinal anesthesia. Proc. Soc. Exp. Biol. Med. 27: 728, 1930.

BRULL, S. J., AND GREENE, N. M.: Time-courses of zones of differential sensory blockade during spinal anesthesia with hyperbaric tetracaine or bupivacaine. Anesth. Analg. 69: 342, 1989.

BRULL, S. J., LIEPONIS, J. V., MURPHY, M. J., GARCIA, R., AND SILVERMAN, D. G.: Acute and long-term benefits of iliac crest donor site perfusion with local anesthetics. Anesth. Analg. 74: 145, 1992.

BURCH, J. C., AND HARRISON, T. R.: The effect of spinal anesthesia on the cardiac output. Arch. Surg. 21: 330, 1930.

BURCH, J. C., AND HARRISON, T. R.: The effect of spinal anesthesia on arterial tone. Arch. Surg. 22: 1040, 1931.

BURCH, J. C., HARRISON, T. R., AND BLALOCK, A.: A comparison of the effects of hemorrhage under ether anesthesia and under spinal anesthesia. Arch. Surg. 21: 693, 1930.

BURSTEIN, C. L.: Postural blood pressure changes during spinal anesthesia: a preliminary experimental report. Anesth. Analg. 18: 132, 1939.

BURTON, A. C.: Role of geometry, of size and shape, in the microcirculation. Fed. Proc. 25: 1753, 1966.

BURTON, K. S., AND JOHNSON, P. C.: Reactive hyperemia in individual capillaries of skeletal muscle. Am. J. Physiol. 223: 517, 1972.

BUTTERWORTH, J. F., IV, AUSTIN, J. C., JOHNSON, M. D., BERRIZBEITIA, L. D., DANCE, G. R., HOWARD, G., AND COHN, L. H.: Effect of total spinal anesthesia on arterial and venous responses to dopamine and dobutamine. Anesth. Analg. 66: 209, 1987.

BUTTERWORTH, J. F., IV, PICCIONE, W., JR., BERRIZBEITIA, L. D., DANCE, G., SHEMIN, R. J., AND COHN, L. H.: Augmentation of venous return by adrenergic agonists during spinal anesthesia. Anesth. Analg. 65: 612, 1986.

CABALUM, T., ZUGAIB, M., LIEB, S., NUWAYHID, B., BRINKMAN, C. R., III, AND ASSALI, N. S.: Effect of dopamine on hypotension induced by spinal anesthesia. Am. J. Obstet. Gynecol. 133: 630, 1979.

CAIN, W. E., AND HAMILTON, W. K.: Central and peripheral venous oxygen saturations during spinal anesthesia. Anesthesiology 27: 209, 1966.

CALLESEN, T., JARNVIG, I., THAGE, B., KRANTZ, T., AND CHRISTIANSEN, C.: Influence of temperature of bupivacaine on spread of spinal analgesia. Anaesthesia 46: 17, 1991.

CANNON, W. B., AND ROSENBLUETH, A.: *The Supersensitivity of Denervated Structures. A Law of Denervation.* New York: The Macmillan Co., 1949.

CAPLAN, R. A., WARD, R. J., POSNER, K., AND CHENEY, F. W.: Unexpected cardiac arrest during spinal anesthesia: a closed claims analysis of predisposing factors. Anesthesiology 68: 5, 1988.

CAPPS: R. B.: A method for measuring tone and reflex constriction of the capillaries, venules, and veins of the human hand with the results in normal and diseased states. J. Clin. Invest. 15: 229, 1936.

CASTENFORS, J., LINDBLAD, L. E., AND MORTASAWI, A.: Effect of dihydroergotamine on peripheral circulation during epidural anaesthesia in man. Acta Anaesth. Scand. 19: 79, 1975.

CERILLI, G. J., AND ENGELL, H. C.: The effect of spinal anesthesia on femoral vein oxygen tension. Surgery 60: 668, 1966.

CERNACEK, P., AND STEWART, D. J.: Immunoreactive endothelin in human plasma: marked elevations in patients in cardiogenic shock. Biochem. Biophys. Res. Commun. 161: 562, 1989.

CHAMBERS, R.: Blood capillary circulation under normal conditions and in traumatic shock. Nature 162: 835, 1948.

CHAMBERS, R., AND ZWEIFACH, B. W.: Topography and function of the mesenteric capillary circulation. Am. J. Anat. 75: 173, 1944.

CHAMBERS, R., AND ZWEIFACH, B. W.: Intercellular cement and capillary permeability. Physiol. Rev. 27: 436, 1947.

CHIEN, S.: Rheology of sickle cells and the microcirculation. N. Engl. J. Med. 311: 1567, 1984.

CO TUI, F. W.: The effect of pathologic states on the minimum lethal dose of procaine intracisternally. J. Pharmacol. Exp. Ther. 50: 51, 1934.

CO TUI, F. W.: Spinal anesthesia: the experimental basis of some prevailing clinical practices. Arch. Surg. 33: 825, 1936.

CO TUI, F. W., AND STANDARD, S.: Experimental studies on subarachnoid anesthesia: paralysis of vital medullary centers. Surg. Gynecol. Obstet. 55: 290, 1932.

COBBOLD, A., FOLKOW, B., KJELLMER, I., AND MELLANDER, S.: Nervous and local chemical control of pre-capillary sphincters in skeletal muscle as measured by changes in filtration coefficient. Acta Physiol. Scand. 57: 180, 1963.

COCKS, T. M., BROUGHTON, A., DIB, M., SUDHIR, K., AND ANGUS, J. A.: Endothelin is blood vessel selective: studies on a variety of human and dog vessels in vitro and on regional blood flow in the conscious rabbit. Clin. Exp. Pharmacol. Physiol. 16: 243, 1989.

COE, A. J., AND REVANÄS, B.: Forum: Is crystalloid preloading useful in spinal anaesthesia in the elderly? Anaesthesia 45: 241, 1990.

COHEN, L. I.: Asystole during spinal anesthesia in a patient with sick sinus syndrome. Anesthesiology 68: 787, 1988.

COLE, F.: Head lowering in treatment of hypotension. J. A. M. A. 150: 273, 1952.

COOK, P. T., DAVIES, M. J., CRONIN, K. D., AND MORAN, P.: A prospective randomised trial comparing spinal anesthesia using hyperbaric cinchocaine with general anaesthesia for lower limb vascular surgery. Anaesth. Intens. Care 14(4): 373, 1986.

COOPER, T., WILLMAN, V. L., AND HERTZMAN, A. B.: Vascular reactivity to epinephrine following sympathectomy. Fed. Proc. 15: 40, 1956.

COVERT, C. R., AND FOX, G. S.: Anaesthesia for hip surgery in the elderly. Can. J. Anaesth. 36: 311, 1989.

CRILE, G. W., AND LOWER, W. E.: Anoci-Association. Philadelphia: W. B. Saunders Co., 1915.

CRONENWETT, J. L., ZELENOCK, G. B., WHITEHOUSE, W. M., JR., STANLEY, J. C., AND LINDENAUER, S. M.: The effect of sympathetic innervation on canine muscle and skin blood flow. Arch. Surg. 118: 420, 1983.

CROWELL, J. W., AND SMITH, E. E.: Determinant of the optimal hematocrit. J. Appl. Physiol. 22: 501, 1967.

CUCCHIARA, R. F., AND RESTALL, C. J. O.: Mephentermine and intravenous fluids for the prevention of hypotension associated with spinal anesthesia. Anesthesiology 39: 109, 1973.

CURBELLO, M. M.: Continuous peridural segmental anesthesia by means of a urethral catheter. Anesth. Analg. 28: 12, 1949.

DALE, H. H., AND RICHARDS, A. N.: The vasodilator action of histamine and of some other substances. J. Physiol. 52: 110, 1918–1919.

DALENS, B. J.: Pediatric Regional Anesthesia. Boca Raton, Florida: CRC Press, 1990.

DANOFF, D. S., AND GREENE, N. M.: Vasodilation and the metabolic response to hemorrhage. Surgery 55: 820, 1964.

DAVIS, M. T., AND GREENE, N. M.: Polarographic studies of skin oxygen tension following sympathetic denervation. J. Appl. Physiol. 14: 961, 1959.

DAVIS, F. M., AND LAURENSON, V. G.: Spinal anaesthesia or general anaesthesia for emergency hip surgery in elderly patients. Anaesth. Intens. Care 9: 532, 1981.

DAVIS, F. M., LAURENSON, V. G., GILLESPIE, W. J., FOATE, J., AND SEAGAR, A. D.: Leg blood flow during total hip replacement under spinal or general anaesthesia. Anaesth. Intens. Care 17: 136, 1989 a.

DAVIS, F. M., LAURENSON, V. G., GILLESPIE, W. J., WELLS, J. E., FOATE, J., AND NEWMAN, E.: Deep vein thrombosis after total hip replacement. J. Bone Joint Surg. 71: 181, 1989 b.

DAVIS, F. M., McDERMOTT, E., HICKTON, C., WELLS, E., HEATON, D. C., LAURENSON, V. G., GILLESPIE, W. J., AND FOATE, J.: Influence of spinal and general anaesthesia on haemostasis during total hip arthroplasty. Br. J. Anaesth. 59: 561, 1987.

DE ANGELIS, J., CHANG, P., KAPLAN, J. H., KUDISH, H., SACKS, S., WENDER, R., BONWELL, P., AND BLUESTONE, D.: Hemodynamic changes during prostatectomy in cardiac patients. Crit. Care Med. 10: 38, 1982.

DE MAREES, H., DE CALEYA, C., HEMPELMANN, G., AND SIPPEL, R.: Der einfluss der spinalanästhesie auf die periphere hamodynamik. Z. Kardiol. 65: 478, 1976.

DEFALQUE, R. J.: Compared effects of spinal and extradural anesthesia upon the blood pressure. Anesthesiology 23: 627, 1962.

DEMEL, R., AND BURKE, J.: Die Regulierbare hohe Ruckenmarksanasthesie. Zentralbl. Chir. *57:* 838, 1930.

DOHI, S., NAITO, H., AND TAKAHASHI, T.: Age-related changes in blood pressure and duration of motor block in spinal anesthesia. Anesthesiology *50:* 319, 1979.

DOMENECH-ALSINA, F.: Les accidents graves immédiats de la rachianesthésie: leur pathogénie et leur traitment. J. Chir. *40:* 371, 1932.

DOUD, E. A., AND ROVENSTINE, E. A.: Changes in the velocity of the blood flow during spinal anesthesia. Anesthesiology *1:* 82, 1940.

DUNER, H., GRANATH, A., AND KLINGENSTROM, P.: The effect of ergotamine on blood pressure and cardiac output during spinal anaesthesia in man. Acta Anaesthesiol. Scand. *4:* 5, 1960.

EATHER, K. F., PETERSON, L. H., AND DRIPPS, R. D.: Studies of the circulation of anesthetized patients by a new method for recording arterial pressure and pressure pulse contours. Anesthesiology *10:* 125, 1949.

ECKENHOFF, J. E., HAFKENSCHIEL, J. H., FOLTZ, E. L., AND DRIVER, R. L.: Influence of hypotension on coronary blood flow, cardiac work, and cardiac efficiency. Am. J. Physiol. *152:* 545, 1948.

ECONOMACOS, G., AND SKOUNTZOS, V.: Clinical aspects of high spinal anaesthesia in urological surgery on 3012 patients. Acta Anaesth. Belg. *31* (Suppl.): 183, 1980.

EDERSTROM, H. E., VERGEER, T., RHODE, R. A., AND AHLNESS, P.: Quantitative changes in foot blood flow in the dog following sympathectomy and motor denervation. Am. J. Physiol. *187:* 461, 1956.

EICHNA, L. W.: Capillary blood pressure in man. Direct measurements in the digits of patients with Raynaud's disease and scleroderma before and after sympathectomy. Am. Heart A. *25:* 812, 1943.

EICHNA, L. W., AND BORDLEY, A., III: Capillary blood pressure in man. Direct measurements in digits of normal and hypertensive subjects during vasoconstriction and vasodilation variously induced. J. Clin. Invest. *21:* 711, 1942.

EICHNA, L. W., AND WILKINS, R. W.: Capillary blood pressure in man. Direct measurements in the digits during induced vasoconstriction. J. Clin. Invest. *21:* 697, 1942.

EIGE, S. A., AND BELL, C.: Pediatric pain management, in BELL, C., HUGHES, C. W., AND OH, T. H., *The Pediatric Anesthesia Handbook.* St. Louis: Mosby-Year Book, Inc., pp. 503–528, 1991.

ELDOR, A., FALCONE, D. J., HAJJAR, D. P., MINICK, C. R., AND WEKSLER, B. B.: Recovery of prostacyclin production by de-endothelialized rabbit aorta. Critical role of neointimal smooth muscle cells. J. Clin. Invest. *67:* 735, 1981.

ELSTEIN, I. D., AND MARX, G. F.: Electrocardiographic changes during cesarean section under regional anesthesia (lett.). Anesth. Analg. *71:* 100, 1990.

ENGEL, D.: The influence of the sympathetic nervous system on capillary permeability. J. Physiol. *99:* 161, 1940.

ERIKSSON, E., AND LISANDER, B.: Change in precapillary resistance in skeletal muscle vessels studied by intravital microscopy. Acta Physiol. Scand. *84:* 295, 1972.

EVANS, C. H.: *Spinal Anesthesia (Subarachnoid Radicular Conduction Block): Principles and Technic.* New York: Paul B. Hoeber, Inc., 1929.

EVANS, C. H.: Possible complications with spinal anesthesia: their recognition and the measures employed to prevent and to combat them. Am. J. Surg. *5:* 581, 1928.

FAGRELL, B., INTAGLIETTA, M., AND ÖSTERGREN, J.: Relative hematocrit in human skin capillaries and its relation to capillary blood flow velocity. Microvasc. Res. *20:* 327, 1980.

FELDER, D. A., LINTON, R. R., TODD, D. P., AND BANKS, C.: Changes in the sympathectomized extremity with anesthesia. Surgery *29:* 803, 1951.

FELDMAN, H. S., ARTHUR, G. R., AND COVINO, B. G.: Cardiovascular effects of total spinal anesthesia following intrathecal administration of bupivacaine with and without epinephrine in the dog. Regional Anesth. *9:* 22, 1984.

FERGUSON, L. K., AND NORTH, J. P.: Observations on experimental spinal anesthesia. Surg. Gynecol. Obstet. *54:* 621, 1932.

FINCH, L., HICKS, P. E., AND PALEY, H. E.: Investigation into the role of spinal alpha adrenoceptors in cardiovascular modulation in rats. Br. J. Pharmacol. *68:* 185P, 1980.

FISCH, S., GILSON, S. B., AND TAYLOR, R. E.: Capillary circulation in human arms studied by venous congestion. A cutaneo-muscular vasomotor reflex. J. Appl. Physiol. *3:* 113, 1950.

FOATE, J. A., HORTON, H., AND DAVIS, F. M.: Lower limb blood flow during transurethral resection of the prostate under spinal or general anaesthesia. Anaesth. Intens. Care *13:* 383, 1985.

FOLKOW, B.: Intravascular pressure as a factor regulating the tone of the small vessels. Acta Physiol. Scand. *17:* 289, 1949.

FOLKOW, B.: Nervous control of blood vessels. Physiol. Rev. *35:* 629, 1955.

FOLKOW, B., AND MELLANDER, S.: Veins and venous tone. Am. Heart J. *68:* 397, 1964.

FOREGGER, R.: Surface temperatures during anesthesia. Anesthesiology *4:* 392, 1943.

FOSTER, A. D., NEUMAN, C., AND ROVENSTINE, E. A.: Peripheral circulation during anesthesia, shock, and hemorrhage: the digital plethysmograph as a clinical guide. Anesthesiology *6:* 246, 1945.

FREEMAN, N. E.: The effect of temperature on the rate of blood flow in the normal and in the sympathectomized hand. Am. J. Physiol. *113:* 384, 1935.

FREEMAN, N. E., AND MONTGOMERY, H.: Lumbar sympathectomy in treatment of intermittent claudication: selection of cases by claudication test with lumbar paravertebral procaine injection. Am. Heart J. *23:* 224, 1942.

FREEMAN, N. E., SHAFER, S. A., SCHECTER, A. E., AND HOLLING, H. E.: The effect of total sympathectomy on the occurrence of shock from hemorrhage. J. Clin. Invest. *17:* 359, 1938.

FREIS, E. D., SCHNAPER, H. W., AND LILIENFIELD, L. S.: Rapid and slow components of the circulation in the human forearm. J. Clin. Invest. *36:* 245, 1957.

FREIS, E. D., STANTON, J. R., AND EMERSON, C. P.: Estimation of relative velocities of plasma and red cells in the circulation of man. Am. J. Physiol. *157:* 153, 1949.

FRIEDLAND, C. K., HUNT, J. S., AND WILKINS, R. W.: Effects of changes in venous pressure upon blood flow in the limbs. Am. Heart J. *25:* 631, 1943.

FRUMIN, M. J., NGAI, S. H., AND WANG, S. C.: Evaluation of vasodilator mechanisms in the canine hind leg: question of dorsal root participation. Am. J. Physiol. *173:* 428, 1953.

FRYE, R. L., BRAUNWALD, E., AND COHEN, E. R.: Studies on Starling's Law of the heart. I. The circulatory response to acute hypervolemia and its modification by ganglionic blockade. J. Clin. Invest. *39:* 1043, 1960.

FUCHS, R. M., RUTLEN, D. L., AND POWELL, W. J., JR.: Effect of dobutamine on systemic capacity in the dog. Circ. Res. *46:* 133, 1980.

FURCHGOTT, R. F.: Role of endothelium in responses of vascular smooth muscle. Circ. Res. *53:* 557, 1983.

FURCHGOTT, R. F., AND ZAWADZKI, J. V.: The obligatory role of endothelial cells in the relaxation of arterial smooth muscle by acetylcholine. Nature *288:* 373, 1980.

GALINDO, A.: Hemodynamic changes in the internal carotid artery produced by total sympathetic block (epidural anesthesia) and carbon dioxide. Anesth. Analg. *43:* 276, 1964.

GALLAGHER, T. M., AND CREAN, P. M.: Spinal anaesthesia in infants born prematurely. Anaesthesia *44:* 434, 1989.

GASKELL, P., AND KRISMAN, A. M.: The brachial to digital blood pressure gradient in normal subjects and in patients with high blood pressure. Can. J. Biochem. Physiol. *36:* 889, 1958.

GERBERSHAGEN, H. V., AND KENNEDY, W. F., JR.: Herzstillstand nach hoher Spinalanaesthesia. Anaesthesist *20:* 192, 1971.

GIASI, R. M., D'AGOSTINO, E., AND COVINO, B. G.: Absorption of lidocaine following sub-arachnoid and epidural administration. Anesth. Analg. 58: 360, 1979.

GILLIES, J.: Anaesthesia for the surgical treatment of hypertension. Proc. R. Soc. Med. 42: 295, 1949.

GILLIES, J.: Anaesthetic factors in the causation and prevention of excessive bleeding during surgical operations. Ann. R. Coll. Surg. Engl. 7: 204, 1950.

GLICK, G., AND BRAUNWALD, E.: Relative roles of the sympathetic and parasympathetic nervous systems in the reflex control of heart rate. Circ. Res. 16: 363, 1965.

GOLDFARB, W., PROVISOR, B., AND KOSTER, H.: Circulation during spinal anesthesia. Arch. Surg. 39: 429, 1939.

GORDH, T.: Postural circulatory and respiratory changes during ether and intravenous anaesthesia: an experimental analysis of the significance of postural changes during anaesthesia with special regard to the value of the head-down posture in resuscitation. Acta Chir. Scand. (Suppl.) 92: 102, 1945.

GORDON, R. J., AND RAVIN, M. B.: Rheology and anesthesiology. Anesth. Analg. 57: 252, 1978.

GORE, R. W.: Pressures in cat mesenteric arterioles and capillaries during changes in systemic arterial blood pressure. Circ. Res. 34: 581, 1974.

GOTO, F., FUJITA, N., AND FUJITA, T.: Cerebrospinal norepinephrine concentrations and the duration of epidural analgesia. Can. J. Anaesth. 37: 839, 1990.

GOTO, F., FUJITA, N., AND FUJITA, T.: Cerebrospinal fluid catecholamine levels and duration of spinal anaesthesia. Can. J. Anaesth. 35: 157, 1988.

GRAHAM, A. J. P., AND DOUGLAS, D. M.: Effect of the head-down position on the circulation in hypotensive states. Lancet 2: 941, 1949.

GRANT, R. T.: Observations on local arterial reactions in the rabbit's ear. Heart 15: 257, 1929–1931.

GRANT, R. T., AND PEARSON, R. S.: The blood circulation in the human limb: observations on the differences between the proximal and distal parts and remarks on the regulation of body temperature. Clin. Sci. 3: 119, 1938.

GRAVES, C. L., AND KLEIN, R. L.: Central venous pressure monitoring during routine spinal anesthesia. Arch. Surg. 97: 843, 1968.

GRAVES, C. L., UNDERWOOD, P. S., KLEIN, R. L., AND KIM, Y. I.: Intravenous fluid administration as therapy for hypotension secondary to spinal anesthesia. Anesth. Analg. 47: 548, 1968.

GRAY, H. T., AND PARSONS, L.: Blood pressure variations associated with lumbar puncture and the induction of spinal anesthesia. Q. J. Med. 5: 339, 1912.

GREEN, H. D., LEWIS, R. N., NICKERSON, N. D., AND HELLER, A. L.: Blood flow, peripheral resistance, and vascular tonus with observations on the relationship between blood flow and cutaneous temperature. Am. J. Physiol. 141: 518, 1944.

GREEN, H. D., AND KEPCHAR, J. H.: Control of peripheral resistance in major systemic vascular beds. Physiol. Rev. 39: 617, 1959.

GREEN, J. F.: Mechanism of action of isoproterenol on venous return. Am. J. Physiol. 232: H152, 1977.

GREENE, N. M.: Hypotensive spinal anesthesia. Surg. Gynecol. Obstet. 95: 331, 1952.

GREENE, N. M.: The pharmacology of local anesthetic agents with special reference to their use in spinal anesthesia. Anesthesiology 16: 573, 1955.

GREENE, N. M.: Blood levels of local anesthesics during spinal and epidural anesthesia. Anesth. Analg. 56: 357, 1979.

GREENE, N. M., AND BACHAND, R. G.: Vagal component of the chronotropic response to baroreceptor stimulation in man. Am. Heart J. 82: 22, 1971.

GREENE, N. M., BUNKER, J. P., KERR, W. S., VON FELSINGER, J. M., KELLER, J. W., AND BEECHER, H. K.: Hypotensive spinal anesthesia: respiratory, metabolic, hepatic, renal, and cerebral effects. Ann. Surg. 140: 641, 1954.

GREGORETTI, S.: Case report. Paroxysmal atrio-ventricular heart block during spinal anesthesia. Regional Anesth. 10: 149, 1985.

GREGORY, R., AND LEVIN, W. C.: Studies on hypertension. V. Effect of high spinal anesthesia on the blood pressure of patients with hypertension and far-advanced renal disease—its possible relationship to the pathogenesis of hypertension. J. Lab. Clin. Med. 30: 1037, 1945.

GREGORY, R., AND LEVIN, W. C.: Studies on hypertension. VII. Mechanism of the fall in arterial pressure produced by high spinal anesthesia in patients with essential hypertension. Arch. Intern. Med. 81: 352, 1948.

GRIFFIN, P. P., GREEN, H. D., YOUMANS, P. L., AND JOHNSON, H. D.: Effects of acute and chronic denervation of the hind leg of the dog on the blood flow responses in the vascular beds of skin and muscle to adrenergic drugs and to adrenergic blockade. J. Pharmacol. Exp. Ther. 110: 93, 1954.

GRIFFITHS, H. W. C., AND GILLIES, J.: Thoracolumbar splanchnicectomy and sympathectomy: anaesthetic procedure. Anaesthesia 3: 134, 1948.

GUEST, S. I., MANN, L. S., AND SEARLES, P. W.: The immediate effects of spinal Pontocaine anesthesia on blood volume in man. Anesthesiology 10: 289, 1949.

GUYTON, A. C., AND HARRIS, J. W.: Peripheral circulatory factors as determinants of cardiac output. Fed. Proc. 10: 57, 1951.

GUYTON, A. C., LINDSEY, A. W., ABERNATHY, B., AND LANGSTON, J. B.: Mechanism of increased venous return and cardiac output caused by epinephrine. Am. J. Physiol. 192: 126, 1958.

HACKEL, D. B., SANCETTA, S. M., AND KLEINERMAN, J.: Effect of hypotension due to spinal anesthesia on coronary blood flow and myocardial metabolism in man. Circulation 13: 92, 1956.

HADDY, F. J., AND GILBERT, R. P.: The relation of a venous-arteriolar reflex to transmural pressure and resistance in small and large systemic vessels. Circ. Res. 4: 25, 1956.

HADENFELDT, H.: Uber die Blutdruckhaltung wahrend der Ruckenmarksbetaubung. Arch. Klin. Chir. 168: 439, 1932.

HALLIGAN, E. J., GIBBS, J. C., JR., GRIECO, R. V., AND MCKEOWN, J. E.: An evaluation of peripheral arteriosclerotic insufficiency utilizing radioactive iodinated human serum albumin. Surg. Gynecol. Obstet. 102: 511, 1956.

HALTER, J. B., AND PFLUG, A. E.: Effect of sympathetic blockade by spinal anesthesia on pancreatic islet function in man. Am. J. Physiol. 239 (Endocrinol. Metab. 2): E150, 1980.

HAMPTON, L. J., AND LITTLE, D. M.: Results of a questionnaire concerning controlled hypotension in anaesthesia. Lancet 264: 1299, 1953 a.

HAMPTON, L. J., AND LITTLE, D. M.: Complications associated with the use of "controlled hypotension" in anesthesia. Arch. Surg. 67: 549, 1953 b.

HARANATH, P. S. R. K., AND VENKATAKRISHNA-BHATT, H.: Studies of cinchocaine and lidocaine administered intro cerebral ventricles of conscious and anaesthetized dogs. Indian J. Med. Res. 56: 217, 1968.

HARNIK, E. V., HOY, G. R., POTOLICCHIO, S., STEWART, D. R., AND SIEGELMAN, R. E.: Spinal anesthesia in premature infants recovering from respiratory distress syndrome. Anesthesiology 64: 95, 1986.

HARRISON, P. V., AND ALLEN, P. R.: Spinal anesthesia in treating leg ulcers. J. Dermatol. Surg. Oncol. 12: 753, 1986.

HEINEKE, H., AND LAEWEN, A.: Experimentelle Untersuchungen uber Lumbalanasthesie. Arch. Clin. Chir. 81: 373, 1906.

HEMMINGSEN, C., POULSEN, J. A., AND RISBO, A.: Prophylactic ephedrine during spinal anaesthesia: double-blind study in patients in ASA groups I–III. Br. J. Anaesth. 63: 340, 1989.

HIGGS, G. A., CARDINAL, D. C., MONCADA, S., AND VANE, J. R.: Microcirculatory effects of prostacyclin (PGI$_2$) in the hamster cheek pouch. Microvasc. Res. 18: 245, 1979.

HILGENBERG, J. C., AND JOHANTGEN, W. C.: Bradycardia after intravenous fentanyl during subarachnoid anesthesia. Anesth. Analg. 59: 161, 1980.

HILKE, H., KANTO, J., MANTYLA, R., KLEIMOLA, T., AND SYVALAHTI, E.: Dihydroergotamine: pharmacokinetics and usefulness in spinal anaesthesia. Acta Anaesthesiol. Scand. 22: 215, 1978.

HILTON, J. G.: Effects of spinal anesthesia and adrenalectomy on blood pressure responses to histamine. Am. J. Physiol. 190: 77, 1957.

HINGSON, R. A., AND HELLMAN, L. M.: Organization of obstetric anesthesia on a 24-hour basis in a large and a small hospital. Anesthesiology 12: 745, 1951.

HINGSON, R. A., AND SOUTHWORTH, J. L.: The use of continuous caudal and continuous spinal analgesia in the diagnosis, prognosis, and rehabilitation of the peripheral vascular diseases of the lower extremities. Milit. Surg. 100: 474, 1947.

HYMAN, C.: Filtration across the vascular wall as a function of several factors. Am. J. Physiol. 142: 671, 1944.

IGNARRO, L. J.: Biological actions and properties of endothelium-derived nitric oxide formed and released from artery and vein. Circ. Res. 65: 1, 1989.

IGNARRO, L. J., BYRNS, R. E., BUGA, G. M., AND WOOD, K. S.: Endothelium-derived relaxing factor (EDRF) released from artery and vein appears to be nitric oxide (NO) or a closely related radical species. Fed. Proc. 46: 644, 1987.

JAMES, F. M., III, AND GREISS, F. C., JR.: The use of inflatable boots to prevent hypotension during spinal anesthesia for cesarean section. Anesth. Analg. 52: 246, 1973.

JANVRIN, S. B., DAVIES, G., AND GREENHALGH, R. M.: Postoperative deep vein thrombosis caused by intravenous fluids during surgery. Br. J. Surg. 67: 690, 1980.

JOHNS, R. A.: Local anesthetics inhibit endothelium-dependent vasodilation. Anesthesiology 70: 805, 1989.

JOHNSON, S. R.: The effect of some anesthetic agents on the circulation in man. Acta Chir. Scandinav. (Suppl.) 158: 9, 1951.

JOHNSTON, J. F. A., AND HENDERSON, V. E.: An experimental enquiry into spinal anesthesia. Anesth. Analg. 11: 78, 1932.

JONNESCO, T.: Remarks on general spinal anaesthesia. Br. Med. J. 2: 1396, 1909.

KANTO, J., MAENPAA, M., MANTYLA, R., SELLMAN, R., AND VALOVIRTA, E.: Effect of age on the pharmacokinetics of diazepam given in conjunction with spinal anesthesia. Anesthesiology 51: 154, 1979.

KAPPAGODA, C. T., LINDEN, R. J., AND SNOW, H. M.: A reflex increase in heart rate from distension of the junction between the superior vena cava and the right atrium. J. Physiol. (Lond.) 220: 177, 1972.

KEHLET, H.: Modification of responses to surgery and anesthesia by neural blockade, in COUSINS, M. J., BRIDENBAUGH, P. O., Neural Blockade in Clinical Anesthesia and Management of Pain. Philadelphia: J. B. Lippincott, Co., 1987.

KENNEDY, W. F., JR., BONICA, J. J., AKAMATSU, T. J., WARD, R. J., MARTIN, W. E., AND GRINSTEIN, A.: Cardiovascular and respiratory effects of subarachnoid block in the presence of acute blood loss. Anesthesiology 29: 29, 1968.

KENNEDY, W. F., JR., EVERETT, G. B., COBB, L. A., AND ALLEN, G. D.: Simultaneous systemic and hepatic hemodynamic measurements during high spinal anesthesia in normal man. Anesth. Analg. 49: 1016, 1970 a.

KENNEDY, W. F., JR., SAWYER, T. K., GERBERSHAGEN, H. U., EVERETT, G. B., CUTLER, R. E., AND BONICA, J. J.: Simultaneous systemic cardiovascular and renal hemodynamic measurements during high spinal anaesthesia in man. Acta Anaesthesiol. Scand. Suppl. 37: 163, 1970 b.

KETY, S. S., KING, B. D., HORVATH, S. M., JEFFERS, W. A., AND HAFKENSCHIEL, J. H.: The effects of an acute reduction in blood pressure by means of differential spinal sympathetic block on the cerebral circulation of hypertensive patients. J. Clin. Invest. 29: 402, 1950.

KHAN, M. T., AND FURCHGOTT, R. F.: Similarities of behavior of nitric oxide (NO) and endothelium-derived relaxing factor in a perfusion cascade bioassay system. Fed. Proc. 46: 385, 1987.

KIM, J. M., AND REED, K.: PvO$_2$ changes in cutaneous veins during regression of spinal anaesthesia. Can. J. Anaesth. 34: 358, 1987.

KIM, J. M., LASALLE, A. D., AND PARMLEY, R. T.: Sympathetic recovery following lumbar epidural and spinal analgesia. Anesth. Analg. 56: 352, 1977.

KING, B. D., AND DRIPPS, R. D.: The use of methoxamine for maintenance of the circulation during spinal anesthesia. Surg. Gynecol. Obstet. 90: 659, 1950.

KLAPP, R.: Experimentelle Studien uber Lumbalanaesthesie. Arch. Klin. Chir. 75: 151, 1905.

KLASSEN, G. A., BRAMWELL, R. S., BROMAGE, P. R., AND ZBOROWSKA-SLUIS, D. T.: Effect of acute sympathectomy by epidural anesthesia on the canine circulation. Anesthesiology 52: 8, 1980.

KLEINERMAN, J., SANCETTA, S. M., AND HACKEL, D. B.: Effects of high spinal anesthesia on cerebral circulation and metabolism in man. J. Clin. Invest. 37: 285, 1958.

KLINGENSTROM, P.: The effect of ergotamine on blood pressure, especially in spinal anaesthesia. Acta Anaesthesiol. Scand. (Suppl.) 4, 1960.

KLOCKE, F. J., ELLIS, A. K., AND ORLICK, A. E.: Sympathetic influences on coronary perfusion and evolving concepts of driving pressure, resistance, and transmural flow regulation. Anesthesiology 52: 1, 1980.

KOCK, M., BLOMBERG, S., EMANUELSSON, H., LOMSKY, M., STROMBLAD, S-O., AND RICKSTEN, S-E.: Thoracic epidural anesthesia improves global and regional left ventricular function during stress-induced myocardial ischemia in patients with coronary artery disease. Anesth. Analg. 71: 625, 1990.

KOSTER, H.: Spinal anesthesia, with special reference to its use in surgery of the head, neck, and thorax. Am. J. Surg. 5: 554, 1928.

KOSTER, H., AND KASMAN, L. P.: Spinal anesthesia for the head, neck, and thorax; its relation to respiratory paralysis. Surg. Gynecol. Obstet. 49: 617, 1929.

KOSTER, H., SHAPIRO, A., AND LEIKENSOHN, A.: Concentration of procaine in the cerebrospinal fluid of the human being after subarachnoid injection. Arch. Surg. 37: 603, 1938.

KREUTZ, J. M., AND MAZUZAN, J. E.: Sudden asystole in a marathon runner: the athletic heart syndrome and its anesthetic implications. Anesthesiology 73: 1266, 1990.

KROGH, A.: Anatomy and Physiology of Capillaries. New Haven, Connecticut: Yale University Press, 1929.

KUNKEL, P., STEAD, E. A., JR., AND WEISS, S.: Blood flow and vasomotor reactions in the hand, forearm, foot, and calf in response to physical and chemical stimuli. J. Clin. Invest. 18: 225, 1939.

KUNSTADT, D., PUNJA, M., CAGIN, N., GERNANDEZ, P., LEVITT, B., AND YUCEOGLU, Y. Z.: Bifascicular block: a clinical and electrophysiologic study. Am. Heart J. 86: 173, 1973.

LABAT, G.: The trend of subarachnoid block. Surg. Clin. North Am. 10: 671, 1930.

LAHNBORG, G., AND BERGSTROM, K.: Clinical and haemostatic parameters related to thromboembolism and low-dose heparin prophylaxis in major surgery. Acta Chir. Scand. 141: 590, 1975.

LAKS, H., PILON, R. N., KLOVENKORN, W. P., ANDERSON, W., MacCALLUM, J. R., AND O'CONNOR, N. E.: Acute hemodilution: its effect on hemodynamics and oxygen transport in anesthetized man. Ann. Surg. 180: 103, 1973.

LANDIS, E. M.: Micro-injection studies of capillary blood pressure in human skin. Heart 15: 209, 1929–1931.

LANDIS, E. M.: Capillary pressure and capillary permeability. Physiol. Rev. 14: 404, 1934.

LEE, J. S.: Determination of lateral pressure in small blood vessels by the microchamber method. J. Appl. Physiol. 10: 329, 1957.

LEE, R. E., AND HOLZE, E. A.: The peripheral vascular system in the bulbar conjunctiva of young normotensive adults at rest. J. Clin. Invest. 29: 146, 1950.

LEIER, C. V., AND UNVERFERTH, D. V.: Dobutamine. Ann. Intern. Med. 99: 490: 1983.

LEVACK, I. D., HOLMES, J. D., AND ROBERTSON, G. S.: Abdominal would perfusion for the relief of postoperative pain. Br. J. Anaesth. 58: 615, 1986.

LEWIS, D. L., AND PALSER, E. G. M.: Changes in blood pressure and respiratory volume following a spinal anaesthetic. Br. Med. J. 1: 1202, 1938.

LEWIS, D. L., AND THOMPSON, W. A. L.: Reduction of post-operative pain. Br. Med. J. 1: 973, 1953.

LEWIS, T.: Observations upon the reaction of the vessels of the human skin to cold. Heart 15: 177, 1929–1931.

LEWIS, T., AND LANDIS, E. M.: Some physiological effects of sympathetic ganglionectomy in the human being and its effect in a case of Raynaud's malady. Heart 15: 151, 1929–1931.

LEWIS, T., AND PICKERING, G. W.: Vasodilation in the limbs in response to warming the body, with evidence for sympathetic vasodilator nerves in man. Heart 16: 33, 1931.

LI, T-H., SHIMOSATO, S., AND ETSTEN, B. E.: Methoxamine and cardiac output in nonanesthetized man and during spinal anesthesia. Anesthesiology 26: 21, 1965.

LI, T-H., SHIMOSATO, S., GAMBLE, C. A., AND ETSTEN, B. E.: Hemodynamics of mephentermine during spinal anesthesia in man. Anesthesiology 24: 817, 1963.

LOESCHKE, H. H., AND KOEPCHEN, H. P.: Versuch zur Lokalisation des Angriffsortes der Atmungs- und Kreisaufwirkung von Novocain im Liquor cerebrospinalis. Pflugers Arch. Ges. Physiol. 266: 628, 1958.

LORHAN, P. H., AND DEVINE, M. M.: Blood volume during low spinal anesthesia. Am. Surg. 18: 179, 1952.

LORHAN, P. H., AND MERRIAM, W.: Spinal anesthesia: analysis of causes of deaths in 716 cases. Surgery 31: 421, 1952.

LOUBSER, P., SUH, K., AND COHEN, S.: Adverse effects of spinal anesthesia in a patient with idiopathic hypertrophic subaortic stenosis. Anesthesiology 60: 228, 1984.

LUFT, J. H.: Fine structure of capillary and endocapillary layer as revealed by ruthenium red. Fed. Proc. 25: 1773, 1966.

LYNN, R. B., SANCETTA, S. M., SIMEONE, F. A., AND SCOTT, R. W.: Observations on the circulation in high spinal anesthesia. Surgery 32: 195, 1952.

MACKEY, D. C., CARPENTER, R. L., THOMPSON, G. E., BROWN, D. L., AND BODILY, M. N.: Bradycardia and asystole during spinal anesthesia: a report of three cases without morbidity. Anesthesiology 70: 866, 1989.

MADSEN, R. E., AND MADSEN, P. O.: Influence of anesthesia form on blood loss in transurethral prostatectomy. Anesth. Analg. 46: 330, 1967.

MAHE, V., AND ECOFFEY, C.: Spinal anesthesia with isobaric bupivacaine in infants. Anesthesiology 68: 601, 1988.

MAJID, P. A., DEFEYTER, P. J. F., VAN DER WALL, E. E., WARDEN, R., AND ROOS, J. P.: Molsidomine in the treatment of patients with angina pectoris: acute hemodynamic effects and clinical efficacy. N. Engl. J. Med. 302: 1, 1980.

MALMQVIST, L-A., BENGTSSON, M., BJORNSSON, G., JORFELDT, L., AND LOFSTROM, J. B.: Sympathetic activity and haemodynamic variables during spinal analgesia in man. Acta Anaesthesiol. Scand. 31: 467, 1987.

MANARA, A. R., SMITH, D. C., AND NIXON, C.: Sedation during spinal anaesthesia: a case for the routine administration of oxygen. Br. J. Anaesth. 63: 343, 1989.

MANN, L. S., AND GUEST, S. I.: Early effects of spinal anesthesia and surgery on blood volume in man. Am. J. Physiol. 161: 239, 1950.

MARK, A. L.: The Bezold-Jarisch reflex revisited: clinical implications of inhibitory reflexes originating in the heart. J. Am. Coll. Cardiol. 1: 90, 1983.

MARX, H., AND SCHOOP, W.: Studies of integral capillary pressure in man by the use of continuous recordings. Angiology 7: 541, 1956.

MASON, D. T.: The autonomic nervous system and regulation of cardiovascular performance. Anesthesiology 29: 670, 1968.

MASON, D. T., AND BARTTER, F. C.: Autonomic regulation of blood volume. Anesthesiology 29: 681, 1968.

MASON, D. T., ZELIS, R., AND AMSTERDAM, E. A.: Action of the nitrites on the peripheral circulation and myocardial oxygen consumption: significance in the relief of angina pectoris. Chest 59: 296, 1971.

MATHER, L. E., RUNCIMAN, W. B., ILSLEY, A. H., CARAPETIS, R. J., AND UPTON, R. N.: A sheep preparation for studying interactions between blood flow and drug disposition. V: The effects of general and subarachnoid anaesthesia on blood flow and pethidine disposition. Br. J. Anaesth. 58: 888, 1986.

MAY, L. G., BENNETT, A., LANE, A. L., FUTCH, E. D., LYNN-SCHOOMER, M., AND GREGORY, R.: Effect of high spinal anesthesia on the cardiac output of normal and hypertensive patients. Am. J. Med. 7: 251, 1949.

MAYROVITZ, H. N., TUMA, R. F., AND WIEDEMAN, M. P.: Relationship between microvascular blood velocity and pressure distribution. Am. J. Physiol. 232: H400, 1977.

McDOWALL, R. J. S., MALCOMSON, G. E., AND McWHAN, I.: The Control of the Circulation of the Blood. London: Dawson, 1956.

McGOWAN, S. W., AND SMITH, G. F. N.: Anaesthesia for transurethral prostatectomy: a comparison of spinal intradural analgesia with two methods of general anaesthesia. Anaesthesia 35: 847, 1980.

McKENZIE, P. J., WISHART, H. Y., GRAY, I., AND SMITH, G.: Effects of anaesthetic technique on deep vein thrombosis: a comparison of subarachnoid and general anaesthesia. Br. J. Anaesth. 57: 853, 1985.

McLEAN, A. P. H., MULLIGAN, G. W., OTTON, P., AND MACLEAN, L. D.: Hemodynamic alterations associated with epidural anesthesia. Surgery 62: 79, 1967.

McMASTER, P. D., HUDACK, S., AND ROUS, P.: The relation of hydrostatic pressure to the gradient of capillary permeability. J. Exp. Med. 55: 203, 1932.

MENSINK, F. J., KOZODY, R., KEHLER, C. H., AND WADE, J. G.: Dose-response relationship of clonidine in tetracaine spinal anesthesia. Anesthesiology 67: 717, 1987.

MILLER, V. M., KOMORI, K., BURNETT, J. C., JR., AND VANHOUTTE, P. M.: Differential sensitivity to endothelin in canine arteries and veins. Am. J. Physiol. 257: H1127, 1989.

MILSTEIN, S., BUETIKOFER, J., LESSER, J., ET AL.: Cardiac asystole: a manifestation of neurally mediated hypotension-bradycardia. J. Am. Coll. Cardiol. 14: 1626, 1989.

MILWIDSKY, H., AND DE VRIES, A.: Regulation of blood pressure during spinal anesthesia: observations on intramuscular pressure and skin temperature. Anesthesiology 9: 258, 1948.

MIYAUCHI, T., YANAGISAWA, M., TOMIZAWA, T., SUGISHATA, Y., SUZUKI, N., FUJINO, M., AJISAKA, P., GOTO, K., AND MASAKI, T.: Increased plasma concentrations of endothelin-1 and big endothelin-1 in acute myocardial infarction (lett.). Lancet 2: 53, 1989.

MODIG, J.: Influence of regional anaesthesia, local anaesthetics and sympathicomimetics on the pathophysiology of deep vein thrombosis. Acta. Chir. Scand. (Suppl.) 550: 119, 1988.

MODIG, J., BORG, T., BAGGE, L., AND SALDEEN, T.: Role of extradural and of general anaesthesia in fibrinolysis and coagulation after total hip replacement. Br. J. Anaesth. 55: 625, 1983.

MODIG, J., BORG, T., KARLSTROM., G., MARIPUU, E., AND SAHLSTEDT, B.: Thromboembolism after total hip replacement: role of epidural and general anesthesia. Anesth. Analg. 62:174, 1983.

MODIG, J., MUSCH, C., OLERUD, S., SALDEEN, T., AND WAERNBAUM, G.: Arterial hypotension and hypoxaemia during total hip replacement: the importance of thromboplastic products, fat embolism and acrylic monomers. Acta. Anaesth. Scand. 19: 28, 1975.

MOIR, D. D.: Blood loss during major vaginal surgery. A statistical study of the influence of general anaesthesia and epidural analgesia. Br. J. Anaesth. 40: 233, 1968.

MONCADA, S., HERMAN, A. G., HIGGS, E. A., AND VANE, J. R.: Differential formation of prostacyclin (PGX or PGI₂) by layers of the arterial wall. An explanation for the anti-thrombotic properties of vascular endothelium. Thromb. Res. 11: 323, 1977.

MORTON, J. J., AND SCOTT, W. J. M.: The measurement of sympathetic vasoconstrictor activity in the lower extremities. J. Clin. Invest. 9: 235, 1930.

MUELLER, R. P., LYNN, R. B., AND SANCETTA, S. M.: Studies of hemodynamic changes in humans following induction of low and high spinal anesthesia. II. The changes in splanchnic blood flow, oxygen extraction and consumption, and splanchnic vascular resistance in humans not undergoing surgery. Circulation 6: 894, 1952.

MURAVCHICK, S., AND JOHNSON, R.: Oxygenation of peripheral tissues in young and elderly patients during spinal anesthesia. Regional Anesth. 11: 7, 1986.

NAKAYAMA, E., NOGUCHI, T., KARUBE, Y., BABA, I., AND HARAGUCHI, M.: Circulation and respiration in anesthesia. I. Circulation and respiration during spinal anesthesia. J. Jpn. Obstet. Soc. (Engl. Ed.) 3: 159, 1956.

NEUMANN, C., FOSTER, A. D., AND ROVENSTINE, E. A.: The importance of compensatory vasoconstriction in unanesthetized areas in the maintenance of blood pressure during spinal anesthesia. J. Clin. Invest. 24: 345, 1945.

NICKERSON, M., AND CARTER, S. A.: Protection against acute trauma and traumatic shock by vasodilators. Can. J. Biochem. 37: 1161, 1959.

NISHIKAWA, T., ANZAI, Y., AND NAMIKI, A.: Asystole during spinal anaesthesia after change from Trendelenburg to horizontal position. Can. J. Anaesth. 35: 406, 1988.

NISHIMURA, N., KAJIMOTO, Y., KABE, T., AND SAKAMOTO, A.: The effects of volume loading during epidural analgesia. Resuscitation 13: 31, 1985.

NOLTE, H.: Physiologie und Pathophysiologie der subarachnoidalen und epiduralen Block-ade. Reg. Anaesth. 1: 3, 1978.

NOWAK, S. J. G.: The urinary excretion of novocaine after spinal anesthesia and the theory of toxic absorption. Anesth. Analg. 12: 232, 1933.

NOWAK, S. J. G., AND DOWNING, V.: Oxygen and carbon dioxide changes in arterial and venous blood in experimental spinal anesthesia. J. Pharmacol. Exp. Ther. 64: 271, 1938.

NUWAYHID, B., VAUGHN, D., BRINKMAN, C. R. III, AND ASSALI, N. S.: Circulatory shock in pregnant sheep. IV. Fetal and neonatal circulatory responses to hypovolemia—influence of anesthesia. Am. J. Obstet. Gynecol. 132: 658, 1978.

NYLIN, G., AND PANNIER, R.: L'Influence de l'orthostatisme et du shock sur la vitesse circula-toire determinée à l'aide du phosphore radioactif. Arch. Internat. Pharmacodyn. 73: 401, 1947.

O'ROURKE, G. W., AND GREENE, N. M.: Autonomic blockade and the resting heart rate in man. Am. Heart J. 80: 469, 1970.

OBERG, B., AND THOREN, P.: Increased activity in left ventricular receptors during hemor-rhage or occlusion of caval veins in the cat.—A possible cause of the vaso-vagal reaction. Acta Physiol. Scand. 85: 164, 1972.

ORR, J. E., LOWE, G. D. O., NIMMO, W. S., WATSON, R., AND FORBES, C. D.: A haemorheolog-ical study of lignocaine. Br. J. Anaesth. 58: 306, 1986.

OSTER, A., AND MADSEN, P. O.: Determination of absorption of irrigation fluid during trans-urethral resection of the prostate by means of radioisotopes. J. Urol. 102: 714, 1969.

OTTON, P. E., AND WILSON, E. J.: The cardiovascular effects of upper thoracic epidural analgesia. Can. Anaesth. Soc. J. 13: 541, 1966.

OVERTON, R. C., AND DEBAKEY, M. E.: Experimental observations on the influence of hypo-thermia and autonomic blocking agents on hemorrhagic shock. Ann. Surg. 143: 439, 1956.

OWEN, H., GALLOWAY, D. J., AND MITCHELL, K. G.: Analgesia by wound infiltration after surgical excision of benign breast lumps. Ann. R. Coll. Surg. Eng. 67: 114, 1985.

OYAMA, T., TANIGUCHI, K., JIN, T., SATONE, T., AND KUDO, T.: Effects of anaesthesia and surgery on plasma aldosterone concentration and renin activity in man. Br. J. Anaesth. *51:* 747, 1979.

OZAKI, N., KAWAKITA, S., AND TODA, N.: Effects of dobutamine on isolated canine cerebral, coronary, mesenteric, and renal arteries. J. Cardiovasc. Pharmacol. *4:* 456, 1982.

PAGE, I. H., TAYLOR, R. D., CORCORAN, A. C., AND MUELLER, L.: Correlation of clinical types with renal function in arterial hypertension. II. The effect of spinal anesthesia. J. A. M. A. *124:* 736, 1944.

PALKAR, N. V., AND CRAWFORD, M. W.: Spinal anaesthesia in prolonged Q-T interval syndrome. Br. J. Anaesth. *58:* 575, 1986.

PALMER, C. M., NORRIS, M. C., GIUDICI, M. C., LEIGHTON, B. L., AND DESIMONE, C. A.: Incidence of electrocardiographic changes during cesarean delivery under regional anesthesia. Anesth. Analg. *70:* 36, 1990.

PALMER, R. M. J., FERRIGE, A. G., AND MONCADA, S.: Nitric oxide release accounts for the biological activity of endothelium-derived relaxing factor. Nature *327:* 524, 1987.

PANNETT, C. A.: Problems of spinal anaesthesia. Lancet *2:* 169, 1933.

PAPPENHEIMER, J. R.: Peripheral circulation. Ann. Rev. Physiol. *14:* 259, 1952.

PAPPENHEIMER, J. R., RENKIN, E. M., AND BORRERO, L. M.: Filtration, diffusion, and molecular sieving through peripheral capillary membranes. Am. J. Physiol. *167:* 13, 1951.

PAPPER, E. M., BRADLEY, S. E., AND ROVENSTINE, E. A.: Circulatory adjustments during high spinal anesthesia. J. A. M. A. *121:* 27, 1943.

PASTORE, J. O., YURCHAK, P. M., JANIS, K. M., MURPHY, J. D., AND ZIR, L. M.: The risk of advanced heart block in surgical patients with right bundle branch block and left axis deviation. Circulation *57:* 677, 1978.

PATEL, J. M., LANZAFAME, R. J., WILLIAMS, J. S., MULLEN, B. V., AND HINSHAW, J. R.: The effect of incisional infiltration of bupivacaine hydrochloride upon pulmonary functions, atelectasis and narcotic need following elective cholecystectomy. Surg. Gynecol. Obstet. *157:* 338, 1983.

PATHAK, C. L.: The fallacy of the Bainbridge reflex. Am. Heart J. *72:* 577, 1966.

PATHAK, C. L.: Autoregulation of chronotropic response of the heart through pacemaker stretch. Cardiology *48:* 45, 1973.

PAYNE, J. P. Hypotensive response to carbon dioxide: the influence of carbon dioxide on the blood pressure response of cats to hypotensive drugs. Anaesthesia *13:* 279, 1958.

PAYNE, R.: Subarachnoid injection of cocaine as a general anesthetic for operations upon the head. Tr. Am. Laryngol. Rhin. Otol. Soc. *7:* 215, 1901.

PEACH, M. J., LOEB, A. L., SINGER, H. A., AND SAYE, J.: Endothelium-derived vascular relaxing factor. 1984 Blood Pressure Council. (Suppl. I): Hypertension *7(3):* I94, 1985 a.

PEACH, M. J., SINGER, H. A., AND LOEB, A. L.: Commentary: mechanisms of endothelium-dependent vascular smooth muscle relaxation. Biochem. Pharmacol. *34:* 1867, 1985 b.

PEARL, R. G., McLEAN, R. F., AND ROSENTHAL, M. H.: Effects of spinal anesthesia on response to main pulmonary arterial distension. J. Appl. Physiol. *64(2):* 742, 1988.

PEREIRA, A. DE, S.: The innervation of the veins: its role in pain, venospasm, and collateral circulation. Surgery *19:* 731, 1946.

PERL, J. I.: Intra-abdominal use of epinephrine in hypotension during spinal anesthesia. Am. J. Surg. *17:* 275, 1932.

PERMUTT, S., AND CALDINI, P.: Regulation of cardiac output by the circuit: venous return, in BAAN, J., NOORDERGRAAF, A., AND RAINES, J., *Cardiovascular System Dynamics.* Cambridge, Massachusetts: MIT Press, 1978.

PETERS, J., KUTKUHN, B., MEDERT, H. A., SCHLAGHECKE, R., SCHUTTLER, J., AND ARNDT, J. O.: Sympathetic blockade by epidural anesthesia attenuates the cardiovascular response to severe hypoxemia. Anesthesiology *72:* 134, 1990.

PFLUG, A. E., AASHEIM, G. M., AND FOSTER, C.: Sequence of return of neurologic function and criteria for safe ambulation following subarachnoid block (spinal anaesthetic). Can. Anaesth. Soc. J. *25:* 133, 1978.

PHEMISTER, D. B., LAESTAR, C. H., EICHELBERGER, L., AND SCHACTER, R. J.: Afferent vasodepressor nerve impulses as a cause of shock tested experimentally by aortic-depressor
nerve stimulation. Ann. Surg. *119:* 26, 1944.

PHILIPOWICZ, I.: Der heutige Stand der Lumbalanasthesie mit Bervcksichtigrnng der neues-
ten Mittle und Verllihren. Zentralbl. Chir. *60:* 2793, 1933.

POLANO, H.: Experimentelle Untersuchungen uber das Verhalten des Minutenvolumens
des menschlichen Herzens Lei Athernarkose, Lumbalanasthesie und nach operativen
Eingrrif. Dtsch. Ztschr. f. Chir. *239:* 505, 1933.

PONTEN, J., BIBER, B., BJURO, T., HENRIKSSON, B-A., HJALMARSON, A., AND LUNDBERG, D.: β-
receptor blockade and spinal anaesthesia. Withdrawal versus continuation of long-term
therapy. Acta. Anaesth. Scand. (Suppl.) *76:* 62, 1982.

PRINZMETAL, M., AND WILSON, C.: The nature of the peripheral resistance in arterial hypertension with special reference to the vasomotor system. J. Clin. Invest. *15:* 63, 1936.

PUGH, L. G. C., AND WYNDHAM, C. L.: The circulatory effects of high spinal anesthesia in
hypertensive and control patients. Clin. Sci. *9:* 189, 1950.

QUILLIGAN, E. J., HENRICKS, C. H., AND HINGSON, R.: Cardiac output. The acute effects of
various anesthetic agents and techniques as measured by the pulse-pressure method.
Anesth. Analg. *36:* 33, 1957.

RACLE, J. P., BENKHADRA, A., POY, J. Y., AND GLEIZAL, B.: Prolongation of isobaric bupivacaine spinal anesthesia with epinephrine and clonidine for hip surgery in the elderly.
Anesth. Analg. *66:* 442, 1987.

RASHKIND, W. J., LEWIS, D. M., HENDERSON, J. B., HEIMAN, D. F., AND DIETRICK, R. B.:
Venous return as affected by cardiac output and total peripheral resistance. Am. J. Physiol. *175:* 413, 1953.

RAWSON, R. O.: A highly sensitive, miniaturized photoelectric plethysmograph. J. Appl.
Physiol. *14:* 1049, 1959.

REINHART, K., DALLINGER-STILLER, G., HEINEMEYER, G., DENNHARDT, R., AND EYRICH, K.:
Respiratorische und schlafinduzierende wirkungen von midazolam i.m. als pramedikation zur regionalanaesthesie. Anaesthesist *32:* 525, 1983.

REPLOGLE, R. L, MEISELMAN, H. J., AND MERRILL, E. W.: Clinical implications of blood rheology studies. Circulation *36:* 148, 1967.

RICE, L., DEMARS, P., CROOMS, J., AND WHALEN, T.: Duration of spinal anesthesia in infants
under one year of age: comparison of three drugs. Anesth. Analg. *66:* S1, 1987.

ROBERTS, F. L., BROWN, E. C., DAVIS, R., AND COUSINS, M. J.: Comparison of hyperbaric
and plain bupivacaine with hyperbaric cinchocaine as spinal anaesthetic agents. Anaesthesia *44:* 471, 1989.

ROBERTSON, D., AND MICHELAKIS, A. M.: Effect of anesthesia and surgery on plasma renin
activity in man. J. Clin. Endocrinol. *34:* 831, 1972.

RODGERS, G. P., SCHECHTER, A. N., NOGUCHI, C. T., KLEIN, H. G., NIENHUIS, A. W., AND
BONNER, R. F.: Periodic microcirculatory flow in patients with sickle-cell disease. N. Engl.
J. Med. *311:* 1534, 1984.

ROEDER, C. A.: Carbon dioxide as an adjunct to spinal anesthesia. Am. J. Surg. *14:* 454,
1931.

ROHSE, W. G., AND RANDALL, W. C.: Functional analysis of sympathetic innervation of
heart. Fed. Proc. *14:* 123, 1955.

ROIZEN, M. F., HORRIGAN, R. W., AND FRAZER, B. M.: Anesthetic doses blocking adrenergic
(stress) and cardiovascular responses to incision—MAC BAR. Anesthesiology *54:* 390,
1981.

ROLBIN, S. H., LEVINSON, G., SHNIDER, S. M., BIEHL, D. R., AND WRIGHT, R. G.: Dopamine
treatment of spinal hypotension decreases uterine blood flow in the pregnant ewe. Anesthesiology *51:* 36, 1979.

ROOME, N. W., KEITH, W. S., AND PHEMISTER, D. B.: Experimental shock: The effect of bleeding after reduction of the blood pressure by various methods. Surg. Gynecol. Obstet. *56:* 161, 1933.

ROVENSTINE, E. A., PAPPER, E. M., AND BRADLEY, S. E.: Circulatory adjustments during spinal anesthesia in normal man with special reference to the autonomy of arterial tone. Anesthesiology *3:* 421, 1942.

RUBANYI, G. M., ROMERO, J. C., AND VANHOUTTE, P. M.: Flow-induced release of endothelium-derived relaxing factor. Am. J. Physiol. *250:* H1145, 1986.

RUBEN, J. E.: Continuous lumbar sympathetic block for the treatment of acute arterial occlusion and other vascular diseases of the lower extremity. Ann. Surg. *131:* 194, 1950.

RUNCIMAN, W. B., ILSLEY, A. H., MATHER, L. E., CARAPETIS, R., AND RAO, M. M.: A sheep preparation for studying interactions between blood flow and drug disposition. I: Physiological profile. Br. J. Anaesth. *56:* 1015, 1984 c.

RUNCIMAN, W. B., MATHER, L. E., ILSLEY, A. H., CARAPETIS, R. J., AND McLEAN, C. F.: A sheep preparation for studying interactions between blood flow and drug disposition. II: Experimental applications. Br. J. Anaesth. *56:* 1117, 1984 a.

RUNCIMAN, W. B., MATHER, L. E., ILSLEY, A. H., CARAPETIS, R. J., AND UPTON, R. N.: A sheep preparation for studying interactions between blood flow and drug disposition. III: Effects of general and spinal anaesthesia on regional blood flow and oxygen tensions. Br. J. Anaesth. *56:* 1247, 1984 b.

RUNCIMAN, W. B., MATHER, L. E., ILSLEY, A. H., CARAPETIS, R. J., AND UPTON, R. N.: A sheep preparation for studying interactions between blood flow and drug disposition. IV: The effects of general and spinal anaesthesia on blood flow and cefoxitin disposition. Br. J. Anaesth. *57:* 1239, 1985.

RUNCIMAN, W. B., MATHER, L. E., ILSLEY, A. H., CARAPETIS, R. J., AND UPTON, R. N.: A sheep preparation for studying interactions between blood flow and drug disposition. VI: Effects of general or subarachnoid anaesthesia on blood flow and chlormethiazole disposition. Br. J. Anaesth. *58:* 1308, 1986.

RUTLEN, D. L., SUPPLE, E. W., AND POWELL, W. J., JR.: The role of the liver in the adrenergic regulation of blood flow from the splanchnic to the central circulation. Yale J. Biol. Med. *52:* 99, 1979.

SAINT-MAURICE, C., AND SCHULTE-STEINBERG, O.: Regional anaesthesia in children. Medi Globe, 1990.

SAKLAD, M.: Studies in spinal anesthesia. Am. J. Surg. *11:* 452, 1931.

SAMII, K., ELMELIK, E., MOURTADA, M. B., DEBEYRE, J., AND RAPIN, M.: Intraoperative hemodynamic changes during total knee replacement. Anesthesiology *50:* 239, 1979.

SANCETTA, S. M., LYNN, R. B., AND SIMEONE, F. A.: Studies of hemodynamic changes in humans following induction of spinal anesthesia. IV. Observations in low spinal anesthesia during surgery. Surg. Gynecol. Obstet. *97:* 597, 1953.

SANCETTA, S. M., LYNN, R. B., SIMEONE, F. A., AND SCOTT, R. W.: Studies of hemodynamic changes in humans following induction of low and high spinal anesthesia. I. General considerations of the problem. The changes in cardiac output, brachial arterial pressure, peripheral and pulmonary oxygen contents and peripheral blood flows induced by spinal anesthesia in humans not undergoing surgery. Circulation *6:* 559, 1952.

SARNOFF, S. J., AND ARROWOOD, J. G.: Differential spinal block. Surgery *20:* 150, 1946.

SARNOFF, S. J., AND ARROWOOD, J. G.: Differential spinal block. II. The reaction of sudomotor and vasomotor fibers. J. Clin. Invest. *26:* 203, 1947.

SARNOFF, S. J., AND FARR, H. W.: Spinal anesthesia in the therapy of pulmonary edema: a preliminary report. Anesthesiology *5:* 69, 1944.

SARNOFF, S. J., AND SIMEONE, F. A.: Vasodilator fibers in the human skin. J. Clin. Invest. *26:* 453, 1947.

SARNOFF, S. J., ARROWOOD, J. G., AND CHAPMAN, W. P.: Differential spinal block. IV. The investigation of intestinal dyskinesia, colonic atony, and visceral afferent fibers. Surg. Gynecol. Obstet. *86:* 571, 1948.

SARNOFF, S. J., MALONEY, J. V., AND WHITTENBERGER, J. L.: Electrophrenic respiration. V. Effect on the circulation of electrophrenic respiration and positive pressure breathing during the respiratory paralysis of high spinal anesthesia. Ann. Surg. *132:* 921, 1950.

SCHILF, E., AND ZIEGNER, H.: Das Wesen der Blutdrucksenkung bei der Lumbalanasthesie. Arch. Klin. Chir. *130:* 352, 1924.

SCHLOSSBERG, T., AND SAWYER, M. E.: Studies of homeostasis in normal, sympathectomized, and ergotamized animals: IV. The effect of hemorrhage. Am. J. Physiol. *104:* 195, 1933.

SCHOTTE, A.: La Prevention et le Traitment des Accidents de la Rachi-anesthesia Emploi de l'Ephedrine et du Carbogene. Presse Med. *41:* 1365, 1933.

SCHUBERTH, O. O.: On the disturbance of the circulation in spinal anaesthesia. Acta Chir. Scand. *78:*(Suppl.) 43, 1936.

SCULCO, T. P., AND RANAWAT, C.: The use of spinal anesthesia for total hip-replacement arthroplasty. J. Bone Joint Surg. *57A*(2): 173, 1975.

SEEVERS, M. H., AND WATERS, R. M.: Respiratory and circulatory changes during spinal anesthesia. J. A. M. A. *99:* 961, 1932 a.

SEEVERS, M. H., AND WATERS, R. M.: Circulatory changes during spinal anesthesia. Anesth. Analg. *11:* 85, 1932 b.

SHARNOFF, J. G., ROSEN, R. L., SADLER, A. H., AND IBARRA-ISUNZA, G. C.: Prevention of fatal pulmonary thromboembolism by heparin prophylaxis after surgery for hip fractures. J. Bone Joint Surg. *58A:* 913, 1976.

SHAW, J. L., STEELE, B. F., AND LAMB, C. A.: Effect of anesthesia on the blood oxygen: II. A study of the effect of spinal anesthesia on the oxygen in the arterial and in the venous blood. Arch. Surg. *35:* 503, 1937.

SHESKEY, M. C., ROCCO, A. G., BIZZARRI-SCHMID, M., FRANCIS, D. M., EDSTROM, H., AND COVINO, B. G.: A dose-response study of bupivacaine for spinal anesthesia. Anesth. Analg. *62:* 931, 1983.

SHIMOSATO, S., AND ETSTEN, B. E.: The role of the venous system in cardiocirculatory dynamics during spinal and epidural anesthesia in man. Anesthesiology *30:* 619, 1969.

SIDI, A., POLLAK, D., FLOMAN, Y., AND DAVIDSON, J. T.: Hypobaric spinal anesthesia in the operative management of orthopedic emergencies in geriatric patients. Isr. J. Med. Sci. *20:* 589, 1984.

SINCLAIR, R., CASSUTO, J., HÖGSTRÖM, S., LINDÉN, I., FAXÉN, A., HEDNER, T., AND EKMAN, R.: Topical anesthesia with lidocaine aerosol in the control of postoperative pain. Anesthesiology *68:* 895, 1988.

SIRCAR, P.: A study of the circulating blood volume under anaesthesia. 3. Spinal anaesthesia. J. Indian Med. Assoc. *21:* 340, 1952.

SIVARAJAN, M., AMORY, D. W., LINDBLOOM, L. E., AND SCHWETTMAN, R. S.: Systemic and regional blood-flow changes during spinal anesthesia in the Rhesus monkey. Anesthesiology *43:* 78, 1975.

SMITH, H. W., ROVENSTINE, E. A., GOLDRING, W., CHASIS, H., AND RANGES, H. A.: The effects of spinal anesthesia on the circulation in normal, unoperated man with reference to the autonomy of the arterioles and especially those of the renal circulation. J. Clin. Invest. *18:* 319, 1939.

SMITH, N. T., AND CORBASCIO, A. N.: The use and misuse of pressor agents. Anesthesiology *33:* 58, 1970.

SMITH, G. G., AND PORTER, W. T.: Spinal anesthesia in the cat. Am. J. Physiol. *38:* 108, 1915.

SMITH, S. M., AND REES, V. L.: The use of prolonged continuous spinal anesthesia to relieve vasospasm and pain in peripheral embolism. Anesthesiology *9:* 229, 1948.

SOBIN, S. S.: The role of the sympathetic nervous system in human arterial hypertension. Cardiac output studies in differential spinal block. Am. J. Med. *6:* 386, 1949.

SOBIN, S. S., AND TREMER, H. M.: Functional geometry of the microcirculation. Fed. Proc. *25:* 1744, 1966.

SOLOFF, L. A., BURNETT, W. E., AND BELLO, C. T.: A study of the comparative value of tetraethylammonium bromide and diagnostic spinal anesthesia in the selection of hypertensive patients for sympathectomy. Am. J. Med. Sci. *216:* 665, 1948.

STEVENS, W. C., CAIN, W. E., AND HAMILTON, W. K.: Circulatory studies during spinal anesthesia. Central and peripheral venous oxygen saturation before and after administration of vasopressors. Anesth. Analg. *47:* 725, 1968.

SVARTLING, N., LEHTINEN, A-M., AND TARKKANEN, L.: The effect of anaesthesia on changes in blood pressure and plasma cortisol levels induced by cementation with methylmethacrylate. Acta Anaesthesiol. Scand *30:* 247, 1986.

SVARTLING, N., PFAFFLI, P., AND TARKKANEN, L.: Methylmethacrylate blood levels in patients with femoral neck fracture. Arch. Orthop. Trauma Surg. *104:* 242, 1985.

Symposium on Active Neurogenic Vasodilation. Fed. Proc. *25:* 1583, 1966.

TAIVAINEN, T.: Comparison of ephedrine and etilefrine for the treatment of arterial hypotension during spinal anaesthesia in elderly patients. Acta Anaesthesiol. Scand. *35:* 164, 1991.

TAIVAINEN, T., TUOMINEN, M., AND ROSENBERG, P. H.: Spinal anaesthesia with hypobaric 0.19% or plain 0.5% bupivacaine. Br. J. Anaesth. *65:* 234, 1990.

TARDIEU, G., TARDIEU, C., AND POCIDALO, J. J.: Anesthesie medullaire totale. Etude hemodynamique. Premiers resultats. J. Physiol. Paris *49:* 390, 1957.

TAYLOR, R. D., BIRCHALL, R., CORCORAN, A. C., AND PAGE, I. H.: Circulatory responses to spinal and caudal anesthesia in hypertension: relation to the effect of sympathectomy. I. Effect on arterial pressure. Am. Heart J. *36:* 221, 1948 a.

TAYLOR, R. D., CORCORAN, A. C., AND PAGE, I. H.: Effects of denervation on experimental renal hypertension. Fed. Proc. *7:* 123, 1948 b.

THISTLEWAITE, J. R., EDISON, T. G., GURENWALD, C., AND HARRISON, I.: Experience with epidural analgesia for sympathetic block. Surgery *33:* 289, 1953.

THOMAS, D. F. M., LAMBERT, W. G., AND WILLIAMS, K. L.: The direct perfusion of surgical wounds with local anaesthetic solution: an approach to postoperative pain? Ann. R. Coll. Surg. Engl. *65:* 226, 1983.

THORBURN, J.: Subarachnoid blockade and total hip replacement: effect of ephedrine on intraoperative blood loss. Br. J. Anaesth. *57:* 290, 1985.

THORBURN, J., LOUDEN, J. R., AND VALLANCE, R.: Spinal and general anaesthesia in total hip replacement: frequency of deep vein thrombosis. Br. J. Anaesth. *52:* 1117, 1980.

TUFFIER, T., AND HALLION, L.: Effets Circulatoires des injections Sous-Arachnoidiennes de Cocaine dans la Region Lombaire. Compt. Rend. Soc. Biol. *52:* 897, 1900.

TUOHY, E. B.: The adaptations of continuous spinal anesthesia. Anesth. Analg. *31:* 372, 1952.

TURAI, S., MIKAI, C., AND TILIPESCU, Z.: Der Einfluss der Spinalanasthesie Auf Gewebsflussikgeits- und Bluthaushalt in der postoperativen Phase. Zentralbl. Chir. *81:* 1645, 1956.

TURK, N. L., AND GLENN, W. W. L.: Cardiac arrest: results of attempted cardiac resuscitation in 42 cases. N. Engl. J. Med. *251:* 795, 1954.

TVERSKOY, M., COZACOV, C., AYACHE, M., BRADLEY, E. L., JR., AND KISSIN, I.: Postoperative pain after inguinal herniorrhaphy with different types of anesthesia. Anesth. Analg. *70:* 29, 1990.

UNDERWOOD, S. M., AND GLYNN, C. J.: Sick sinus syndrome manifest after spinal anaesthesia. Anaesthesia *43:* 307, 1988.

URMEY, W. F., AND LAMBERT, D. H.: Spinal anesthesia associated with reversal of myocardial ischemia. Anesth. Analg. *65:* 908, 1986.

VALENTIN, N., LOMHOLT, B., JENSEN, J. S., HEJGAARD, N., AND KREINER, S.: Spinal or general anaesthesia for surgery of the fractured hip? A prospective study of mortality in 578 patients. Br. J. Anaesth. *58:* 284, 1986.

VAN GRONDELLE, A., WORTHEN, G. S., ELLIS, D., ET AL.: Altering hydrodynamic variables influences PGI$_2$ production by isolated lungs and endothelial cells. J. Appl. Physiol. 57: 388, 1984.

VANE, J. R., ANGGARD, E. E., AND BOTTING, R. M.: Regulatory functions of the vascular endothelium. N. Engl. J. Med. 323: 27, 1990.

VANHOUTTE, P. M.: The end of the quest? Nature 327: 459, 1987.

VEHRS, G. R.: Heart beat and respiration in total novocaine analgesia. Northwest Med. 30: 256, 1931.

VEHRS, G. R.: Spinal Anesthesia: Technic and Clinical Application. St. Louis: The C. V. Mosby Co., 1934.

VENKATARAMAN, K., MADIAS, J. E., AND HOOD, W. B., JR.: Indications for prophylactic preoperative insertion of pacemakers in patients with right bundle branch block and left anterior hemiblock. Chest 68: 501, 1975.

VENN, P. J. H., SIMPSON, D. A., RUBIN, A. P., AND EDSTROM, H. H.: Effect of fluid preloading on cardiovascular variables after spinal anaesthesia with glucose-free 0.75% bupivacaine. Br. J. Anaesth. 63: 682, 1989.

VIEGAS, O. J., RAVINDRAN, R. S., AND STRAUSBURG, B. J.: Attenuation of cardiovascular responses following spinal blockade in patients treated with propranolol. Regional Anesth. 8: 61, 1983.

VOELKEL, N. F., GERBER, J. G., McMURTRY, I. F., NIES, A. S., AND REEVES, J. T.: Release of vasodilator prostaglandin, PGI$_2$, from isolated rat lung during vasoconstriction. Circ. Res. 48: 207, 1981.

WARD, R. J., BONICA, J. J., FREUND, F. G., AKAMATSU, T., DANZIGER, F., AND ENGLESSON, S.: Epidural and subarachnoid anesthesia: cardiovascular and respiratory effects. J. A. M. A. 191: 275, 1965.

WARD, R. J., DANZIGER, F., AKAMATSU, T., FREUND, F., AND BONICA, J. J.: Cardiovascular response of oxygen therapy for hypotension of regional anesthesia. Anesth. Analg. 45: 140, 1966 a.

WARD, R. J., KENNEDY, W. F., JR., BONICA, J. J., MARTIN, W. E., TOLAS, A. G., AND AKAMATSU, T.: Experimental evaluation of atropine and vasopressors for the treatment of hypotension of high subarachnoid anesthesia. Anesth. Analg. 45: 621, 1966 b.

WARREN, J. V., WALTER, C. W., ROMANO, J., AND STEAD, E. A., JR.: Blood flow in the hand and forearm after paravertebral block of the sympathetic ganglia. Evidence against sympathetic vasodilator nerves in the extremities of man. J. Clin. Invest. 21: 665, 1942.

WASSERMAN, F., BELLET, S., AND SAICHEK, R. P.: Post-operative myocardial infarction. N. Engl. J. Med. 252: 967, 1955.

WEBB, G., SCHEINFELD, W., AND COLIN, H.: The importance in surgery of the blood circulation time. Ann. Surg. 104: 460, 1936.

WEBB-PEPLOE, M. M., AND SHEPHERD, J. T.: Veins and their control. N. Engl. J. Med. 278: 317, 1968.

WEINHEIMER, G., DOOLEY, D. J., CAZZONELLI, M., AND OSSWALD, H.: Aging and endothelin-1 induced vascular contractions. Experientia 46: 1008, 1990.

WEISS, S., PARKER, F., JR., AND ROBB, G. P.: A correlation of the hemodynamics, function, and histologic structure of the kidney in malignant arterial hypertension with malignant nephrosclerosis. Ann. Intern. Med. 6: 1599, 1933.

WENGER, C. B., STEPHENSON, L. A., AND DURKIN, M. A.: Effect of nerve block on response of forearm blood flow to local temperature. J. Appl. Physiol. 61: 227, 1986.

WETSTONE, D. L., AND WONG, K. C.: Sinus bradycardia and asystole during anesthesia. Anesthesiology 41: 87, 1974.

WHELAN, E., WOOD, A. J. J., SHAY, S., AND WOOD, M.: Lack of effect of spinal anesthesia on drug metabolism. Anesth. Analg. 69: 307, 1989.

WHITE, J. C.: Diagnostic blocking of sympathetic nerves to extremities with procaine. A test to evaluate benefit of sympathetic ganglionectomy. J. A. M. A. 94: 1382, 1930.

WILKINSON, P. L., TYBERG, J. V., MOYERS, J. R., AND WHITE, A. E.: Correlates of myocardial oxygen consumption when afterload changes during halothane anesthesia in dogs. Anesth. Analg. 59: 233, 1980.

WILLENKIN, R. L., AND GREENE, N. M.: Skeletal muscle oxygen tension and metabolism during induced hypotension and during vasopressor administration. Anesthesiology 24: 168, 1963.

WILLIAMS, J. F., JR., GLICK, G., AND BRAUNWALD, E.: Studies on cardiac dimensions in intact unanesthetized man. V. Effects of nitroglycerin. Circulation 32: 767, 1965.

WILSON, H., ROOME, N. W., AND GRIMSON, K.: Complete sympathectomy: observations of certain vascular reactions during and after complete exclusion of the sympathetic nervous system in dogs. Ann. Surg. 103: 498, 1936.

WRIGHT, A. D.: Spinal anaesthesia with special reference to operations above the diaphragm. Proc. R. Soc. Med. 24: 1930–1931.

YANAGISAWA, M., KURIHARA, H., KIMURA, S., ET AL.: A novel potent vasoconstrictor peptide produced by vascular endothelial cells. Nature 332: 411, 1988.

YASUOKA, S., AND YAKSH, T. L.: Effects on nociceptive threshold and blood pressure of intrathecally administered morphine and alpha-adrenergic agonist. Neuropharmacology 22: 309, 1983.

ZIMMERMAN, B. G., ABBOUD, F. N., AND ECKSTEIN, J. W.: Comparison of the effects of sympathomimetic amines upon venous and total vascular resistance in the foreleg of the dog. J. Pharmacol. Exp. Ther. 139: 290, 1963.

ZWEIFACH, B. W.: Direct observation of the mesenteric circulation in experimental animals. Anat. Rec. 120: 277, 1954 a.

ZWEIFACH, B. W.: Transcript of the Fourth Conference on Shock and Circulatory Homeostasis. New York: The Josiah Macy, Jr., Foundation, 1954 b.

ZWEIFACH, B. W., AND INTAGLIETTA, M.: Fluid exchange across the blood capillary interface. Fed. Proc. 25: 1784, 1966.

ZWEIFACH, B. W., AND METZ, D. B.: Selective distribution of blood through the germinal vascular bed of mesenteric structures and skeletal muscle. Angiology 6: 282, 1955.

ZWEIFACH, B. W., LEE, R. E., AND HYMAN, C.: Omental circulation in morphinized dogs subjected to graded hemorrhage. Ann. Surg. 120: 232, 1944.

CHAPTER 3

Pulmonary Ventilation and Hemodynamics

One of the main advantages of properly managed spinal anesthesia for surgery below the level of the umbilicus is the ability to achieve both sensory blockade and profound muscular relaxation with little or no impairment of the respiratory muscles. In this respect, spinal anesthesia may offer some particular advantages over general anesthesia (Table 3.1). For surgery above this level, however, the concentrations of local anesthetic agent in the subarachnoid space necessary for higher levels of anesthesia may also block the motor fibers of the intercostal nerves. At one time it was assumed that a level of anesthesia high enough to produce intercostal paralysis would decrease pulmonary ventilation in proportion to the number of intercostal nerves blocked (Gray and Parsons, 1912; Bower, et al., 1926, 1932; Seevers and Waters, 1932 a, b). However, reports giving actual measurements of pulmonary mechanics during spinal anesthesia in humans have shown that such is not the case.

Muscles of Respiration and Pulmonary Mechanics

The literature contains at least two studies that have elucidated the individual contribution of the diaphragm and intercostal muscles to maintenance of the normal ventilatory capacity, as well as the interrelationship among these muscles. The first such study by De Troyer, et al. (1981) investigated the differential function of the two embryologically and anatomically distinct muscles of the diaphragm, the costal part (originating from myoblasts in the lateral body wall), and the crural part (developing from the dorsal mesentery of the esophagus). In their study in dogs, the authors demonstrated that when the abdominal wall was open, stimulation of the costal part of the diaphragm increased the dimensions of the lower thorax, while stimulation of the crural part decreased these dimensions. In the intact (unopened) abdomen, stimulation of the costal diaphragm increased thoracic dimensions, lung

201

Table 3.1.
Various Reported Benefits and Disadvantages of Properly Administered Spinal and General Anesthesia on the Respiratory System

Spinal Anesthesia	General Anesthesia
Benefits	Benefits
Avoids airway manipulation	Provides control of difficult airway
Avoids inhibition of ciliary function	Provides access for pulmonary toilet
Avoids intraoperative patient oversedation and improves postoperative ambulation and pulmonary function	Provides bronchodilation via potent inhaled anesthetics
Provides postoperative anesthesia or analgesia without sedation, decreasing "splinting" and atelectasis	Facilitates some surgery by allowing use of muscle relaxant agents and decreases operative time
Decreases hypercoagulability and incidence of pulmonary embolism	Improves patient acceptance and comfort for upper abdominal and thoracic surgery
Improves postoperative oxygenation	Disadvantages
Decreases need for postoperative analgesia, minimizing risk of apnea	Slower recovery to full consciousness
Decreases incidence of postoperative pulmonary infection	Airway manipulation may induce bronchospasm
Disadvantages	Inhibits ciliary function
Diminishes ability to cough	Anesthesia and analgesia are relatively short-lived, leading to "splinting"
Increases incidence of urinary retention	High-risk patients may require postoperative mechanical ventilation
May be associated with weakness or paralysis of muscles of respiration	

volume, and abdominal pressure; stimulation of the crural diaphragm increased abdominal pressure, abdominal dimensions and lung volume, but had no effect on lower rib cage dimensions. The authors concluded that in dogs, the costal diaphragm is arranged in series with the intercostal and accessory muscles of inspiration (i.e., they work synergistically), and that they have a direct inspiratory action on the lower thorax. Alternatively, the crural diaphragm is arranged in parallel (i.e., it has little or no net effect on the thorax as long as the abdominal pressure is allowed to increase) and, therefore, it has an expiratory action. The authors thus established that the costal and crural parts of the diaphragm have different innervation and different actions on the chest wall.

The second study that investigated the function of the muscles of respiration is by Hecker, et al. (1989), who reported the effect of intercostal nerve blockade on respiratory mechanics in seven healthy male volunteers. These authors produced intercostal nerve (ICN) blockade from T_{6-12}, and abdominal wall paralysis was documented electromyographically; then, pulmonary function tests and hypercapnic ventilatory responses to exercise were recorded. The only change induced by ICN blockade was a minimal (17.6%) decrease in peak expiratory flows, from 11.23 ± 1.8 to 9.25 ± 2.5 L/sec. The authors concluded that ICN blockade "does not exert a clinically significant adverse effect on pulmonary mechanics and that ventilatory function is well maintained even at extremes of ventilatory demand." Other studies have examined pulmonary function and mechanics during clinical spinal anesthesia.

Effects of Spinal Anesthesia on Pulmonary Function Parameters

In subjects with normal pulmonary function and levels of spinal anesthesia high enough to block intercostal nerves, but not enough to produce phrenic paralysis, Schuberth (1936) found no significant change in respiratory rate or tidal volume in 29 patients with sensory levels of anesthesia involving mid-thoracic or upper thoracic dermatomes. Similarly, Johnson (1951) found no change in the respiratory rate of six patients who did not receive supplemental barbiturates and who had sensory blockade to the third or fourth thoracic segment. He did, however, report a slight decrease (10 percent) in tidal and minute volumes. Whether such a change in only six patients is statistically significant is doubtful. In a detailed analysis of the effect of spinal anesthesia on ventilatory volumes, Egbert, et al. (1961) found no change in respiratory rate during spinal anesthesia in 20 subjects with sensory levels of T_{2-6}, and a slight increase in tidal volume. This increase (from 464 ± 115 to 483 ± 99 ml) was not statistically significant. Nor were these authors able to detect a significant change in inspiratory capacity during anesthesia, the average preanesthetic value decreasing slightly from 3.47 ± 0.56 to 3.35 ± 0.63 L.

Egbert, et al. (1961), also noted in their patients a significant decrease in expiratory reserve volume (from 0.74 ± 0.41 to 0.50 ± 0.27 L), as did Freund, et al. (1967). Askrog, et al. (1964) studied six patients with sensory levels of T_{4-6} and found that resting respiratory minute volume increased slightly in four patients, remained unchanged in one, and decreased in one (because of a decrease in respiratory rate). Tidal volumes remained unchanged, but total lung capacity decreased by about 8 percent during anesthesia, from baseline levels of 6.3 ± 1.4 to 5.8 ± 1.4 L. The reduction in total lung capacity was proportional to the decrease in all other respiratory parameters (inspiratory reserve volume, expiratory reserve volume, and residual volume) with the exception of tidal volume (Fig. 3.1). Although statistically significant, the decrease in total lung capacity observed by these authors was not of clinical significance inasmuch as alveolar gas exchange remained unimpaired (see below). Studying 10 patients undergoing lower extremity orthopedic surgery under bupivacaine spinal anesthesia with T_2-T_{10} levels, Steinbrook,

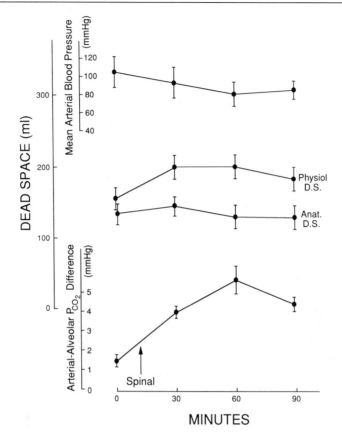

Figure 3.1. Average changes in mean arterial blood pressure, respiratory dead space, and arterial-end tidal (arterial-alveolar) carbon dioxide tension difference during high spinal anesthesia in six patients. Physiol. D.S. and Anat. D.S. denote physiologic and anatomic dead space, respectively. (Reproduced with permission from Askrog, V. F., Smith, T. C., and Eckenhoff, J. E. Changes in pulmonary ventilation during spinal anesthesia. Surg. Gynec. Obstet. *119:* 563, 1964.)

et al. (1988) likewise found that induction of spinal anesthesia was not associated with any significant change in maximal inspiratory pressure, vital capacity, or resting end-tidal carbon dioxide levels. A similar lack of effect of spinal anesthesia ($T_2–T_{11}$) on minute ventilation, tidal volume, respiratory rate, or mean inspiratory flow rate was reported by Steinbrook and Concepcion in 1991, while Eisele, *et al.* (1968) found no change in minute ventilation in 4 patients undergoing T_1 spinal anesthesia. These studies suggest that in normal patients, mid- or even high-thoracic levels of spinal anesthesia have little, if any, effect on resting ventilatory mechanics. Any changes that may occur during spinal anesthesia are more likely to affect expiratory ability, especially forced expiration, rather than inspiratory ability.

That expiratory, rather than inspiratory ability is affected preferentially by spinal anesthesia (Table 3.2) was demonstrated by Axelsson and Widman (1985) in a clinical report in which three patients with T_{2-3} spinal anesthetic levels had difficulty coughing. In 1991, Harrop-Griffiths, et al. studied 20 patients undergoing cesarean section under regional (spinal or epidural) anesthesia. In the 10 patients undergoing spinal anesthesia (mean "block height" was thoracic dermatome 3.8 ± 1.1; medians not provided), the authors used the maximum expiratory pressure (PE_{max}) as the best indicator of a patient's ability to cough, and found this to decrease significantly (by 23 percent) after induction of spinal anesthesia (60 mmHg in the supine position before, and 46 mmHg after, block).

Although there is no uniform agreement on which respiratory function test is the best indicator of the ability to cough, all other parameters tested by Harrop-Griffiths, et al. showed some decrease after induction of spinal (and also epidural) anesthesia (Table 3.2). The authors concluded that although the changes in respiratory parameters may not be significant enough in normal healthy patients, inadvertently high levels of spinal anesthesia in patients "who have preexisting pulmonary disease" may result in significant further impairment of pulmonary function. A similar depression of expiratory function induced by spinal anesthesia was reported by Pitkanen (1987), who showed an 11 percent decrease in peak expiratory flow (PEF) when the anesthetic level was T_8, and a 17 percent reduction when the level was at T_4 (Table 3.2).

Several studies have demonstrated that high thoracic spinal anesthesia may be associated with some degrees of impairment of inspiratory capacity. Freund, et al. (1967) reported a modest (8 percent) decrease in inspiratory capacity during spinal anesthesia with sensory levels to T_2. Similarly, Axelsson and Widman (1985) also reported that 20 percent of their patients with spinal anesthesia to a T_{2-10} level had their inspiratory capacity (measured as the circumference of the lower thoracic cage) reduced to 45–70 percent of baseline values. In their study, the respiratory deflections recorded from the lower thoracic cage decreased particularly in patients with high spinal (T_{2-3}) anesthetic levels.

In 1985, Hedenstierna and Löfstrom compared respiratory function following major lower extremity surgery in patients who had received either spinal or general anesthesia. They found that 18 hr postoperatively, forced vital capacity (FVC, measured by spirometry), forced expiratory volume in 1 sec (FEV_1), and functional residual capacity (FRC, measured by multiple-breath nitrogen washout) decreased significantly below preoperative values in patients who had spinal or general anesthesia. The authors suggested that spinal anesthesia was associated with slight hypoventilation, which "may have contributed to impaired gas

Table 3.2.
Effects of Spinal Anesthesia on Pulmonary Function

Reference	Level of Sensory Denervation (Mean, Range)	Pulmonary Parameter	Parameter Change	Laboratory Tests	Test Change	Comments
Harrop-Griffiths, et al. (1991)	$T_{3.8}$ (±1.1) (unknown sensory modality tested)	FVC FEV_1 PEF PE_{max}	$\rightarrow$ $\rightarrow$ $\rightarrow$ $\rightarrow$			PE_{max} used as index of cough effectiveness. Study conducted in pregnant patients
Steinbrook and Concepcion (1991)	T_2–T_{11}	VT RR MV MIFR VT	No Δ No Δ No Δ No Δ No Δ	$P_{ET}CO_2$	$\rightarrow$	Breath-to-breath variability of ventilation increased with spinal anesthesia
Gauthier, et al. (1990)	T_5 (T_3–T_8)	MIFR	No Δ			MIFR used as index of respiratory drive ($L\cdot sec^{-1}$)
Welborn, et al. (1990)	Adequate for inguinal hernia repair (pediatrics)					Spinal only group: no patients with apnea. Spinal plus sedation: 89% incidence of apnea or bradycardia
Bailey, et al. (1989)	"High spinal"			Pulse oximetry	$\rightarrow$	Labored breathing, marked retractions, and arterial desaturation to 85% in a formerly premature infant
Steinbrook, et al. (1988)	T_2–T_{10}	MIP VC	No Δ No Δ	$P_{ET}CO_2$	No Δ	
Kim and Reed (1987)	$\geq T_{10}$ T_{11-12} T_4 T_8			P_vO_2 P_vO_2 ABG ABG	$\leftarrow$ No Δ No Δ No Δ	P_vO_2 increased during sympathectomy due to opening of arteriovenous anastomoses
Pitkanen (1987)		PEF PEF	$\downarrow$ (-17%) $\downarrow$ (-11%)			
Cook, et al. (1986)	T_{10} and above			ABG (PaO_2)	$\rightarrow$	8.5% intraoperative incidence of PaO_2 <90 mmHg
Muravchick and Johnson (1986)	T_1–T_{11} (mean $T_{6.7}$)	IC	$\rightarrow$	T_cPO_2	No Δ	T_cPO_2 measured in young (29.8 ± 1.4 yr) and elderly (72.1 ± 1.6 yr) patients
Axelsson and Widman (1985)	T_{6-7}; T_9 (T_{2-10}) (pinprick)					Measured thoracic respiratory deflections
Hedenstierna and Löfstrom (1985)	T_8 (T_3–T_{10}) (unknown sensory modality tested)	FVC FEV_1 FRC ERV	$\rightarrow$ $\rightarrow$ $\rightarrow$ No Δ			Parameters measured 18 hr postoperatively; patients also received intrathecal morphine, 0.3 mg

Study	Sensory level	Measure	Change	Comments
Sheskey, et al. (1983) Sinclair, et al. (1982)	Cervical sensory level C4 (analgesia)			No patients had "difficulty in ventilation" Patient had "no trouble maintaining spontaneous breathing"
Davis and Laurenson (1981)	Not reported	ABG (PaO$_2$)	→	PaO$_2$ maintained for 24 hr postoperatively, then decreased below baseline
McKenzie, et al. (1980)	Not reported	ABG (PaO$_2$) ABG (PaCO$_2$)	No Δ No Δ	No PaO$_2$ change in spinal group, significant decrease in PaO$_2$ in general anesthesia group. Mortality 4 wk postoperatively: 10.2% in spinal, 15.7% in general anesthesia groups
Catenacci and Sampathachar (1969)	T$_{4-10}$	ERV VC IC; PaO$_2$ (N) PaO$_2$ (O) PaCO$_2$	Variable Variable →; No Δ ← No Δ	PaO$_2$ (N) = arterial PO$_2$ in non-obese patients. No change in PaCO$_2$ regardless of presence of obesity (O). All patients received premedication prior to spinal anesthesia
Paskin, et al. (1969)	T$_8$–C$_5$	VC MMEF Peak flow; PaO$_2$ PaCO$_2$	→ ↔ →; No Δ No Δ	Both CO$_2$ production and O$_2$ uptake decreased significantly during spinal anesthesia
Eisele, et al. (1968)	T$_1$	MV P$_{ET}$CO$_2$	No Δ Δ	
Freund, et al. (1967)	T$_{2,3}$ ± 1.8 (pinprick), T$_{5.1}$ ± 2.4 (motor)	IV ERV MV VT	→ → Variable No Δ	
Askrog, et al. (1964)	T$_{4-6}$	TLC MIF MMEF; PaCO$_2$	→ → →; →	MV increased in 4, unchanged in 1, and decreased in 1 patient
Lynn, et al. (1952)	"High spinal" (T$_2$)	MVO$_2$ PaO$_2$	→ No Δ	MVO$_2$ = oxygen consumption
Sancetta, et al. (1952)	High spinal Low spinal	MVO$_2$ MVO$_2$	→ →	Oxygen consumption decreased more in the "high spinal" group

Abbreviations: ABG, arterial blood gases; ERV, expiratory reserve volume (L); FEV$_1$, forced expiratory volume in 1 sec (L·sec^{-1}); FRC, functional residual capacity (L); FVC, forced vital capacity (L); IC, inspiratory capacity (L); MIF, maximum inspiratory flow; MIFR, maximum inspiratory flow rate (L·sec^{-1}); MIP, maximal inspiratory pressure; MMEF, mid-maximum expiratory flow rate (L·sec^{-1}); MV, minute ventilation; MVO$_2$, oxygen consumption; PaCO$_2$, arterial carbon dioxide tension; PaO$_2$, arterial oxygen tension; P$_{ET}$O$_2$, end-tidal oxygen tension; P$_v$O$_2$, venous oxygen tension; PE$_{max}$, maximum expiratory pressure; PEF, peak expiratory flow rate; RR, respiratory rate; T$_c$PO$_2$, transcutaneous oxygen tension; TLC, total lung capacity (L); VC, vital capacity (L); VT, tidal volume.

distribution and ventilation-perfusion matching." It should be noted, however, that all patients undergoing spinal anesthesia also received 0.3 mg morphine intrathecally; this may explain the slight degree of postoperative hypoventilation. Nevertheless, one of the major findings of this study was the reduced FRC in patients undergoing either spinal anesthesia or general inhalation anesthesia (Table 3.2).

Effects of Spinal Anesthesia on Pulmonary Function in Disease States

The effects of spinal anesthesia on pulmonary ventilation in patients with pulmonary disease have also been studied. Paskin, et al. (1969) studied nine unpremedicated patients with chronic obstructive pulmonary disease severe enough to produce abnormal pulmonary function tests but not severe enough to be associated with abnormal arterial blood gas tensions. Pulmonary function tests were performed before and during mid- or high thoracic sensory levels of spinal anesthesia while breathing room air. They found (Table 3.3) a statistically significant increase in mid-maximum expiratory flow rates and a statistically significant decrease in peak expiratory flow rates during anesthesia. Both carbon dioxide production and oxygen uptake also decreased significantly. The former decreased more than the latter, leading to a reduction in the respiratory quotient. Changes in respiratory gas exchange were not, however, sufficient to affect arterial carbon dioxide tension (P_aCO_2) or arterial oxygen tension (P_aO_2). Other tests of pulmonary mechanics were unaffected by anesthesia.

While spinal anesthesia has singularly little effect on resting pulmonary ventilation in patients with chronic obstructive pulmonary disease, high spinal anesthesia may affect more significantly the pulmonary function of patients who have normal lungs but are grossly obese. Catenacci and Sampathachar (1969) studied 16 unpremedicated patients, 8 normal and 8 obese, before and during spinal anesthesia with sensory levels of T_{4-10}. The obese patients averaged 47 percent above ideal body weight (range 25 percent to 86 percent). The normal patients showed no significant changes in inspiratory capacity, tidal volume, or arterial blood gas tensions during anesthesia; however, expiratory reserve volume decreased in six of the eight patients and increased in two. With equal levels of spinal anesthesia, all obese patients evidenced diminished inspiratory capacity, but had no changes in expiratory reserve volume.

Heavy cigarette smoking also alters the effect of spinal anesthesia on ventilatory mechanics (Aldrete, et al., 1973). In both moderate and heavy smokers (15–30 and over 30 pack-year history, respectively), FVC, FEV_1,

Table 3.3.
Effect of Spinal Anesthesia on Pulmonary Function in Patients with Chronic Obstructive Pulmonary Disease (Mean ± SD)[a]

Parameter	Before Anesthesia	During Anesthesia	Average Change
Vital capacity (L)	2.56 ± 0.74	2.09 ± 0.40	−0.5 ± 0.5
Dead space (L)[b]	0.279 ± 0.057	0.319 ± 0.71	+0.040 ± 0.049
Minute volume ($L \cdot min^{-1} \cdot m^{-2}$)	5.9 ± 2.5	5.4 ± 1.8	−0.4 ± 1.1
Tidal volume (L)	0.543 ± 0.127	0.553 ± 0.115	+0.010 ± 0.069
FEV_1 (L)	1.16 ± 0.40	1.09 ± 0.30	−0.07 ± 0.17
FEV_1 (% of vital capacity)	47.2 ± 11.0	53.2 ± 14.0	+6.0 ± 9.5
Mid-maximum expiratory flow ($L \cdot sec^{-1}$)	0.47 ± 0.14	0.61 ± 0.31[c]	+0.178 ± 0.24[c]
Maximum voluntary ventilation ($L \cdot min^{-1}$)	52.1 ± 27.7	43.3 ± 17.6	−8.8 ± 12.2
Peak expiratory flow ($L \cdot min^{-1}$)	166 ± 79	116 ± 54[c]	−50.2 ± 37.7[c]
CO_2 production ($ml \cdot min^{-1}$)	114.3 ± 42.2	99.3 ± 28.7[c]	−15.0 ± 14.7[c]
O_2 uptake ($ml \cdot min^{-1}$)	130.0 ± 15.6	118.1 ± 9.9[c]	−10.8 ± 8.4[c]
Respiratory quotient	0.91 ± 0.17	0.83 ± 0.19[c]	−0.05 ± 0.06[c]
V_D/V_T (%)[b]	53.1 ± 7.0	58.2 ± 5.0	+5.1 ± 7.7
Q_s/Q_T (%)	11.3 ± 9.9	10.1 ± 11.5	−2.04 ± 3.72
PaO_2 (mmHg)	85.0 ± 16.5	86.5 ± 16.9	+1.2 ± 10.3
$PaCO_2$ (mmHg)	36.8 ± 6.5	37.2 ± 5.4	+0.56 ± 3.7
pH	7.42 ± 0.04	7.43 ± 0.04	+0.01 ± 0.03

Abbreviations: FEV_1, forced expiratory volume in 1 sec; Q_s/Q_T, shunt fraction; $PaCO_2$, arterial carbon dioxide tension; PaO_2, arterial oxygen tension; V_D/V_T, respiratory dead space to tidal volume ratio.
[a] Reproduced with permission from Paskin, S., Rodman, T., and Smith, T. C.: Effect of spinal anesthesia on the pulmonary function of patients with chronic obstructive pulmonary disease. Ann. Surg. *169*: 35, 1979.
[b] Includes apparatus dead space of 60 ml.
[c] Statistically significant change.

forced expiratory flow rates, and forced mid-expiratory flow rates were adversely affected with levels of spinal anesthesia above T_{10}. These tests of pulmonary function were unaffected in both nonsmokers and light smokers (less than 15 pack-year history) with spinal levels above T_{10}. With spinal levels below T_{10}, pulmonary function tests were not affected regardless of smoking history.

Several reports have investigated the relationship between spinal anesthesia (and the sympathectomy it produces) and bronchospasm in patients at risk (i.e., asthmatics). Shnider and Papper (1961) were among the first to report the incidence of wheezing in patients during a two-and-a-half-year period in which 55,696 surgical procedures were performed. The authors found that in 14 actively wheezing patients undergoing regional (spinal or epidural) anesthesia, wheezing worsened in 1 patient following induction of anesthesia, and remained the same in the other 13 patients. In 159 patients with history of asthma but without active wheezing at the time of induction of regional (spinal or epidural) anesthesia, 3 (1.9 percent) developed wheezing during anesthesia. In contrast, 19 (6.4 percent) of patients undergoing general anesthesia with endotracheal intubation developed wheezing. Similarly, the frequency of bronchospasm during spinal anesthesia has been reported more recently as being low (Mallampati, 1981; McGough and Cohen, 1990). The regulation of bronchomotor tone and the possible mechanisms by which bronchospasm may develop during anesthesia were reviewed by Aviado (1975). One of the mechanisms postulated was that the sympathectomy produced by spinal anesthesia might remove the bronchodilating effects of the sympathetic nervous system (i.e., circulating epinephrine) (Mallampati, 1981). Though an attractive hypothesis, one questions why such cases of bronchospasm are not reported more frequently, considering that asthma and bronchospastic disorders are reported in up to 4 percent of the population.

Although changes in normal minute ventilatory capacity induced by high thoracic spinal anesthesia have been reported only infrequently in adults, Bailey, et al. (1989) reported respiratory distress and arterial oxygen desaturation in a former premature infant inadvertently given high spinal anesthesia. The possibility of increased susceptibility of former preterm infants undergoing spinal anesthesia to postoperative apnea was investigated by Welborn, et al. (1990). Thirty-six former preterm infants having inguinal hernias repaired were studied: 16 had general anesthesia, 9 had spinal anesthesia plus sedation with ketamine, and 11 had spinal anesthesia without sedation. Thirty-one percent of infants given general anesthesia and 89 percent of infants undergoing spinal anesthesia with ketamine sedation developed postoperative prolonged apnea or apnea with bradycardia. In sharp contrast, none of the infants undergoing spinal anesthesia without sedation developed these postoperative sequelae. Satisfactory results and lack of complications in high-risk infants (because of prematurity or presence of neonatal respiratory distress) also have been reported in 36 infants by Abajian, et al. (1984). In a more recent study of 20 infants, Harnik, et al. (1986), concluded that spinal anesthesia "may avoid the increased incidence of postoperative respiratory complications associated with general anesthesia." As discussed in Chapter 2, however, all infants undergoing anesthesia (spinal or general) should have intensive perioperative monitoring.

Resting pulmonary ventilation is little affected even by high sensory levels of spinal anesthesia for two reasons. First, the diaphragm can compensate for decreases in ventilation resulting from intercostal paralysis. This compensatory mechanism is aided by the concurrent paralysis of the abdominal wall muscles. The diaphragm is thereby able to descend into the abdominal cavity during inspiration with less resistance. Furthermore, as described previously (p. 202), the diaphragm and the inter-costal muscles operate on the rib cage to generate pressure as though they were arranged in series (i.e., additive function) (DeTroyer, *et al.*, 1981). Paralysis of only one of these muscles, therefore, is expected to have little influence on overall performance. Second, similar to the zone of differential blockade that exists between sensory and sympathetic lev-els during spinal anesthesia (Chapter 1), there also is a zone of differen-tial blockade between sensory and motor levels, since large motor fibers are more resistant to local anesthetics than smaller sensory fibers. Walts, *et al.* (1964) used electromyophonic techniques to record the presence or absence of intercostal muscle activity during tetracaine spinal anesthesia. Walts, *et al.* found that at a time when the spinal segmental anesthesia to touch averaged $T_{4.4}$, the level of motor blockade averaged $T_{6.2}$, or a mean difference of 1.8 spinal segments (median data not provided). Using electromyographic techniques, Freund, *et al.* (1967) found the av-erage difference between sensory (pinprick) and motor levels to be 2.8 dermatomes (median data not provided). The difference between their results and those reported by Walts, *et al.* is most likely the result of differences in the technique of measuring the level of sensory blockade (touch vs. pinprick).

Effects of Spinal Anesthesia on Pulmonary Blood Flow

Although resting pulmonary ventilation remains unchanged even during high spinal anesthesia, changes in pulmonary blood flow might still produce abnormalities of oxygen uptake and carbon dioxide elimina-tion. Such changes in pulmonary blood flow could involve changes in either or both total alveolar blood flow and its distribution. A change in total alveolar blood flow might also cause a change in pulmonary arterial pressure. This would depend, on the one hand, on the possible effect of spinal anesthesia on pulmonary vascular resistance, a function of pulmo-nary arterial and arteriolar vasomotor tone, and pulmonary capillary pressure (including the effect of left atrial pressure). On the other hand, the change may depend on the effect of spinal anesthesia on pulmonary arterial blood flow, that is, right ventricular output. Pulmonary arterial pressure would not be altered by decreased right ventricular output if pulmonary vascular resistance increased proportionately. Pulmonary ar-terial pressure would also remain unchanged if right ventricular output were to increase and pulmonary vascular resistance were to decrease simultaneously and proportionately. In the former instance, total alveo-lar blood flow would decrease, while in the latter instance it would increase, even though pulmonary arterial pressures remained the same in both instances. Pulmonary arterial pressures are therefore unreliable indices of total alveolar blood flow. It is nonetheless instructive to review the effects of spinal anesthesia on pulmonary arterial pressure.

Sancetta, et al. (1952), for example, found in five nonoperative subjects who did not receive vasopressors during spinal anesthesia with sensory levels below T_4, that mean pulmonary arterial pressure decreased from an average of 18.4 mmHg before, to an average of 15.2 mmHg during, anesthesia (a 17.4 percent decrease). During higher levels of spinal anesthesia in five other subjects, mean pulmonary arterial pressure decreased from 14.9 to 9.8 mmHg (a 34.2 percent decrease). Similarly, Duner, et al. (1960) found that when sympathetic outflow was blocked to T_4 by spinal anesthesia, mean pulmonary arterial pressure decreased an average of 3.0 mmHg in three patients, and increased 2 mmHg in one patient. Lynn, et al. (1952), compared the effects of spinal anesthesia on pulmonary arterial pressure in nonoperative and operative patients. Interestingly, the decrease was greater in 18 nonoperative patients (14.9–8.9 mmHg, i.e., a decrease of 40 percent) than in 10 operative patients (13.8 to 10.2 mmHg, a decrease of only 26 percent). This difference may partially be explained by the fact that, unlike nonoperative subjects, patients undergoing operations had intravenous barbiturate sedation or even general anesthesia and, in some cases, also had artificial ventilation. It is also reasonable to expect that the higher levels of endogenous catecholamines in operative patients (due to surgical stress) may have contributed to this difference. A decrease in pulmonary arterial pressure during operations under spinal anesthesia was noted in a third report by the same group of investigators (Sancetta, et al., 1953), as well as by Bergenwald, et al. (1972). The latter authors found that in 10 nonoperative subjects, mean pulmonary arterial pressure decreased from an average level of 15.0 ± 4.6 mmHg before anesthesia to 12.4 ± 3.9 mmHg during sensory levels of spinal anesthesia high enough to be associated with total sympathetic block. Samii, et al. (1979), however, found no change in mean pulmonary arterial pressure during T_{10} levels of spinal anesthesia.

The above data indicate that mid- or high thoracic levels of spinal anesthesia are characteristically associated with a decrease in mean pulmonary arterial pressure. This decrease in pressure could be due to diminution of either pulmonary flow or pulmonary vascular resistance, or to a decrease in both. There are only two reports on the effects of spinal anesthesia on pulmonary vascular resistance in humans. In Johnson's report (1951), no change was found in five patients who had sensory levels of T_{3-4}. All patients, however, were given ephedrine preanesthetically, obscuring the effects of spinal anesthesia on pulmonary vascular resistance. In the second report, Samii, et al. (1979) studied two groups of five patients during low thoracic levels of anesthesia. None of the patients received vasopressors. In one group, pulmonary vascular resistance decreased 0.7 mmHg·min^{-1}·L^{-1}·m^{-2} (from 3.6 ± 0.3 to 2.9 ± 0.4 mmHg·min^{-1}·L^{-1}·m^{-2}); and in the other, resistance decreased 0.5 mmHg·min^{-1}·L^{-1}·m^{-2} (from 3.4 ± 0.6 to 2.9 ± 0.3). More recently, other authors have investigated changes in pulmonary vascular resistance, though not in humans. In an elegant study performed in dogs during halothane anesthesia, Pearl, et al. (1988) investigated the effects of total spinal anesthesia (TSA) on pulmonary hemodynamics following pulmonary artery distension by an inflatable balloon. Although control hemodynamic measurements were not made prior to induction of halothane anesthesia, the addition of TSA during halothane general anesthesia had little effect on pulmonary vascular resistance (PVR), while TSA alone (without general anesthesia) resulted in an increase in PVR from 295 ± 42 to 351 ± 58 dynes·sec·cm^{-5} (Table 3.4). In this study, general anesthesia, TSA, or the combination of the two had little effect on mean pulmonary arterial pressure (Table 3.4) (Pearl, et al., 1988). The cardiovascular effects of local anesthetic absorbed into the blood were minimized in this investigation by the use of chloroprocaine, the rapid metabolism of which by pseudocholinesterases results in low plasma concentrations (Chapter 2).

An alternative, albeit less precise means of obtaining information on pulmonary vascular resistance is use of data already reported by Sancetta, et al. (1952) to calculate pulmonary arterial flow (i.e., the ratio of mean pulmonary arterial pressure to cardiac output). These measurements can be extracted from data in studies in which both pulmonary arterial pressure and cardiac output were measured simultaneously. For example, in the study by Sancetta, et al. (1952), the data from five patients

Table 3.4.
Effects of Anesthesia on Pulmonary Hemodynamics

Parameter	Halothane[a]	Halothane + TSA	TSA
P$_{pa}$ (mmHg)	14.3 ± 0.8	13.6 ± 1.3	14.4 ± 1.6
CO (L·min^{-1})	2.6 ± 0.4	1.8 ± 0.3	1.8 ± 0.2
PVR (dynes·sec·cm^{-5})	291 ± 40	295 ± 42	351 ± 58
MAP (mmHg)	107 ± 9	81 ± 7	112 ± 12
CVP (mmHg)	4.1 ± 0.6	4.6 ± 0.9	4.9 ± 0.7
SVR (dynes·sec·cm^{-5})	3,573 ± 620	3,893 ± 643	5,000 ± 818
HR (beats·min^{-1})	134 ± 10	92 ± 3	91 ± 5

Adapted from Pearl, R. G., McLean, R. F., and Rosenthal, M. H.: Effects of spinal anesthesia on response to main pulmonary arterial distension. J. Appl. Physiol. 64: 742, 1988.
Abbreviations: CO, cardiac output; CVP, mean central venous pressure; HR, heart rate; MAP, mean systemic arterial pressure; P$_{pa}$, mean pulmonary arterial pressure; PVR, pulmonary vascular resistance; SVR, systemic vascular resistance; TSA, total spinal anesthesia.
[a] General anesthesia with halothane.

who had low spinal anesthesia show that "resistance" decreased from an average preanesthetic level of 3.2 (pulmonary artery pressure of 18.4 mmHg, cardiac output of 5.7 L·min^{-1}) to 2.9 during anesthesia (pressure 15.2 mmHg, output 5.1 L·min^{-1}). In six subjects studied by the same authors in 1953, "resistance" was 3.2 (pressure 14.1 mmHg, output 4.4 L·min^{-1}) before, and 2.7 (pressure 11.9 mmHg, flow 4.4 L·min^{-1}) during, low spinal anesthesia.

During high spinal anesthesia, similar retrospective calculations indicated that "resistance" averaged 1.9 (pressure 11.0 mmHg, output 5.7 L·min^{-1}) before, and 2.4 (pressure 9.0 mmHg, output 3.7 L·min^{-1}) during, anesthesia in the four patients reported by Duner, et al. (1960). In five subjects with high spinal anesthesia reported by Sancetta, et al. (1952), comparable figures were 3.1 (pressure 14.8 mmHg, output 4.7 L·min^{-1}) before, and 2.6 (pressure 8.4 mmHg, flow 3.2 L·min^{-1}) during, high spinal anesthesia. In the 18 nonoperative subjects reported by Lynn, et al. (1952), the calculated "resistance" averaged 3.2 before (pressure 14.9 mmHg, output 4.6 L·min^{-1}) and 2.8 (pressure 8.9 mmHg, flow 3.2 L·min^{-1}) during, high (T$_3$ or higher) spinal anesthesia. Lynn, et al. (1952) also studied five operative patients during high spinal anesthesia combined with general anesthesia and controlled positive pressure ventilation. In these patients, "resistance" averaged 2.4 (pressure 12.4 mmHg, flow 5.2 L·min^{-1}) before induction of spinal anesthesia; following induction of anesthesia, "resistance" doubled to 4.9, because as pressure decreased to 8.9 mmHg, output decreased relatively more, to 1.8 L·min^{-1}. Finally, in 10 patients studied by Bergenwald, et al. (1972), "resistance" decreased from 2.4 (pressure 15.0 mmHg, flow 6.3 L·min^{-1}) before anesthesia to 2.1 (pressure 12.4 mmHg, output 6.0 L·min^{-1}) during T$_{1-3}$ sensory levels of spinal anesthesia.

Results obtained by retrospective calculation of pulmonary vascular resistance for the operative cases reported by Lynn, et al. (1952) are not necessarily accurate because their patients were given general anesthesia plus controlled positive pressure ventilation, either or both of which might have caused the increase in resistance. However, five of the remaining six studies mentioned above in which calculations were made suggest that pulmonary arterial "resistance" decreases slightly during both high and low spinal anesthesia. The exception, the study by Duner, et al. (1960), could be explained by the significant decrease in mean blood pressure from preanesthetic levels of 71 mmHg to levels of 35 mmHg after induction of T$_2$ spinal anesthesia. This was associated with a statistically significant decrease in cardiac output from 4.2 L·min^{-1} to 1.6 L·min^{-1}. If data from this patient are excluded, the calculated pulmonary "resistance" would remain unchanged (1.8) following induction of high spinal anesthesia. The fact remains, nevertheless, that in five of the six reports in which "resistance" has been calculated retrospectively, a decrease occurred during spinal anesthesia; this suggests that resistance to blood flow through the pulmonary artery may be decreased by spinal anesthesia. This possibility is supported by the more exactly derived data of Samii, et al. (1979) (see below). However, reasons why pulmonary resistance decreases during spinal anesthesia, if in fact it does, have not yet been determined.

The tendency for PVR to decrease might reflect changes in pulmonary vasomotor tone, changes in pulmonary capillary pressure, or changes in blood viscosity secondary to changes in pulmonary arterial flow (Chapter 2). Samii, et al. (1979) are the only authors who measured pulmonary (capillary) wedge pressure while investigating the effects of spinal anesthesia on pulmonary vascular resistance in humans. In one of two patient groups, in which patients with a mean age of 69 years were undergoing knee replacement without the use of bone cement, and with T_{10} levels of spinal anesthesia, the authors found capillary wedge pressures to increase, from 7.5 ± 1.8 mmHg before, to 9.8 ± 0.6 mmHg during spinal anesthesia. In the other group, with a mean age of 63 years and undergoing knee replacement with use of bone cement, wedge pressures increased from 7.1 ± 1.2 mmHg before, to 7.8 ± 1.2 mmHg during spinal anesthesia, even before cementing. Why the pulmonary capillary wedge pressure increased with such low levels of spinal anesthesia may be due to one of several reasons. First, all patients had atropine and diazepam premedication, and were receiving a continuous intravenous infusion of diazepam. Second, all patients also had received intravascular volume expansion with 830–860 ml of blood following induction of spinal anesthesia. Third, and just as important, following induction of spinal anesthesia, pulmonary wedge pressures were measured while the lower extremity tourniquet had been inflated for a considerable length of time (85 min), which may have resulted in changes in pressure due to tourniquet pain, excessive catecholamines, etc. These same factors may apply in these authors' study to the calculation of pulmonary vascular "resistance," which decreased during T_{10} spinal anesthesia by an average of 17 percent and 15 percent in the two patient groups, respectively (3.5 ± 0.3 to 2.9 ± 0.4; and 3.4 ± 0.6 to 2.9 ± 0.3).

It is tempting to relate any possible decrease in pulmonary vascular resistance during spinal anesthesia to vasodilation of pulmonary resistance vessels associated with sympathetic denervation. However, this would be purely speculative in the absence of data on the effects of thoracic sympathetic denervation without concurrent changes in either pulmonary arterial blood flow or pulmonary capillary pressure. Indeed, sympathetic nerves appear to exert little if any effect on the tone of pulmonary resistance vessels (Tkachenko, et al., 1969). Furthermore, changes in resistance as calculated above are not related to the level of sensory anesthesia. This would not be expected to be the case if high thoracic levels of sympathetic denervation altered pulmonary vascular resistance by producing pulmonary vasodilation. If high levels of denervation did produce pulmonary vasodilation, resistance would be expected to decrease only during high levels of spinal anesthesia, rather than during both high and low levels.

Effects of Spinal Anesthesia on Gas Exchange

Decreases in total alveolar blood flow, regardless of etiology, may be associated with decreases in arterial oxygenation. Changes in the distribution of alveolar blood flow may also alter arterial oxygenation through changes in the normal ratio of alveolar ventilation to alveolar perfusion. Changes in either or both total alveolar blood flow and its distribution, if significant enough, would be associated with decreased arterial oxygen tension and an increase in alveolar-arterial oxygen tension gradient. It is therefore appropriate to review in some detail reports on the effects of spinal anesthesia on arterial oxygenation.

There are many reports concerning arterial oxygenation during spinal anesthesia. Some early authors, such as Weiss, et al. (1933), found very slight increases (0.6 and 0.3 volumes percent) in the arterial blood oxygen content of patients following induction of spinal anesthesia, without any apparent increase in the concentration of oxygen in the inspired air (FIO_2). Shaw, et al. (1937) reported a similar change in dogs during spinal anesthesia. Five of eight animals had increases in arterial oxygen content, the mean increase being 1.3 volumes percent. In these animals, as in the patients reported by Weiss, et al., there was no increase in arterial oxygen capacity. Thus, the increased content was the result of increased saturation (i.e., tension).

The increases in arterial oxygenation reported by Weiss, et al. and Shaw, et al. are difficult to explain. The increased arterial oxygen saturation during hypotensive spinal anesthesia reported by Greene, et al. (1954) was undoubtedly because their patients were breathing higher than normal concentrations of oxygen. Other workers have not found any change in arterial oxygenation during spinal anesthesia. Burch and Harrison (1930) as well as Nakayama, et al. (1956) and Tardieu, et al. (1957) were unable to detect any changes in dogs. McClure, et al. (1939) found arterial oxygen content, capacity, and saturation to be normal in 8 of 10 patients, and below normal in 2 (levels before induction of anesthesia were not measured). Kety, et al. (1950) found the mean arterial oxygen content in 17 patients breathing room air to be 17.0 volumes percent before, and 16.9 volumes percent during, differential spinal block.

Despite the above, most investigators who have measured arterial oxygenation have observed slight reductions in arterial oxygen content. Seevers and Waters (1932 a, b) reported significant decreases in arterial oxygen content in dogs during spinal anesthesia, but the data are reported in such a manner that it is not possible to determine quantitative values. Decreases in arterial oxygenation, though slight, have been reported rather consistently during spinal anesthesia, however, when the concentration of oxygen in the inspired air remains constant. Schuberth (1936), for example, found the mean arterial oxygen content in 29 patients to be 14.5 ± 0.5 volumes percent before induction of spinal anesthesia and 12.6 ± 0.5 during anesthesia (sensory levels usually at mid-thoracic or high-thoracic levels). Nowak and Downing (1938) observed in seven cats an association between spinal anesthesia and a slight decrease in arterial oxygen carrying capacity (15.1 to 12.5 volumes percent), with no changes in oxygen saturation (90.3 percent to 90.8 percent). Using an oximeter attached to the ear in 25 patients, Latterell and Lundy (1949) found that arterial oxygen saturation decreased by an average of 1.0 percent during spinal anesthesia. This decrease in oximetric saturation was not confirmed, however, when the authors measured oxygen saturation directly in 17 arterial blood samples. The Van Slyke technique used showed the average arterial oxygen saturation to be 95.5 percent before and 95.3 percent during anesthesia. There was no correlation with either height of anesthesia, or presence or absence of intercostal nerve block. Johnson (1951) found a slight decrease in the average oxygen content of arterial blood in six patients during high spinal blockade who did not receive supplemental barbiturates. The figures were 18.1 volumes percent before and 17.5 volumes percent during anesthesia. Similar results were reported by Nowak and Downing (1938). In 1986, Muravchick and Johnson investigated the effects of spinal anesthesia with a mean level of $T_{6.7}$ (range T_1–T_{11}, medians not provided) on transcutaneous tissue oxygen tension (T_cPO_2) in both young and elderly patients. They found that induction of spinal anesthesia was not associated with any significant changes in T_cPO_2, regardless of patients' age.

One of the most complete series of studies of arterial blood oxygenation during spinal anesthesia was reported by Sancetta, et al. (Sancetta, et al., 1952, 1953; Lynn, et al., 1952; Hackel, et al., 1956; Kleinerman, et al., 1958). The results are summarized in Table 3.5. Their data indicate that regardless of sensory level, spinal anesthesia has no significant effect on arterial oxygen content, capacity, or saturation. However, a slight decrease in content can be detected, which, while probably not statistically significant in itself, occurs consistently enough to be considered a regular rather than a fortuitous effect. This decrease is accompanied by an equally slight decrease in oxygen carrying capacity, so that there is practically no change in oxygen saturation. Similar maintenance of oxy-

Table 3.5.
Arterial Oxygenation During Spinal Anesthesia (Average Figures from the Literature)

Reference	Oxygen Content (vol %)		Oxygen Capacity (vol %)		Oxygen Saturation (%)		Remarks
	Before	During	Before	During	Before	During	
Sancetta, et al. 1952	13.1	12.9	14.5	14.4	89.9	89.2	5 patients, low spinal
	13.1	12.5	14.4	13.8	91.5	90.5	5 patients, high spinal
Lynn, et al. 1952	15.2	14.3	16.5	15.5	91.8	91.9	10 operative cases
	15.4	14.7	16.7	16.1	92.7	91.8	18 nonoperative cases
Sancetta, et al. 1953	14.6	14.2	15.7	15.4	91.9	91.9	6 patients; operative
Hackel, et al. 1956	14.6	13.4	—	—	—	—	—
Kleinerman, et al. 1958	15.9	15.7	—	—	93	93	9 patients; total sympathetic block

gen saturation near baseline values (94 percent–95 percent) following induction of mid- to high-thoracic spinal anesthesia has been reported by Manara, et al. (1989).

Reports indicating that spinal anesthesia has no significant effect on arterial oxygenation are supplemented by observations on the effect of spinal anesthesia on arterial oxygen tension. De Jong (1965) studied 10 patients having surgery performed under spinal anesthesia. They found that, with no sedatives or narcotics being administered during anesthesia, arterial partial pressure of oxygen (pO_2) decreased in four patients, increased in four, and remained unchanged in four when compared to pO_2 levels following premedication but prior to induction of anesthesia (FIO_2 was kept constant). The mean change was a decrease of 1.1 mmHg. Bonica, et al. (1966), on the other hand, reported a slight, but unspecified increase in arterial pO_2 during spinal anesthesia in seven non-operative subjects. Ward, et al. (1965) found an increase as well, averaging 14.9 mmHg in 14 patients. Similarly, the subjects studied by Kennedy, et al. (1968) showed elevations of arterial pO_2, ranging from 3 percent to 9 percent above control levels. Particularly interesting was the observation (Catenacci and Sampathachar, 1969) in eight obese patients that arterial pO_2 increased significantly from 70.5 mmHg before induction of spinal anesthesia, to 78.0 mmHg during anesthesia, in the absence of any change in FIO_2. Eight thin patients with equal levels of spinal anesthesia studied simultaneously showed no change in arterial pO_2.

James and Fisher (1969), however, recorded decreases in arterial pO_2 from 417 mmHg prior to spinal anesthesia to 335 mmHg during anesthesia. Their 11 patients (5 with weights less than, and 6 with weights more than, those predicted from their height and age) had spinal anesthesia after induction of halothane-oxygen general anesthesia with spontaneous respiration (inspired oxygen concentration was not reported); the supplemental oxygen delivered could explain the high arterial pO_2 levels present before administration of spinal anesthesia. The fact that these patients also had general anesthesia, plus the fact that data from eight patients were pooled with data from three patients undergoing epidural anesthesia, make these results difficult to interpret.

Wishart (1971) also studied arterial pO_2 levels when spinal anesthesia was administered during general anesthesia. He, too, observed a decrease in arterial pO_2 following induction of spinal anesthesia. With an FIO_2 of 0.5 during general anesthesia, arterial pO_2 decreased from 157 to 130 mmHg after 1 hr of spinal anesthesia. Ravin (1971) reported arterial oxygen tensions in emphysematous patients during T_{6-11} sensory levels of spinal anesthesia that were similar to those observed in emphysematous patients undergoing comparable types of surgery during halothane-nitrous oxide-oxygen anesthesia, FIO_2 being the same (0.4) in both groups. Furthermore, induction of spinal or general anesthesia was not associated with changes in arterial pO_2 from baseline preanesthetic levels. The data of Ravin do not, of course, prove whether spinal anesthesia is associated with maldistribution of alveolar blood flow during spinal anesthesia and an increase in alveolar-arterial pO_2 gradient. The results suggest that if ventilation-to-perfusion mismatch does occur with spinal anesthesia, it is no greater than that observed during general anesthesia. On the other hand, Cabalum, et al. (1979) found statistically significant decreases in arterial pO_2 in experimental animals breathing room air during high spinal anesthesia. Finally, McKenzie, et al. (1980) found no change in arterial pO_2 in 49 geriatric patients (average age 76.8 years) undergoing surgical correction of femur fractures under spinal anesthesia.

The above data lead to the following conclusions: (a) High spinal anesthesia is not associated with clinically significant changes in arterial oxygenation. (b) Minor increases in alveolar-arterial pO_2 gradients may occur during high spinal anesthesia due to decreases in alveolar blood flow or maldistribution of alveolar blood flow. However, increases in alveolar-arterial pO_2 gradients that occur during spinal anesthesia are not of clinical significance. (c) Under certain conditions, arterial pO_2 may increase during spinal anesthesia. Anxiety-induced hyperventilation may increase arterial pO_2 slightly; if so, arterial carbon dioxide tension (pCO_2) decreases (Kennedy, et al., 1968; Steinbrook and Concepcion, 1991). Arterial pO_2 may also increase during spinal anesthesia in obese patients (Catenacci and Sampathachar, 1969). This may represent restoration toward normal of alveolar ventilation-to-perfusion ratios that were abnormal preanesthetically because of obesity.

It should also be noted that regional, including high spinal, anesthesia has no demonstrable effect on hypoxic pulmonary vasoconstriction. As a rule, general anesthetics inhibit hypoxic pulmonary vasoconstriction, which shunts blood flow away from hypoxic or nonventilating alveoli to better ventilated alveoli. By inhibiting this local vasoconstriction, general anesthetics may worsen the balance between ventilation and perfusion, by permitting perfusion of nonventilated or poorly ventilated alveoli. Since local pulmonary hypoxic vasoconstriction is not neurally mediated by pathways through the subarachnoid space, spinal anesthesia does not affect flow distribution when alveolar hypoventilation exists. Therefore, spinal anesthesia will not worsen an already impaired alveolar oxygen uptake due to intrapulmonary shunting.

Unlike arterial oxygenation, arterial pCO_2 is primarily determined by alveolar ventilation and is nearly independent of blood flow. While measurements of pCO_2 provide little information on pulmonary blood flow, they are sensitive indices of alveolar ventilation. Decreases in alveolar ventilation that are not sufficient to alter arterial oxygenation may reduce carbon dioxide excretion. That the sympathetic block produced by spinal anesthesia itself has no effect on arterial pCO_2 is supported by the observation that total epidural sympathetic block does not alter arterial pCO_2 in experimental animals (Greene and Phillips, 1957). In humans as well, total preganglionic sympathetic block does not adversely affect alveolar ventilation as measured by arterial pCO_2 levels or by end-tidal pCO_2 levels (Eisele, et al., 1968). Kety, et al. (1950) produced differential spinal sympathetic block in 15 patients and found that the average arterial pCO_2 actually decreased slightly from the control level of 43 to 38 mmHg as a result of spontaneous hyperventilation. Greene, et al. (1954) reported alveolar ventilation to be adequate during clinical spinal anesthesia. Although their patients were under light general anesthesia when given high levels of spinal blockade as part of a study of "hypotensive spinal" anesthesia, respirations were neither assisted nor controlled. No abnormal elevations of arterial pCO_2 were seen in any of the patients. Thus, it may be assumed that spinal anesthesia per se had little affect on alveolar ventilation. In 22 cases, the average arterial pCO_2 was 36.6 mmHg before anesthesia. During anesthesia, it averaged 39.4 mmHg, a figure below the accepted normal level of 40 mmHg, comparing favorably with the not infrequently high arterial pCO_2 found during spontaneous respiration with general anesthesia.

De Jong (1965) has also confirmed that arterial pCO_2 remained normal during surgery performed under spinal anesthesia. Of 10 patients who received premedication but no other drugs following the induction of anesthesia, de Jong found that arterial pCO_2 increased above preanesthetic control values in three subjects, decreased in five, and remained unchanged in two. The mean change was an increase of 0.3 mmHg. Similar reports by Catenacci and Sampathachar (1969), Wishart (1971), McKenzie, et al. (1980), Cabalum, et al. (1979) and Steinbrook, et al. (1988) confirm that in both humans and experimental animals alveolar ventilation remains unaffected even during high levels of spinal anesthesia, so that arterial pCO_2 does not change. Indeed, arterial pCO_2 does not change during spinal anesthesia even in patients who are likely to develop alveolar hypoventilation. Catenacci and Sampathachar (1969) found no change in arterial pCO_2 with T_{4-10} levels of anesthesia in the eight obese patients they studied. Ravin (1971) found no significant change in arterial pCO_2 in 10 patients with chronic obstructive pulmonary disease during T_{6-11} levels of anesthesia.

A decrease in arterial pCO_2 during spinal anesthesia usually is caused by hyperventilation, including that associated with apprehension. This is most evident in nonoperative subjects undergoing spinal anesthesia without premedication with hypnotics or barbiturates (Kleinerman, et al., 1958; Askrog, et al., 1964; Ward, et al., 1965; Kennedy, et al., 1968). The average decrease under these conditions usually ranges from 2 to 6 mmHg. Anxiety related to "impending surgery" has been proposed as the reason for the decrease in resting end-tidal pCO_2 ($P_{ET}CO_2$) reported by Steinbrook and Concepcion (1991) in 11 unpremedicated patients. The same group of investigators also reported a slight (but statistically significant) decrease in resting end-tidal pCO_2 from a preanesthetic level of 40 ± 3 mmHg, to 38 ± 3 mmHg during T_{2-10} spinal anesthesia (Steinbrook, et al., 1988). Inadequate sensory levels of anesthesia also cause hyperventilation and hypocarbia.

Increases in pCO_2 during spinal anesthesia are most frequently due to simultaneous administration of narcotics or sedatives. However, not all sedatives depress respiration during spinal anesthesia; when used to supplement spinal anesthesia in elderly males undergoing prostatic surgery, diazepam, in doses averaging 20 mg, had no significant effect on arterial pCO_2 (Pearce, 1974). No mention is made in that study, however, about arterial oxygen saturation. Furthermore, it must be emphasized that in a recent study of 14 cases of sudden cardiac arrest in healthy patients undergoing spinal anesthesia, one of the two patterns of management that have been implicated as contributors to this occurrence has been the "intraoperative use of sufficient sedation to produce a comfortable-appearing, sleep-like state in which there was no spontaneous verbalization" (Caplan, et al., 1988). The danger of oversedation with benzodiazepines during spinal anesthesia, despite the availability of the antagonist flumazenil, has recently been reemphasized (Halim, et al., 1990; Manara, et al., 1989; Reinhart, et al., 1983). For this reason, Manara, *et al.* (1989) have recommended that supplementary oxygen "should be administered routinely to patients receiving sedatives during spinal anesthesia."

The absence of carbon dioxide retention during operative spinal anesthesia also extends into the postoperative period. Hamilton and Devine (1957) found that in five "spinals" (actually, two patients with lumbar epidural blocks and three patients with spinal anesthesia) average arterial pCO_2 in the immediate postoperative period with the blocks still in effect was 27.1 mmHg. Comparable figures in patients who had other anesthetics were as follows: 34.2 mmHg in those who had ether, 39.3 mmHg in patients who had cyclopropane, and 44.3 mmHg in those who had nitrous oxide plus intravenous anesthetics. In these cases, the difference in postoperative arterial pCO_2 levels between general and spinal anesthesia can be ascribed to the continued respiratory depression associated with general anesthetics. It is not clear why the patients with spinal anesthetics had such low levels of arterial pCO_2 postoperatively at a time when analgesia was still present. McKenzie, *et al.* (1980) found normal arterial pCO_2 levels 1 hr after conclusion of surgery performed under spinal anesthesia. Arterial pCO_2 levels were significantly greater (5.16 kilopascals (kPa)) during general anesthesia (nitrous oxide-halothane plus succinylcholine with spontaneous respiration) than during spinal anesthesia (4.36 kPa). However, these differences disappeared 60 min after completion of surgery, at which time both types of anesthesia were associated with eucapnia. Thus, after an hour or more postoperatively, there is usually no difference in arterial pCO_2 in patients given either spinal or general anesthesia (Linderholm and Norlander, 1958).

Askrog, *et al.* (1964) studied the effect of spinal anesthesia on intrapulmonary distribution of inspired air to determine if gas exchange was impaired secondary to maldistribution of alveolar ventilation even though tidal volume and minute volume were unaffected. These authors found that in all six patients studied, respiratory dead space increased (Fig. 3.1) from values averaging 154 ± 21 ml before, to 201 ± 22 ml during anesthesia; this represented a 31 percent increase. Anatomic dead space was unaffected by this increase, remaining constant, while alveolar dead space increased. This resulted from an increase in the ratio between respiratory dead space and tidal volume (V_D/V_T), from an average value of 0.30, to 0.41. Despite these changes in alveolar dead space, arterial pCO_2 did not increase; rather, it decreased slightly from control levels of 35.8 ± 1.4 to 32.3 ± 3.1 mmHg during anesthesia. The changes were accompanied, however, by an increase in the normal arterial-end tidal pCO_2 gradient of 1.4 ± 0.6 mmHg preanesthetically, and by an increase of 5.6 ± 1.2 mmHg during anesthesia. These changes in respiratory dead space, arterial-alveolar pCO_2 difference, and V_D/V_T ratio probably were not accompanied by significant changes in arterial pCO_2. A possible explanation is that changes in arterial pCO_2 were compensated for by simultaneous slight decreases in vascular perfusion of normally ventilated alveoli.

Effects of Spinal Anesthesia on Respiratory Drive

It is apparent that spinal anesthesia does not affect ventilation by reducing gas exchange even with sensory levels of anesthesia high enough to produce intercostal paralysis. However, ventilatory inadequacy can and does occur during spinal anesthesia in the following circumstances: (a) reduced diaphragmatic excursions due to either intra-abdominal packs and retractors or to improper positioning of the patient (extreme Trendelenburg position, prone position without proper support, etc.); (b) phrenic nerve paralysis; and (c) central respiratory failure. The occurrence of the latter two, although infrequent, results in sudden respiratory arrest during spinal anesthesia. True phrenic paralysis is the rarer of the two, because there is only a slight chance that the anesthetic will reach the phrenic nerve roots in concentrations sufficient to paralyze the phrenics. Even with cervical levels of sensory anesthesia (Sheskey, et al., 1983; Sinclair, et al., 1982) or in intentionally produced "total" spinal anesthesia with complete sensory blockade, including cranial nerves (Chapter 1), phrenic paralysis rarely occurs. This is because large motor fibers are more resistant than the smaller sensory ones to the effects of local anesthetic agents. While primary phrenic paralysis certainly can occur, it rarely causes respiratory arrest during clinical spinal anesthesia.

The most frequent cause of apnea during spinal anesthesia is failure of the respiratory center, which, rather than resulting from direct action of the local anesthetic on the brainstem (Chapter 1), is caused by inadequate medullary blood flow secondary to a severe reduction in cardiac output. Ischemia of the respiratory center is therefore one of the most frequent causes of respiratory arrest during spinal anesthesia. This is demonstrated by the fact that cardiac arrest is associated with apnea in the vast majority of cases of arrest during anesthesia; after cardiac output is restored, spontaneous respirations return, unless there has been widespread damage to the central nervous system. Therefore, treatment of respiratory arrest during spinal anesthesia requires, first, maintenance of venous return to provide adequate cardiac output. This entails use of the head-down position. Second, the patient's lungs should be ventilated with 100 percent oxygen. By itself, however, artificial ventilation will prove useless without adequate cardiac output. Treatment of respiratory arrest during spinal anesthesia in the head-down position with artificial ventilation ensures safe management of the few cases caused by true phrenic paralysis. Using the same method for those cases in which apnea is due to ischemic paralysis of the brainstem assures adequate alveolar ventilation along with the highest possible cardiac output under conditions of total sympathetic block. If, as may happen, asystole occurs during apnea (Caplan, *et al.*, 1988), cardiac resuscitation must be instituted immediately.

Effects of Anesthetic Technique on Postoperative Outcome

A word should also be said about the influence of the type of anesthesia on the frequency of postoperative pulmonary complications. A frequent clinical impression holds that fewer postoperative pulmonary complications accompany spinal anesthesia than general anesthesia. While there are anecdotal reports substantiating this impression (e.g., Washburn, 1933), there are as many anecdotal reports suggesting the opposite to be the case (Brown, 1931; Brown and Debenham, 1932; Lyford, 1942 a, b; McKittrick, *et al.*, 1931). Age, sex, physical condition, smoking habits of the patient, the nature and site of the operation performed, the skill of the anesthesiologist and standards of preoperative and postoperative management are all factors that, alone or in combination, influence the occurrence of postoperative pulmonary complications. That the anesthetic agent or technique may not determine the frequency of postoperative pulmonary complications was first proposed many years ago by King (1933). He recorded an incidence of postoperative pulmonary complications of 12.4 percent in 2069 patients subjected to laparotomy or herniorrhaphy following ether anesthesia, and an incidence of 16.7 percent in 425 patients following similar operations performed under spinal anesthesia. Further breakdown of King's data supports the fact that the type of anesthesia did not affect significantly the incidence of postoperative pulmonary complications. In King's study, their incidence in male patients (who were all having the same operation (herniorrhaphy) and were between the ages of 20 and 60 years) was 11.1 percent following ether anesthesia (108 patients) and 13.6 percent following spinal anesthesia (110 patients).

King's conclusions were confirmed by Dripps and Deming (1946) who also graphically demonstrated the importance of skill and care in managing the patient before, during and after surgery. Their patients were divided into two groups. The first consisted of those having upper abdominal surgery in whom no special measures were taken to avoid postoperative pulmonary complications. Of the 90 patients given general anesthesia in this group, 11.1 percent developed postoperative pulmonary complications. Only 4.2 percent of the 144 patients (having the same type of surgery) under spinal anesthesia developed postoperative complications. In the second group, all patients were afforded an intensive and meticulously planned program designed to prevent pulmonary complications. This included standard procedures such as postural drainage, attention to oral hygiene, preventing accumulation of pharyngeal or tracheal secretions, and hyperventilation. Such a regime reduced the incidence of postoperative pulmonary complications to 4.1 percent in 343 patients who received general anesthesia. The incidence following spinal anesthesia remained essentially the same (5.0 percent in 543 cases). Similar results have been reported by Urbach, et al. (1964). In a group of 514 patients, all of whom had the same operation (inguinal herniorrhaphy) and received the same high quality of postoperative care, Urbach, et al. found the incidence of postoperative respiratory complications to be the same for both spinal anesthesia and general anesthesia.

However, the literature also contains studies that have shown that spinal anesthesia is indeed associated with a lower incidence of major pulmonary complications such as pulmonary embolism, when compared with general anesthesia. Over 30 years ago, Sevitt and Gallagher (1961) demonstrated that at postmortem, up to 83 percent of patients who died following hip (femoral neck) fracture had evidence of deep vein thrombosis (DVT); 46 percent of these patients had further evidence of pulmonary thromboembolism. There is strong evidence that regional anesthesia (spinal as well as epidural) may be associated with a significantly lower risk of DVT (Chapter 2). Thus, the incidence of pulmonary embolism likewise may be lowered. Nygaard (1936) and Minster (1964) also reported a somewhat lower incidence of respiratory complications after spinal anesthesia than after general anesthesia. Perhaps also related to the lower incidence of pulmonary embolism is the fact that some authors have demonstrated that operations performed under spinal anesthesia are associated with a lower postoperative mortality than similar operations performed under general anesthesia (McLaren, et al., 1978; McKenzie, et al., 1980).

That cellular immunity measured by lymphocyte transformation is equally depressed for a week postoperatively by both spinal and general anesthesia (Kent and Geist, 1975) might be a manifestation of the fact that susceptibility to pulmonary (and other) infections appears to be related not just to the type of anesthesia, but to surgery per se. On the other hand, unlike general anesthesia, spinal anesthesia is not associated with postoperative depression of neutrophil random migration and chemotaxis (Stanley, et al., 1978). Also, following spinal anesthesia, there is an increase in the total white blood cell and polymorphonuclear cell counts (Stanley, et al., 1978). However, the clinical significance of both these observations is still obscure (Chapter 6).

While spinal anesthesia may in some settings significantly decrease the incidence of postoperative respiratory complications, certain respiratory diseases may make the use of spinal anesthesia unwise. This is particularly true if the level of anesthesia must be high in order to provide satisfactory operating conditions. Chief among these are chronic bronchitis and bronchiectasis associated with a cough productive of significant amounts of sputum. Patients with these diseases must be able to maintain an effective cough during spinal anesthesia to clear their secretions, particularly in the supine position. Although in normal subjects or those with preexisting pulmonary disease, resting ventilation is not significantly altered by spinal anesthesia, the ability to hyperventilate and cough effectively may be seriously impaired by high spinal anesthesia. Egbert, et al. (1961), for example, found that while 20 healthy subjects with sensory levels of anesthesia to T_{2-6} maintained normal resting tidal volumes, the ability to produce maximal flow of respiratory gases was impaired. This impairment was demonstrated by a significant diminution in vital capacity (from 4.05 ± 0.81 to 3.73 ± 0.72 L). Similarly, Askrog, et al. (1964) found that high levels of spinal anesthesia decreased maximum breathing capacity from levels of 69.8 ± 10.6 L·min^{-1} before anesthesia, to 52.9 ± 10.2 L·min^{-1} during anesthesia. Perhaps more importantly, high levels of spinal anesthesia impair the ability to generate peak intrathoracic pressures, both positive and negative. The theoretical effects of sympathetic denervation produced by high thoracic spinal anesthesia in asthmatic patients have already been discussed (pp. 209–210).

Egbert, et al. (1961) found that the maximum intrapulmonary positive pressure their subjects were able to generate during forced exhalation averaged 87 ± 21 mmHg following premedication but prior to anesthesia. Following induction of spinal anesthesia with sensory levels of T_{2-6}, the same subjects were able to produce a maximum intrapulmonary pressure during forced exhalation of only 41 ± 22 mmHg. This reduction was associated with comparable changes in intra-abdominal pressures. Maximum intrarectal pressures during forced exhalation averaged 53 ± 20 mmHg before spinal anesthesia, and 7 ± 11 mmHg during anesthesia. The changes in peak ventilatory pressures (Egbert, et al., 1961) were not associated with changes in 1-sec timed inspiratory or expiratory capacities (as a percent of tidal volume). However, they were accompanied by significant decreases in maximum inspiratory flow rates, from control levels of 3.11 ± 0.36 L·sec^{-1} preanesthetically, to levels of 2.46 ± 0.38 L·sec^{-1} during anesthesia (Askrog, et al., 1964).

Paskin, et al. (1969) also demonstrated in patients with chronic obstructive pulmonary disease that, although resting ventilation remained adequate to maintain arterial blood gas tensions at preanesthetic levels, mid- or high thoracic levels of spinal anesthesia were associated with significant decreases in peak expiratory flow rates (Table 3.3). High spinal anesthesia affects forced exhalation because it causes paralysis of abdominal muscles. If abdominal muscles are not fully functional, forced exhalation is inevitably impaired. Consequently, high spinal anesthesia may severely handicap patients with bronchitis, bronchiectasis, or a productive cough, by weakening their ability to generate enough positive pressure during forced exhalation to clear their secretions. Spinal anesthesia may also adversely affect inhalation, especially inspiratory capacity in obese patients, and, thus, decrease vital capacity (Catenacci and Samphathachar, 1969). This occurs because the diaphragm cannot compensate for intercostal paralysis when its descent into the abdominal cavity is impeded by a sufficiently large mass of intraabdominal fat.

The inability to cough normally during operations performed under spinal anesthesia persists into the postoperative period, although splinting (to prevent incisional pain) may affect the postoperative ability to cough as much as the type of anesthesia itself. Egbert, *et al.* (1962) quantitated the ability of patients to cough postoperatively following lower extremity surgery or following herniorrhaphy performed under either general (cyclopropane or ether) or spinal anesthesia, by measuring maximal intrarectal pressure during coughing. Rectal pressures remained far below preoperative control values during the first 2 hr in the recovery room. The depression was greater following herniorrhaphy than after surgery on the lower extremities, and greater following general anesthesia than following spinal anesthesia. Since patients in both groups were awake, the incisional pain caused by the effort of coughing probably contributed to the differences observed. The inability to cough and to generate peak intrathoracic pressures may handicap patients with bronchitis or bronchiectasis as well as patients with other types of preexisting respiratory disease such as emphysema. While such patients may be able to ventilate adequately under resting conditions, they may be unable to compensate for increased ventilatory demands during periods of stress while under spinal anesthesia.

An exception to the above was observed by Giesecke, *et al.* (1968). These authors found that pulmonary ventilation in geriatric patients with chronic lung disease may actually improve during spinal anesthesia when patients are placed in the extreme lithotomy position. All 18 patients studied by Giesecke, *et al.* had significant preexisting pulmonary disease; this was indicated by an average preanesthetic forced vital capacity 65 percent of predicted normal, and by the fact that patients were able to exhale only 45 percent of their total forced vital capacity during the first 0.5 sec of forced exhalation. Following induction of spinal anesthesia to levels adequate for perineal prostatectomy, pulmonary function did not change significantly from preanesthetic control values while the patients remained in the supine position. However, after changing to the exaggerated lithotomy (Young's) position, pulmonary function showed significant improvement, evidenced by a greater ability to move air during the early part (first 0.5 sec) of forced expiration, even though there was no change in the total volume of air moved (forced vital capacity). As the authors suggest, the improvement was probably the result of elevation of the end-exhalational position of the diaphragm and "assisted" return of the diaphragm to the resting position by the weight of the abdominal viscera, combined with flexion of the thighs on the abdomen. This position therefore exerts the same effect as an "emphysema belt" to aid exhalation.

REFERENCES

ABAJIAN, J. C., MELLISH, R. W. P., BROWNE, A. F., PERKINS, F. M., LAMBERT, D. H., AND MAZUZAN, J. E., JR.: Spinal anesthesia for surgery in the high-risk infant. Anesth. Analg. 63: 359, 1984.

ALDRETE, J. A., WOODWARD, S. T., AND TURK, L. H.: Influence of cigarette smoking on the changes produced by spinal anesthesia on expiratory forced volumes and flow rates. Anesth. Analg. 52: 809, 1973.

ASKROG, V. F., SMITH, T. C., AND ECKENHOFF, J. E.: Changes in pulmonary ventilation during spinal anesthesia. Surg. Gynecol. Obstet. 119: 563, 1964.

AVIADO, D. M.: Regulation of bronchomotor tone during anesthesia. Anesthesiology 42: 68, 1975.

AXELSSON, K., AND WIDMAN, G. B.: A comparison of bupivacaine and tetracaine in spinal anaesthesia with special reference to motor block. Acta Anaesthesiol. Scand. 29: 79, 1985.

BAILEY, A., VALLEY, R., AND BIGLER, R.: High spinal anesthesia in an infant. Anesthesiology 70: 560, 1989.

BERGENWALD, L., EKLUND, B., KAIJSER, L., KLINGENSTROM, P., AND WESTERMARK, L.: Haemodynamic effects of dihydroergotamine during spinal anaesthesia in man. Acta Anaesthesiol. Scand. 16: 235, 1972.

BONICA, J. J., KENNEDY, W. F., JR., WARD, R. J., AND TOLAS, A. G.: A comparison of the effects of high subarachnoid and epidural anaesthesia. Acta Anaesthesiol. Scand. (Suppl.) 23: 429, 1966.

BOWER, J. O., WAGONER, G., AND CLARK, J. H.: Clinical and experimental investigation in spinal anesthesia. Anesth. Analg. 5: 95, 1926.

BOWER, J. O., CLARK, J. H., WAGONER, G., AND BURNS, J. C.: Spinal anesthesia; a summary of clinical and experimental investigations with practical deductions. Surg. Gynecol. Obstet. 54: 882, 1932.

BROWN, A. L.: Postoperative pulmonary atelectasis; analysis of four hundred and ninety-seven cases. Arch. Surg. 22: 976, 1931.

BROWN, A. L., AND DEBENHAM, M. W.: Postoperative pulmonary complications: study of their relative incidence following inhalation anesthesia and spinal anesthesia. J. A. M. A. 99: 209, 1932.

BURCH, J. C., AND HARRISON, T. R.: The effect of spinal anesthesia on the cardiac output. Arch. Surg. 21: 330, 1930.

CABALUM, T., SUGAIB, M., LIEB, S., NUWAYHID, B., BRINKMAN, C. R., III, AND ASSALI, N. S.:

Effect of dopamine on hypotension induced by spinal anesthesia. Am. J. Obstet. Gynecol. *133:* 630, 1979.

CAPLAN, R. A., WARD, R. J., POSNER, K., AND CHENEY, F. W.: Unexpected cardiac arrest during spinal anesthesia: a closed claims analysis of predisposing factors. Anesthesiology *68:* 5, 1988.

CATENACCI, A. J., AND SAMPATHACHAR, K. R.: Ventilatory studies in the obese patient during spinal anesthesia. Anesth. Analg. *48:* 48, 1969.

COOK, P. T., DAVIES, M. J., CRONIN, K. D., AND MORAN, P.: A prospective randomised trial comparing spinal anaesthesia using hyperbaric cinchocaine with general anaesthesia for lower limb vascular surgery. Anaesth. Intens. Care *14:* 373, 1986.

DAVIS, F. M., AND LAURENSON, V. G.: Spinal anaesthesia or general anaesthesia for emergency hip surgery in elderly patients. Anaesth. Intens. Care *9:* 352, 1981.

DE TROYER, A., SAMPSON, M., SIGRIST, S., AND MACKLEM, P. T.: The diaphragm: two muscles (lett.). Science *213:* 237, 1981.

DE JONG, R. H.: Arterial carbon dioxide and oxygen tensions during spinal block. J. A. M. A. *191:* 608, 1965.

DRIPPS, R. B., AND DEMING, M. V.: Postoperative atelectasis and pneumonia: diagnosis, etiology, and management based upon 1,240 cases of upper abdominal surgery. Ann. Surg. *124:* 94, 1946.

DUNER, H., GRANATH, A., AND KLINGENSTROM, P.: The effect of ergotamine on blood pressure and cardiac output during spinal anaesthesia in man. Acta Anaesthesiol. Scand. *4:* 5, 1960.

EGBERT, L. D., LAVER, M. B., AND BENDIXEN, H. H.: The effect of site of operation and type of anesthesia upon the ability to cough in the postoperative period. Surg. Gynecol. Obstet. *115:* 295, 1962.

EGBERT, L. D., TAMERSOY, K., AND PEAS, T. C.: Pulmonary function during spinal anesthesia: the mechanism of cough depression. Anesthesiology *22:* 882, 1961.

EISELE, J., TRENCHARD, D., BURKI, N., AND GUZ, A.: The effect of chest wall block on respiratory sensation and control in man. Clin. Sci. *35:* 23, 1968.

FREUND, F. G., BONICA, J. J., WARD, R. J., AKAMATSU, T. J., AND KENNEDY, W. F., JR.: Ventilatory reserve and level of motor block during high spinal and epidural anesthesia. Anesthesiology *28:* 834, 1967.

GAUTHIER, R. A., CHUNG, F., DYCK, B., ROMANELLI, J. R., AND CHAPMAN, K. R.: Does spinal anaesthesia interact with sedation to alter ventilatory responses? Can. J. Anaesth. *37:* S38, 1990.

GIESECKE, A. H., JR., CALE, J. O., AND JENKINS, M. T.: The prostate, ventilation, and anesthesia. J. A. M. A. *203:* 389, 1968.

GRAY, H. T., AND PARSONS, L.: Blood pressure variations associated with lumbar puncture and the induction of spinal anesthesia. Q. J. Med. *5:* 339, 1912.

GREENE, N. M., AND PHILLIPS, A. D'E.: Metabolic response of dogs to hypoxia in the absence of circulating epinephrine and norepinephrine. Am. J. Physiol. *189:* 475, 1957.

GREENE, N. M., BUNKER, J. P., KERR, W. S., VON FELSINGER, J. M., KELLER, J. W., AND BEECHER, H. K.: Hypotensive spinal anesthesia: respiratory, metabolic, hepatic, renal, and cerebral effects. Ann. Surg. *140:* 641, 1954.

HACKEL, D. B., SANCETTA, S. M., AND KLEINERMAN, J.: Effect of hypotension due to spinal anesthesia on coronary blood flow and myocardial metabolism in man. Circulation *13:* 92, 1956.

HALIM, B., SCHNEIDER, I., CLAEYS, M. A., AND CAMU, F.: The use of midazolam and flumazenil in locoregional anaesthesia: an overview. Acta Anaesthesiol. Scand. *34:* 42, 1990.

HAMILTON, W. K., AND DEVINE, J. C.: The evaluation of respiratory adequacy in the immediate postoperative period. Surg. Gynecol. Obstet. *105:* 229, 1957.

HARNIK, E. V., HOY, G. R., POTOLICCHIO, S., STEWART, D. R., AND SIEGELMAN, R. E.: Spinal anesthesia in premature infants recovering from respiratory distress syndrome. Anesthesiology 64: 95, 1986.

HARROP-GRIFFITHS, A. W., RAVALIA, A., BROWNE, D. A., AND ROBINSON, P. N.: Regional anaesthesia and cough effectiveness: a study in patients undergoing Caesarean section. Anaesthesia 46: 11, 1991.

HECKER, B. R., BJURSTROM, R., AND SCHOENE, R. B.: Effect of intercostal nerve blockade on respiratory mechanics and CO_2 chemosensitivity at rest and exercise. Anesthesiology 70: 13, 1989.

HEDENSTIERNA, G., AND LÖFSTROM, G.: Effect of anaesthesia on respiratory function after major lower extremity surgery. Acta Anaesthesiol. Scand. 29: 55, 1985.

JAMES, M. L., AND FISHER, A.: Blood gas changes during spinal and epidural analgesia. Anaesthesia 24: 511, 1969.

JOHNSON, S. R.: The effect of some anaesthetic agents on the circulation in man. Acta Chir. Scandinav. Suppl. 158: 1951.

KENNEDY, W. F., JR., BONICA, J. J., AKAMATSU, T. J., WARD, R. J., MARTIN, W. E., AND GRINSTEIN, A.: Cardiovascular and respiratory effects of subarachnoid block in the presence of acute blood loss. Anesthesiology 29: 29, 1968.

KENT, J. R., AND GEIST, S.: Lymphocyte transformation during operations with spinal anesthesia. Anesthesiology 42: 505, 1975.

KETY, S. S., KING, B. D., HORVATH, S. M., JEFFERS, W. A., AND KAFKENSCHIEL, J. H.: The effects of an acute reduction in blood pressure by means of differential spinal sympathetic block on the cerebral circulation of hypertensive patients. J. Clin. Invest. 29: 402, 1950.

KIM, J. M., AND REED, K.: PvO_2 changes in cutaneous veins during regression of spinal anaesthesia. Can. J. Anaesth. 34: 358, 1987.

KING, D. S.: Postoperative pulmonary complications: part played by anesthesia as shown by 2 years study at Massachusetts General Hospital. Anesth. Analg. 12: 243, 1933.

KLEINERMAN, J., SANCETTA, S. M., AND HACKEL, D. B.: Effects of high spinal anesthesia on cerebral circulation and metabolism in man. J. Clin. Invest. 37: 285, 1958.

LATTERELL, K. E., AND LUNDY, J. S.: Oxygen and carbon dioxide content of arterial blood before and during spinal analgesia. Anesthesiology 10: 677, 1949.

LINDERHOLM, H., AND NORLANDER, O.: Carbon dioxide tension and bicarbonate content of arterial blood in relation to anaesthesia and surgery. Acta Anaesthesiol. Scand. 2: 1, 1958.

LYFORD, J., III: Postoperative infections of respiratory tract in relation to inhalation and spinal anesthesia: a study of 631 cases. Arch. Surg. 44: 35, 1942 a.

LYFORD, J., III: Preoperative and postoperative infections of the respiratory tract in relation to inhalation and spinal anesthesia. Arch. Surg. 44: 41, 1942 b.

LYNN, R. B., SANCETTA, S. M., SIMEONE, F. A., AND SCOTT, R. W.: Observations on the circulation in high spinal anesthesia. Surgery 32: 195, 1952.

MALLAMPATI, S. R.: Bronchospasm during spinal anesthesia. Anesth. Analg. 60: 839, 1981.

MANARA, A. R., SMITH, D. C., AND NIXON, C.: Sedation during spinal anaesthesia: a case for the routine administration of oxygen. Br. J. Anaesth. 63: 343, 1989.

McCLURE, R. D., HARTMAN, F. W., SCHNEDORF, J. G., AND SCHELLING, V.: Anoxia: a source of possible complications in surgical anesthesia. Ann. Surg. 110: 835, 1939.

McGOUGH, E. K., AND COHEN, J. A.: Unexpected bronchospasm during spinal anesthesia. J. Clin. Anesth. 2: 35, 1990.

McKENZIE, P. J., WISHART, H. Y., DEWARD, K. M. S., GRAY, I., AND SMITH, G.: Comparison of the effects of spinal anaesthesia and general anaesthesia on postoperative oxygenation and perioperative mortality. Br. J. Anaesth. 52: 49, 1980.

McKITTRICK, L. S., McCLURE, W. L., AND SWEET, R. H.: Spinal anesthesia in abdominal surgery. Surg. Gynecol. 52: 898, 1931.

McLAREN, A. D., STOCKWELL, M. C., AND REID, V. T.: Anaesthetic techniques for surgical correction of fractured neck of femur. A comparative study of spinal and general anaesthesia in the elderly. Anaesthesia 33: 10, 1978.

MINSTER, J. J.: Comparison of anesthetic methods in elective surgery. Arch. Surg. 88: 728, 1964.

MURAVCHICK, S., AND JOHNSON, R.: Oxygenation of peripheral tissues in young and elderly patients during spinal anesthesia. Regional Anesth. 11: 7, 1986.

NAKAYAMA, E., NOGUCHI, T., KARUBE, Y., BABA, I., AND HARAGUCHI, M.: Circulation and respiration in anesthesia. I. Circulation and respiration during spinal anesthesia. J. Jpn. Obstet. Soc. (Engl. ed.) 3: 159, 1956.

NOWAK, S. J. G., AND DOWNING, V.: Oxygen and carbon dioxide changes in arterial and venous blood in experimental spinal anesthesia. J. Pharmacol. Exp. Ther. 64: 271, 1938.

NYGAARD, K. K.: Routine spinal anaesthesia in a provincial hospital, with a comparative study of postoperative complications following spinal and general ether anaesthesia. Acta Chir. Scand. 78: 379, 1936.

PASKIN, S., RODMAN, T., AND SMITH, T. C.: Effect of spinal anesthesia on the pulmonary function of patients with chronic obstructive pulmonary disease. Ann. Surg. 169: 35, 1969.

PEARCE C.: The respiratory effects of diazepam supplementation of spinal anaesthesia in elderly males. Br. J. Anaesth. 46: 439, 1974.

PEARL, R. G., MCLEAN, R. F., AND ROSENTHAL, M. H.: Effects of spinal anesthesia on response to main pulmonary arterial distension. J. Appl. Physiol. 64: 742, 1988.

PITKANEN, M. T.: Body mass and spread of spinal anesthesia with bupivacaine. Anesth. Analg. 66: 127, 1987.

RAVIN, M. B.: Comparison of spinal and general anesthesia for lower abdominal surgery in patients with chronic obstructive pulmonary disease. Anesthesiology 35: 319, 1971.

REINHART, K., DALLINGER-STILLER, G., HEINEMEYER, G., DENNHARDT, R., AND EYRICH, K.: Respiratorische und Schlafinduzierende Wirkungen von Midazolam i.m. als Pramedikation zur Regionalanaesthesie. Anaesthesist 32: 525, 1983.

SAMII, K., ELMELIK, E., MOURTADA, M. B., DEBEYRE, J., AND RAPIN, M.: Intraoperative hemodynamic changes during total knee replacement. Anesthesiology 50: 239, 1979.

SANCETTA, S. M., LYNN, R. B., AND SIMEONE, F. A.: Studies of hemodynamic changes in humans following induction of spinal anesthesia. IV. Observations in low spinal anesthesia during surgery. Surg. Gynecol. Obstet. 97: 597, 1953.

SANCETTA, S. M., LYNN, R. B., SIMEONE, F. A., AND SCOTT, R. W.: Studies of hemodynamic changes in humans following induction of low and high spinal anesthesia. I. General considerations of the problem. The changes in cardiac output, brachial arterial pressure, peripheral and pulmonary oxygen contents and peripheral blood flows induced by spinal anesthesia in humans not undergoing surgery. Circulation 6: 559, 1952.

SCHUBERTH, O. O.: On the disturbance of the circulation in spinal anaesthesia. Acta Chir. Scand. (Suppl.) 43: 78, 1936.

SEEVERS, M. K., AND WATERS, R. M.: Respiratory and circulatory changes during spinal anesthesia. J. A. M. A. 99: 961, 1932 a.

SEEVERS, M. K., AND WATERS, R. M.: Circulatory changes during spinal anesthesia. Anesth. Analg. 11: 85, 1932 b.

SEVITT, S., AND GALLAGHER, N.: Venous thrombosis and pulmonary embolism, a clinicopathological study in injured and burned patients. Br. J. Surg. 48: 475, 1961.

SHAW, J. L., STEELE, B. F., AND LAMB, C. A.: Effect of anesthesia on the blood oxygen: II. A study of the effect of spinal anesthesia on the oxygen in the arterial and in the venous blood. Arch. Surg. 35: 503, 1937.

SHESKEY, M. C., ROCCO, A. G., BIZZARRI-SCHMID, M., FRANCIS, D. M., EDSTROM, H., AND COVINO, B. G.: A dose-response study of bupivacaine for spinal anesthesia. Anesth. Analg. 62: 931, 1983.

SHNIDER, S. M., AND PAPPER, E. M.: Anesthesia for the asthmatic patient. Anesthesiology 22: 886, 1961.

SINCLAIR, C. J., SCOTT, D. B., AND EDSTROM, H. H.: Effect of the Trendelenberg position on spinal anaesthesia with hyperbaric bupivacaine. Br. J. Anaesth. 54: 497, 1982.

STANLEY, T. K., HILL, G. E., AND HILL, H. R.: The influence of spinal and epidural anesthesia on neutrophil chemotaxis in man. Anesth. Analg. 57: 567, 1978.

STEINBROOK, R. A., AND CONCEPCION, M.: Respiratory effects of spinal anesthesia: resting ventilation and single-breath CO_2 response. Anesth. Analg. 72: 182, 1991.

STEINBROOK, R. A., CONCEPCION, M., AND TOPULOS, G. P.: Ventilatory responses to hypercapnia during bupivacaine spinal anesthesia. Anesth. Analg. 67: 247, 1988.

TARDIEU, G., TARDIEU, C., AND POCIDALO, J. J.: Anesthésie médullaire totale. Etude hémodynamique, premiers résultats. J. Physiol. (Paris) 49: 390, 1957.

TKACHNEKO, B. I., KRASILNIKOV, V. G., POLENOV, S. A., AND CHERNJAVSKAJA, G. V.: Responses of resistance and capacitance vessels at various frequency electrical stimulation of sympathetic nerves. Experientia 25: 38, 1969.

URBRACH, K. F., LEE, W. R., SHEELY, L. L., LANG, F. L., AND SHARP, R. P.: Spinal or general anesthesia for inguinal hernia repair? J. A. M. A. 190: 25, 1964.

WALTS, L. F., KOEPKE, G., AND MARGULES, R.: Determination of sensory and motor levels after spinal anesthesia with tetracaine. Anesthesiology 25: 634, 1964.

WARD, R. J., BONICA, J. J., FREUND, F. G., AKAMATSU, T. J., DANZIGER, F., AND ENGLESSON, S.: Epidural and subarachnoid anesthesia: cardiovascular and respiratory effects. J. A. M. A. 191: 275, 1965.

WASHBURN, F. H.: What we have learned from five hundred spinal anesthesias. N. Engl. J. Med. 209: 345, 1933.

WEISS, S., PARKER, F., JR., AND ROBB, G. P.: A correlation of the hemodynamics, function, and histologic structure of the kidney in malignant arterial hypertension with malignant nephrosclerosis. Ann. Intern. Med. 6: 1599, 1933.

WELBORN, L. G., RICE, L. J., HANNALLAH, R. S., BROADMAN, L. M., RUTTIMANN, U. E., AND FINK, R.: Postoperative apnea in former preterm infants: prospective comparison of spinal and general anesthesia. Anesthesiology 72: 838, 1990.

WISHART, H. Y.: Blood gas changes in patients undergoing high spinal nerve block. Anaesthesia 26: 87, 1971.

CHAPTER 4

Hepatic Function

The effect of spinal anesthesia and surgery on liver function is a complex matter about which few if any categorical statements can be made. The following is presented as an analysis of some of the more important aspects of the problem.

Tests of Hepatic Function in Anesthesia and Surgery

The liver has a number of different functions including the synthesis of biologically vital substances, the storage of various materials, the biotransformation of xenobiotics, and the excretion of waste products. No single test can measure accurately the ability of the liver to perform all of its various functions. Abnormalities of hepatic excretion, for example, may be detected by certain tests which, while they are reliable for this specific purpose, give no information regarding the ability of the liver to synthesize substances such as albumin, globulin, prothrombin, etc. Therefore, before discussing the effects of anesthesia and surgery on hepatic function, function tests must be evaluated with respect to their suitability for the study of such a problem. The tests most appropriate for studying infectious hepatitis are not necessarily the best for studying the effects of anesthesia and surgery on the liver.

Reports on the effects of anesthesia and surgery on hepatic function reveal that most authors have relied on a single test without attempting to determine which of the many tests available might be the best. The considerable range of single tests employed by different authors has, in many cases, rendered the results conflicting and confusing. However, in 1942, Schmidt, *et al.*, employed a group of tests (hippuric acid excretion, bromsulfalein retention, prothrombin time, and serum amylase levels) in their study of the effects of anesthesia and surgery on liver function. They came to the conclusion that of all the tests, prothrombin time and hippuric acid excretion were the "most satisfactory." Unfortunately, they failed to support this opinion with data sufficiently detailed to allow for statistical evaluation. In a similar study, Pohle (1948) also employed a number of liver function tests, but did not try to determine which was the most reliable. His results, although presented in detail are arranged in a way that precludes such a determination. The most definitive investigation of the relative values of function as means of assessing the effects of anesthesia and surgery on the liver is that reported by Fairlie, *et al.*, in 1951. These authors studied 34 patients all of whom had normal hepatic function preoperatively. Operations consisted of procedures on the pelvis or lower extremities. Anesthesia consisted of cyclopropane, gas-oxygen-ether, or spinal. Each patient was subjected to a battery of tests before operation and again on the first, third, and fifth postoperative days. The tests were designed primarily to evaluate the excretory and synthesizing abilities of the liver and included the bromsulfalein retention test, the intravenous hippuric acid excretion test, and determinations of serum bilirubin, plasma prothrombin time, serum alkaline phosphatase, the ratio of serum cholesterol to cholesterol esters, and urinary urobilinogen. On the basis of their results the authors concluded that the bromsulfalein retention test was the most useful single test for evaluating the effects of anesthesia and surgery on liver function. Analysis of the data reveals, however, that even the bromsulfalein retention test is not an entirely reliable index of the frequency and of the degree to which anesthetics may depress liver function. Of 34 patients in the series, only 2 showed no postoperative abnormality in any of the liver function tests employed. The other 32 patients showed abnormalities in one or more of the tests at some time during the postoperative period. Some of the function tests proved to be of less value than others. The ratio of cholesterol esters to total cholesterol, for example, varied considerably after anesthesia and surgery with no significant trend being discernible. Prothrombin time was not significantly changed post-operatively and was also considered an unreliable index of hepatic function following anesthesia and operation. Similarly, postoperative alkaline phosphatase levels showed little change. They became elevated above the normal level of 4.5 Bodansky units in only 2 of 25 patients in whom this determination was made. The hippuric acid excretion test was of some value, but it often gave confusing results. Of 26 patients given this test with results being given in sufficient detail to allow analysis, 13 had normal and 13 had abnormal rates of hippuric acid excretion preoperatively in spite of the fact that all had "normal" livers and no renal disease that might interfere with excretion. Of the 13 patients with normal preoperative hippuric acid excretion, 7 showed depressed excretion below the normal limit of 1.0 g/hr, while 6 showed either no change or an increase after surgery and anesthesia. Among the 13 patients who had subnormal rates of hippuric acid excretion before anesthesia and surgery, 4 showed a further impairment postoperatively but 9 excreted hippuric acid at the same or even a higher rate than before. Determination of serum bilirubin levels proved more reliable than did the hippuric acid test. Of 34 patients in whom serum bilirubin determinations were made, 10 showed elevations above the normal level of 0.7 mg% at some point during the postoperative period.

The most sensitive tests in this series for assessing postoperative hepatic function proved to be measurements of urinary urobilinogen and of the degree of retention of intravenously administered bromsulfalein. Fifteen of the 32 patients in whom urinary urobilinogen studies were carried out showed more than 1.0 Ehrlich units in 2-hr specimens of urine at some time after anesthesia and surgery. The bromsulfalein retention test was even more sensitive. Eighteen of 34 patients in whom this test was carried out postoperatively showed abnormal retention of the dye (more than 5% in 45 minutes). But even this test had definite limitations and did not invariably reflect an hepatic dysfunction that was indicated by other tests. Of 16 patients who showed no postoperative abnormality of bromsulfalein retention, 5 showed above-normal levels of urinary urobilinogen, and 4 showed above-normal levels of bilirubin. In 8 of the 16 patients the rate of excretion of hippuric acid was slower after than before operation; in 6 it changed from normal to abnormal; and in 2 from abnormal to more abnormal. Only 2 of the 16 patients with normal postoperative bromsulfalein retention showed no change in any other postoperative liver function test performed.

Blood levels of enzymes have also been used more recently as measures of hepatic function. Particularly valuable are serum levels of glutamic oxaloacetic transaminase (SGOT), ornithine carbamyl transferase (SOCT), and glutamic pyruvic transaminase (SGPT). SGOT is also referred to as aspartate aminotransferase (AST), while SGPT is also referred to as alanine aminotransferase (ALT). While these enzymes are of demonstrated value in the general medical evaluation of liver function, they reflect primarily the integrity of hepatic cell membranes in terms of their permeability to substances that under normal conditions exist mostly intracellularly. Most, though not all, of the enzymes (SGOT, SOCT, and SGPT) exist within liver cells where they play essential roles in the metabolic syntheses of a variety of important biologic compounds. Injury to hepatic cell membranes is associated with an increase in their permeability. Normal intracellular biologic substances then leak across the damaged membranes and appear in plasma in unusually large amounts. Cell membrane damage may be extensive enough to allow escape of hepatic intracellular constituents in amounts that can be measured in systemic blood. Such damage is assumed to also disrupt hepatic cell functions other than those metabolic steps dependent on normal concentrations of SGOT, SOCT, and SGPT, including, for example, excretion of waste products and biotransformation of xenobiotics. The most frequent causes of loss of integrity of hepatic cell membranes include infection, viral and bacterial, hypoxia or anoxia, and certain toxins. For this reason, serum levels of hepatic isoenzymes are so useful in the medical diagnosis of certain types of hepatic diseases. They are early harbingers of microscopic histologic damage. Hepatic function can also, however, be impaired in the presence of normal hepatic cell membrane permeability and, thus, without increases in serum levels of hepatic isoenzymes. This type of hepatic dysfunction can be associated with anesthesia and surgery in the absence of infections, anoxia, and hepatotoxins.

The above considerations should be taken into account when discussing the effects of anesthesia on liver function. Serum levels of hepatic isoenzymes are not indicative of all types of hepatic dysfunction, including those seen most often in modern anesthesia practice, which no longer uses patently obvious hepatic poisons. Also to be borne in mind is the fact that there are no epidemiologically and biostatistically sound studies comparing the usefulness of serum enzyme levels to that of older hepatic function studies in evaluating hepatic dysfunction associated with anesthesia and surgery. In fact, some of the older methods for evaluating postoperative hepatic dysfunction may be more useful for this particular purpose. In the absence of such a comparison, some of the older tests, perhaps especially bromsulfalein excretion, are included in the following discussion because it has been shown to be a highly reliable test of liver function under these conditions, even though, as emphasized above, there is no one test that can determine accurately the frequency or extent of all changes in liver function. The following discussion also includes a considerable amount of data on the effect of anesthetics on liver function based on studies of what today are considered to be paleoanesthetics, for example, ether and cyclopropane. Such data are not quaint and irrelevant. They are included because of the wealth of information generated in earlier times when the effects of anesthesia and surgery on liver function was a topic of great interest and priority. Such a wealth of information has not been produced on this subject since the introduction of general anesthetics now in general use. Besides, spinal anesthesia, our subject, had the same effect on liver function 40 years ago that it has today.

Although it is a valuable index of the effect of anesthesia on liver function, it should be noted that the rate of excretion of bromsulfalein is related to hepatic blood flow as well as to the functional adequacy of the parenchymal cells (Mendeloff, 1949). For example, in a series of nine patients the average retention of bromsulfalein was 5.1% before spinal anesthesia, while it was 18.9% in the first postoperative hour (Tyler, et al., 1954). Decreased excretion in the immediate postoperative period is probably due to changes in hepatic blood flow rather than to decreased cellular function. It is unlikely, however, that any changes in this liver function test that persist well into the convalescent period represent continuing changes in hepatic blood flow. Instead, they probably represent changes in hepatic function.

Effects of Spinal Anesthesia and Surgery on Normal Liver Function

Accepting with caution the interpretation of liver function tests, it is now appropriate to discuss the influence of spinal anesthesia and surgery on normal liver function. The parts played by the site of operation and preexisting liver disease will be considered later.

The effects of spinal anesthesia and surgery on liver function were first assessed by modern liver function tests in 1938 by Coleman. Using the bromsulfalein retention test, he reported on a series of 100 patients given different types of anesthesia for a variety of surgical procedures. Eight of the 100 patients were given spinal anesthesia. Preoperatively all eight had normal bromsulfalein retention tests, but after operation four of them showed abnormal retention. The rate of bromsulfalein excretion was normal by the seventh postoperative day in all patients. Also in 1938, Boyce and McFetridge (1938 b), using the hippuric acid excretion test reported on a series of patients (number unspecified) having spinal anesthesia for herniorrhaphy or appendectomy. They found, following spinal anesthesia and surgery, that hippuric acid excretion decreased on the average by 49%. In 1942, Schmidt, et al. used the same test for the same purpose. In 21 patients given spinal anesthesia for various surgical procedures, these investigators found that in 3, the hippuric acid excretion was below normal on either the first or second postoperative day. Preoperatively, the average hippuric acid excretion by the 21 patients was 5.23 g in 4 hr. Excluding, for reasons that are not clear, 2 patients that had the most marked impairment of hippuric acid excretion postoperatively, Schmidt, et al., found the average amount excreted to be 4.83 g in 4 hr, a decrease of 7%. Engstrand and Friberg (1945) also reported on postoperative liver function, using the hippuric acid excretion as the sole test. The value of their extensive report is unfortunately somewhat diminished because many of their "spinal" cases were also given ether, cyclopropane, or nitrous oxide plus an intravenous barbiturate. Among 36 patients whose liver function was studied following spinal anesthesia, all but 6 received supplemental general anesthesia. Those six patients given only spinal anesthesia all evidenced a postoperative decrease in hippuric acid excretion, including some as low as zero. In view of this and the fact that the average decrease in blood pressure in the 6 patients was 30% (range: 15–60% decrease), these authors claim that "with a normal blood pressure perlsain [i.e., spinal] anesthesia does not give rise to a reduction in liver function" does not appear substantiated. Furthermore, in the patients who received both spinal and supplemental general anesthesia, subnormal postoperative hippuric acid excretion also was the rule.

In 1948, Pohle studied more extensively the effect of anesthesia and surgery on liver function, employing, for the first time, a large series of tests rather than relying on any single one. Only nine patients given spinal anesthesia were studied. Six of the nine patients showed postoperative decreases in hepatic function by one or more of the tests used. None showed any significant change in thymol turbidity. In one patient, the icteric index was abnormally elevated, three showed abnormal cephalin flocculation tests, three showed significant prolongations of prothrombin time, and four exhibited abnormally high bromsulfalein retention.

Pohle's report did not provide information on individual patients and so left unanswered the question as to what was the relationship among tests when only one of them was abnormal postoperatively. He also gave no information on the time relationships of the changes that occurred. Such information was supplied in 1951 by Fairlie, *et al.* They studied 10 patients having spinal anesthesia and undergoing the following procedures: vaginal hysterectomy, perineorrhaphy, or inguinal herniorrhaphy. This particular selection was designed to limit the possibility that varying the site of surgery would influence the results. Their findings are summarized in Table 4.1. Other tests such as cephalin flocculation, thymol turbidity and flocculation, and zinc sulfate turbidity, were also performed in a limited number of patients but were not continued because of their uniform failure to demonstrate significant change. As mentioned above, the bromsulfalein retention test and the urinary urobilinogen levels were found to be the most sensitive indices of postoperative hepatic function. None of the other tests indicated any significant changes in mean postoperative values even though an occasional individual value was outside the normal range. On the first postoperative day, the average bromsulfalein retention for all 10 cases was 6.2%. With the upper limit of normal retention being 5%, 5 of the 10 patients evidenced abnormal retention on the first postoperative day, with values ranging from 6% to 19%. By the third postoperative day, the average dye retention had returned to 5.0%, although it was still above normal limits in five of the patients. On the fifth postoperative day, the average value for bromsulfalein retention was again normal, and it was above normal in only one patient. In all, 6 of 10 patients showed abnormal dye retention at some time in the postoperative period. In contrast to the tendency of the bromsulfalein retention to become abnormal early in

Table 4.1.
Effect of Spinal Anesthesia and Lower Abdominal Surgery on Normal Liver Function[a,b]

Liver Function Test	Preoperative	Postoperative		
		First Day	Third Day	Fifth Day
Bromsulfalein (% retention)	2.5 ± 0.51	6.2 ± 1.63	5.0 ± 1.14	3.8 ± 0.96
Hippuric acid excretion (g in 1 hr)	0.90 ± 0.11	1.04 ± 0.12	0.83 ± 0.18	0.98 ± 0.12
Serum bilirubin (mg/100 ml)	1.10 ± 0.23	1.03 ± 0.20	0.62 ± 0.06	0.59 ± 0.04
Prolongation of plasma prothrombin time (sec)	1.3 ± 0.39	1.8 ± 0.63	2.1 ± 0.56	1.9 ± 0.46
Urine urobilinogen (Ehrlich units/2 hr)	0.57 ± 0.10	0.56 ± 0.08	0.62 ± 0.09	1.45 ± 0.42
Serum alkaline phosphatase (Bodansky units/100 ml)	2.7 ± 0.43	2.6 ± 0.46	2.5 ± 0.52	2.2 ± 0.56
Cholesterol esters (% of total cholesterol)	59 ± 3.0	57 ± 2.8	59 ± 5.5	60 ± 6.4

[a] Mean ± SEM.
[b] Reproduced with permission from Fairlie, *et al.*, N. Engl. J. Med. *244:* 615, 1951.

the postoperative period, and to return to normal relatively rapidly, the urinary urobilinogen remained at normal levels in the immediate postoperative period but tended to become abnormal on about the fifth day. On the first and third postoperative days none of the patients had a level of urinary urobilinogen above the normal value of 1.0 Ehrlich units per 2 hr, while on the fifth postoperative day four of the six patients tested showed values above 1.0 Ehrlich unit, the mean being 1.45 Ehrlich units for all six patients.

The findings of Coleman (1938), Pohle (1948), and Fairlie, *et al.* (1951) on the postoperative changes in bromsulfalein retention were confirmed by Lynn, *et al.* (1952). Among 20 normal patients operated on under spinal anesthesia, abnormal bromsulfalein retention was observed in 9. Lynn, *et al.* related these findings to the level of sensory block attained, since only 1 of 11 patients given "low" spinal anesthesia showed abnormal dye retention, while 8 of 9 patients given "high" spinals showed such a change. Whether this difference in incidence was attributable to the level of spinal anesthesia or to the fact that the site and type of operation were different in the two groups will be discussed on pp. 246–248.

Comparison of the Effects of Spinal Anesthesia and of Other Anesthetics on Liver Function

Having established that spinal anesthesia and surgery are frequently followed by impaired hepatic function, it is pertinent to discover whether this occurs more or less frequently and whether it is more or less severe in patients given spinal anesthesia than in patients given other types of anesthesia. However, again we encounter a wealth of relatively old information comparing the effects of spinal anesthesia on liver function with effects of no longer used general anesthetics and a paucity of similar comparisons since the introduction of modern halogenated inhalation anesthetics and narcotic intravenous anesthetics. The older data, nevertheless, deserve close scrutiny and analysis if for no other reason than their completeness outlines so well the multiple factors involved in making such comparisons, factors as relevant today as they were in the past and, therefore, relevant in our understanding today of the frequency and the extent to which anesthesia may affect function of the liver.

Among the first to evaluate the effects of different anesthetics on liver function were Cantarow, *et al.* (1935). Using serum bilirubin levels and retention of bromsulfalein as measures of hepatic function, they studied 60 patients both before and within 24 hr after cholecystectomy. Preoperatively, 41 of the 60 patients had normal function as determined by the two tests. Of these 41 patients, slightly more than half showed postoperative increases in serum bilirubin and in bromsulfalein retention. All the operations were performed under gas-oxygen-ether, local infiltration, or spinal anesthesia. The authors were not primarily interested in the influence of anesthesia on hepatic function and hence did not report the numbers of patients having the different types of anesthesia. Nevertheless, they came to the conclusion that there was no correlation between the type of anesthesia and the frequency of abnormal postoperative values for serum bilirubin or bromsulfalein excretion. Boyce and McFetridge (1938 b) examined the same problem using the rate of hippuric acid excretion as a measure of postoperative liver function. Reporting on an unstated number of cases, they arrived at a conclusion different from that of Cantarow, *et al.* (1935). Boyce and McFetridge found that herniorrhaphies and appendectomies performed under spinal anesthesia were associated with an average decrease in hippuric acid excretion of 49%, while similar operations performed under ether or under ethylene were associated with reductions of 25% and 21%, respectively. From these findings, they concluded that hepatic function was more impaired after spinal anesthesia than after ether or ethylene. In the same year, Coleman (1938) published a report whose findings agreed more with those of Cantarow, *et al.* than with those of Boyce and McFetridge. Using the bromsulfalein retention test, Coleman found that 25 of 49 patients receiving nitrous oxide–ether anesthesia had abnormal retention of dye postoperatively, compared to only four of the eight patients studied after spinal anesthesia with similar findings. All of Coleman's patients given spinal anesthesia had normal rates of bromsulfalein excretion by the seventh postoperative day, while 8 of the 49 patients receiving nitrous oxide-ether anesthesia evidenced abnormal rates of excretion on the third day. Furthermore, it was not until the 13th postoperative day that the levels had returned to normal. In view of the small number of patients studied after spinal anesthesia, Coleman did not attach much significance to the slight differences noted between spinal and nitrous oxide-ether anesthesia. The only anesthetic found by Coleman to be associated with an abnormally high incidence of postoperative liver damage was tribromoethanol (Avertin). Ten of 13 patients given tribomoethanol evidenced abnormal bromsulfalein retention postoperatively. A third report which also appeared in 1938 agreed with the findings of Coleman and Cantarow, *et al.*, that the anesthetic agent had little influence on postoperative liver function. This investigation by Gray, *et al.* (1938), examined effects of surgery and anesthesia on the postoperative concentration of bile acids. Although only 11 patients were studied, and only 1 had spinal anesthesia, the others receiving cyclopropane, ether or ethylene, the authors concluded that the postoperative decrease in the concentration of bile acids was not related to the type of anesthetic administered.

Schmidt, *et al.* (1942) published a report concluding that the hippuric acid test was the most satisfactory for testing postoperative liver function. The authors also stated that with spinal anesthesia there was less postoperative derangement of hippuric acid excretion than with certain other anesthetics. They based this conclusion on the fact that 18 of 21 patients given spinal anesthesia for procedures varying from uterine curettage to cholecystectomy showed normal hippuric acid excretion on the first postoperative day, while all 16 patients given open-drop ether exhibited a severe depression of hippuric acid excretion at this time. The investigators found no delay in hippuric acid excretion following local anesthesia for thyroidectomies, herniorrhaphies, and skin grafting. However, the combination of tribromoethanol and ethylene resulted in excretion that was retarded more than with spinal anesthesia, but less than with ether. Unfortunately, it is difficult to use the data of these authors for objective evaluation of the effects of different anesthetics on liver function, not only because of the wide difference in the operations being performed, but also because two patients who showed severe depression of hippuric acid excretion postoperatively were eliminated from the spinal anesthetic group.

Engstrand and Friberg (1945), who also used the hippuric acid excretion test, observed that while ether was associated with considerable postoperative hepatic dysfunction, both cyclopropane and spinal anesthesia were comparatively harmless. Although presented in detail, analysis of their data is difficult because of the fact that many patients given spinal anesthesia also received supplemental general anesthetics. The results suggest, however, that all the anesthetics used were followed by a postoperative diminution in excretion of hippuric acid and that there is no statistically significant difference between them in this regard. Including only those patients for whom complete information is available, and taking as the point of reference the lowest postoperative value reported for hippuric acid excretion, the following analysis can be made: all six patients given spinal anesthesia alone showed a decrease in postoperative hippuric acid excretion (averaging 47%). Of 26 patients given spinal plus an intravenous barbiturate or nitrous oxide, 24 showed a postoperative decrease in hippurate excretion (averaging 58%). In three patients given spinal supplemented by ether or cyclopropane, hippurate excretion was reduced an average of 93%. Of the six patients given cyclopropane alone, hippurate excretion decreased in five patients, the decrease averaging 27%. Nitrous oxide-ether or ether alone were administered to 13 patients, in 11 of whom the hippurate excretion decreased postoperatively, the average decrease being 61%. Five of six patients given intravenous barbiturate plus nitrous oxide showed an average postoperative decrease in hippuric acid excretion of 37%. Because of the small number of cases in certain categories and the wide individual variations encountered within the categories, the standard deviations in this study are too large to allow any statistical comparison beyond stating that all anesthetics can decrease postoperative hippuric acid excretion.

Keeton, *et al.* (1948) conducted a carefully designed and extensive study of metabolism in the convalescent period which included an evaluation of the effects of spinal and inhalation (ether) anesthesia. In this investigation, conditions were controlled more rigidly than in any preceding work on the same subject, and hence the results are especially valuable. Not only were the methods of anesthesia taken into account, but also the type of operation remained constant, and, unique among such reports, there was rigid control of dietary factors as well as ambulation in the postoperative period. The authors reported on 13 patients given spinal anesthesia and 9 patients given ether anesthesia, all for inguinal herniorrhaphy. Presentation of data depended upon a complex index, the details of which need not be described here, but the results indicated that spinal anesthesia caused significantly ($P = 0.005$) less elevation of postoperative urinary urobilinogen than did ether anesthesia. The authors also found that while spinal anesthesia was associated with a slight increase in prothrombin activity, ether anesthesia was attended by a slight decrease, the difference between the two groups being statistically significant ($P = 0.016$). These effects of anesthesia on prothrombin have also been reported by Borgstrom (1943). Keeton, et al. (1948) also compared the ratio of cholesterol esters to total cholesterol. They found that on the day after cholecystectomy patients had a significant diminution in the level of cholesterol esters. There was, however, no difference between those levels in the patients having had spinal anesthesia and the patients who had ether anesthesia. Following cholecystectomy there was also a slight decrease in total serum proteins (the albumin/globulin ratio remaining unchanged), although there was no significant difference which could be attributed to the type of anesthesia.

Also in 1948, Pohle published the results of an investigation of a variety of liver function tests following different types of anesthesia. Unfortunately, for the purpose of comparative assessment, the operations were very diverse in character and location, and, equally unfortunate, only nine of the patients studied had spinal anesthesia. Six of the nine patients showed postoperative hepatic dysfunction. Similar dysfunction was found after operation in 11 of 20 patients given chloroform, in 18 of 20 patients given ether, in 12 of 20 patients given cyclopropane, in 5 of 9 patients given thiopental, and interestingly enough, in contrast to Coleman's experience, in only 7 of 21 patients given tribomoethanol.

The icteric index rose approximately 15% in all of Pohle's patients regardless of the type of anesthesia, with the exception of those given chloroform, in whom there was a 30% increase. The bromsulfalein retention test was positive in 40% of the patients, excluding those given tribromoethanol. Only 10% of these patients showed a delay in excretion. The cephalin flocculation test became abnormal in 10% of the patients who were given thiopental or tribromoethanol, in 20% of those who were given chloroform, and in 30% of those who had ether, cyclopropane, or spinal anesthesia.

Pohle's work was confirmed and supplemented by the detailed observations of Fairlie, et al. (1951). As already mentioned, this group studied 34 patients, all of whom underwent comparable operations involving the pelvis, perineum, inguinal area, or lower extremities under cyclopropane, gas-oxygen-ether, or spinal anesthesia. The results, summarized in Table 4.2, showed a significant increase in bromsulfalein retention following surgery. This increase was most marked in the first postoperative day. There was, however, no significant difference in rate of excre-

Table 4.2.
Liver Function Tests in Normal Patients Having Similar Operations Under Different Anesthetics[a,b]

Type of Anesthesia	No. Patients	Preoperative	Postoperative Day		
			First	Third	Fifth
Bromsulfalein retention (%)					
Spinal	10	2.5 ± 0.51	6.2 ± 1.63	5.0 ± 1.14	3.8 ± 0.96
Gas-oxygen-ether	13	2.8 ± 0.44	5.6 ± 1.57	5.4 ± 1.71	6.0 ± 1.88
Cyclopropane	11	2.1 ± 0.37	6.9 ± 1.90	6.1 ± 3.06	6.5 ± 3.91
Hippuric acid excretion (gm·hr^{-1})					
Spinal	9	0.90 ± 0.11	1.04 ± 0.12	0.83 ± 0.18	0.98 ± 0.12
Gas-oxygen-ether	11	1.00 ± 0.12	0.95 ± 0.16	0.85 ± 0.11	0.96 ± 0.18
Cyclopropane	10	0.95 ± 0.14	0.82 ± 0.15	1.06 ± 0.07	1.07 ± 0.10
Serum bilirubin (mg%)					
Spinal	10	1.10 ± 0.23	1.03 ± 0.20	0.62 ± 0.06	0.59 ± 0.04
Gas-oxygen-ether	13	0.69 ± 0.06	0.73 ± 0.06	0.59 ± 0.08	0.54 ± 0.11
Cyclopropane	11	0.77 ± 0.09	0.85 ± 0.13	0.57 ± 0.07	0.50 ± 0.06
Prolongation of plasma prothrombin time (sec)					
Spinal	10	1.3 ± 0.39	1.8 ± 0.63	2.1 ± 0.56	1.9 ± 0.46
Gas-oxygen-ether	13	0.6 ± 0.27	2.7 ± 0.94	2.5 ± 0.78	2.6 ± 0.82
Cyclopropane	11	1.2 ± 0.40	1.4 ± 0.29	2.2 ± 0.70	2.0 ± 0.32
Urine urobilinogen (units·2 hr^{-1})					
Spinal	9	0.57 ± 0.10	0.56 ± 0.08	0.62 ± 0.09	1.45 ± 0.42
Gas-oxygen-ether	13	0.41 ± 0.04	0.80 ± 0.15	0.68 ± 0.10	0.84 ± 0.19
Cyclopropane	11	0.53 ± 0.06	0.96 ± 0.25	0.77 ± 0.24	0.97 ± 0.32
Serum alkaline phosphatase (units·100 ml^{-1})					
Spinal	7	2.7 ± 0.43	2.6 ± 0.46	2.5 ± 0.52	2.2 ± 0.56
Gas-oxygen-ether	9	2.0 ± 0.30	1.9 ± 0.17	2.5 ± 0.36	2.8 ± 0.52
Cyclopropane	9	2.4 ± 0.34	1.9 ± 0.31	2.3 ± 0.19	1.8 ± 0.10
Cholesterol esters (% of total cholesterol)					
Spinal	7	59 ± 3.0	57 ± 2.8	59 ± 5.5	60 ± 6.4
Gas-oxygen-ether	10	61 ± 3.7	57 ± 1.3	52 ± 3.2	53 ± 8.5
Cyclopropane	8	53 ± 4.8	57 ± 3.3	55 ± 3.1	48 ± 4.4

[a] Average ± SEM.
[b] Reproduced with permission from Fairlie, et al., N. Engl. J. Med. 244: 615, 1951.

tion between the three types of anesthesia, a finding that agreed with those of Coleman and Pohle.

Unlike the marked reduction in postoperative hippuric acid excretion described by Boyce and McFetridge (1938 b), Schmidt, *et al.* (1942), and Engstrand and Friberg (1945), Fairlie, *et al.* (1951) were unable to find any significant change following any of the three types of anesthesia. The probable reasons for the discrepancy between the results of Fairlie, *et al.*, and those of earlier investigators are that Fairlie, *et al.* gave the hippuric acid intravenously rather than orally, they eliminated patients with coexisting renal disease from the study, and restricted the range of operations performed.

The figures for serum bilirubin shown in Table 4.2 do not indicate any postoperative increase. With respect to prothrombin time, however, there was a moderate prolongation following all anesthetics, although the authors did not consider this statistically significant. Nor were the increases in urinary urobilinogen observed by Fairlie, *et al.* as marked as those noted by Keeton, *et al.*, despite urinary urobilinogen having proved to be a valuable measurement of postoperative liver dysfunction in certain patients. The changes in alkaline phosphatase and cholesterol esters shown in Table 4.2 were not of clinical significance.

Lamentably scarce, as mentioned above, are more recent studies that utilize modern tests of liver function to compare the effects of modern inhalation halogenated anesthetics with those of spinal anesthesia on postoperative liver function. Beckman, *et al.* (1966), did, however, compare the effects of spinal anesthesia with sensory levels to T_{10} (5 patients) with the effects of halothane (15 patients) and ether (4 patients) using serum enzyme levels as indices of liver function. All patients had comparable types of surgery. In all patients SOCT values increased to above preoperative levels, usually starting on the third postoperative day, and reaching a maximum 1 week postoperatively. In approximately two thirds of the patients, SOCT values reached pathologic levels at some time in the postoperative period. SGOT and SGPT, on the other hand, did not exhibit any characteristic pattern of change, and in no instance did they reach pathologic levels postoperatively. There was no significant difference between the three types of anesthetics. The same group of investigators subsequently reported (Brohult and Gillquist, 1969) that in nine patients given halothane anesthesia for renal angiography, SOCT levels remained unchanged postoperatively. On the other hand, 26 patients given spinal anesthesia for a variety of operations in the lower abdomen had slight increases in SOCT levels following surgery. The elevations were significantly greater in 8 patients who experienced intra-anesthetic hypotension than they were in the 18 patients who remained normotensive. The increase in postoperative SOCT levels following spinal anesthesia unaccompanied by hypotension were comparable to the increases observed in an additional 10 patients who had a variety of intra- and extra-abdominal procedures performed under halothane anesthesia. These data emphasize the role that surgery plays in determining changes in postoperative liver function tests, as discussed below. These data also indicate that when comparable types of surgery are performed, changes in postoperative serum enzyme levels are similar following spinal anesthesia and halothane anesthesia.

In summary, a review of published reports relating postoperative hepatic function to anesthesia, when combined with an evaluation of the statistical validity of these reports, reveals that spinal anesthesia and surgery may be, and frequently are, followed by impaired function in a previously normal liver. There is, however, no proof that the effects of spinal anesthesia are quantitatively or qualitatively any different from those associated with general anesthesia.

Influence of Type of Operative Procedure on Postoperative Liver Function

One might expect that extensive surgical procedures would be followed by more frequent and more severe degrees of postoperative liver dysfunction than are minor operations. This point, although of considerable theoretical importance in any study of the effects of anesthesia on liver function, has unfortunately received little attention from those who have looked at the problem as a whole. Boyce and McFetridge (1938 a) were the first to attempt to determine the role played by the type of surgery. Studying patients undergoing cholecystostomy, cholecystectomy, or choledochostomy under various types of anesthesia, they concluded that postoperative hepatic function was most impaired after choledochostomy, and least impaired after cholecystostomy. However, the possibility that the pathologic conditions necessitating choledochostomy are also more frequently associated with liver disease than are those requiring cholecystectomy, makes an evaluation difficult. In 1945, Engstrand and Friberg compared hepatic function following gastrectomy and cholecystectomy and concluded that postoperative hepatic function as determined by the hippuric acid excretion test was more impaired after gastrectomy than after cholecystectomy. Because the changes following biliary tract surgery were mild, the authors claimed that "cholecystectomy with cholangiography does not affect normal liver function." Operations in other parts of the abdomen as well as extraperitoneal procedures were not studied in large enough numbers to allow comparisons.

Keeton, et al. (1948) investigated the relationship between the site of operation and the degree of postoperative hepatic dysfunction as part of a larger study of convalescence. They compared two blood chemistries related to liver function after two types of surgery. The chemical determinations selected were total serum proteins and the ratio of cholesterol esters to total cholesterol. Keeton, *et al.* found that the percentage of cholesterol esters was less after both inguinal herniorrhaphy and cholecystectomy. The decrease was the same for both operations and was unrelated to the type of anesthesia employed. Total serum proteins also decreased following both types of surgery, but the decrease was more marked after cholecystectomy. The reduction in total protein following cholecystectomy was not accompanied by any change in the albumin/globulin ratio; it was slightly more pronounced after ether than after spinal anesthesia.

The problem was investigated more extensively by French, *et al.* (1952) and by Fairlie, *et al.* (1951). The measurements of bromsulfalein retention found by these two groups of investigators following three different types of operations all performed under the same type of anesthesia (gas-oxygen-ether) are summarized in Table 4.3. Unfortunately, none of the upper abdominal procedures was carried out under spinal anesthesia. However, it is evident that, under gas-oxygen-ether anesthesia, gastrectomy is associated with greater postoperative retention of bromsulfalein than are hysterectomy, herniorrhaphy, and vein stripping, while cholecystectomy is followed by even more dye retention than is gastrectomy. The same pattern was also seen when the three types of operation were performed under cyclopropane anesthesia. In fact, there was no difference between the results obtained following three different types of surgery performed under cyclopropane anesthesia and the same three types performed under gas-oxygen-ether. It may be assumed, therefore, that the degree of postoperative hepatic dysfunction following spinal anesthesia or, indeed, following general anesthesia, is also related

Table 4.3.
Bromsulfalein Retention (%) Following Different Types of Surgery Performed Under Gas-Oxygen-Ether Anesthesia[a,b]

Type of Operation	No. Patients	Preoperative	Postoperative Day		
			First	Third	Fifth
Hysterectomy hernia repair, vein stripping	13	2.8 ± 0.44	5.6 ± 1.57	5.4 ± 1.71	6.0 ± 1.88
Gastrectomy	10	3.6 ± 1.12	10.9 ± 1.69	9.2 ± 1.89	6.9 ± 1.89
Cholecystectomy	13	4.3 ± 0.9	17.1 ± 2.97	25.0 ± 4.86	23.0 ± 5.94

[a] Mean retention (%) ± SEM.
[b] Abstracted with permission from Fairlie, *et al.*, N. Engl. J. Med. *244:* 615, 1951, and from French, *et al.*, Ann. Surg. *135:* 145, 1952.

to the type of surgery being performed. It should be pointed out, however, that the increased bromsulfalein retention following gastrectomy (Table 4.3) is not due to an increase in the degree of postoperative abnormal hepatic function occurring in individual patients, but rather to an increase in the frequency with which moderate degrees of bromsulfalein retention occur. Abnormal dye retention is more common after cholecystectomy than after operations on the lower abdomen or limbs, but the extent of this retention remains essentially the same in both groups. For example, following hernia repairs, vein stripppings, or hysterectomies performed under gas-oxygen-ether anesthesia, six of the patients showed no abnormal bromsulfalein dye retention postoperatively. In the seven patients who did show retention of dye exceeding 5%, the average peak retention was 13.2%, the greatest being 23%. Of 10 patients who underwent gastrectomy, only 2 showed no increase in bromsulfalein retention. The other eight patients did show changes, the average peak retention being 15.4% and the maximum, 22%. The difference, therefore, between the two groups of patients lies in the frequency of abnormal retention of bromsulfalein rather than in the extent of the retention in individual cases. This, however, does not appear to be so following cholecystectomy. Here, both the frequency and extent of abnormal dye retention are increased. After cholecystectomy, only 1 of 13 patients failed to show an abnormal bromsulfalein test, and while the average peak retention was 35.4%, the maximal retention was 60%. Two factors are of significance in the explanation of the difference between the cholecystectomy series and the gastrectomy series. The first is that patients having cholecystectomies have subclinical hepatic damage more frequently than patients having gastrectomies. Second, there is greater risk of trauma to the liver and biliary passage during cholecystectomy than during gastrectomy. That abdominal operations are associated with histologic changes in the liver has long been recognized. In 1949, for example, Zamcheck, et al. found no histologic changes in liver biopsies obtained immediately after laparotomy in six patients. In 15 other patients liver specimens were obtained just prior to closure of the peritoneum following the completion of gastrectomy or cholecystectomy. In every instance there was evidence of acute inflammation, and microscopically there was capsular or subcapsular inflammation, focal collections of polymorphonuclear leukocytes about the central vein, and necrosis of liver cells. Such histologic changes following operative trauma may well explain some of the differences in postoperative hepatic function observed in a group of patients after inguinal herniorrhaphy and those who have had an upper abdominal operation. But histologic changes due to local trauma during surgery do not explain the fact that cup arthroplasty of the hip may be followed by liver dysfunction similar to that observed following gastrectomy (French, et al., 1952). Similarly, craniotomies and hemipelvectomies are followed by hepatic dysfunction (Greene, *et al.*, 1954) which is more pronounced than that found after perineorrhaphy. This would suggest that, as a general rule, radical operations cause greater postoperative changes in liver function than do less invasive or extensive procedures.

Effects of Spinal Anesthesia and Surgery on the Abnormal Liver

It has been shown that, for patients with normal liver, postoperative changes in liver function are related primarily to the site and extent of the operation. Similar operations performed under different types of anesthesia are followed by essentially the same changes in hepatic function. However, in patients whose liver function is abnormal before operation, does the type of anesthesia influence the extent of postoperative liver dysfunction? In 1935, Cantarow, *et al.* considered this problem; they were unable to demonstrate any difference in postoperative liver function tests between patients with preoperative abnormalities and patients in whom the tests have been normal before operation. Of 19 patients with either abnormal bromsulfalein tests or abnormal serum bilirubin levels prior to surgery, 10 showed a postoperative increase in serum bilirubin and 11 showed an increased retention of bromsulfalein. On the other hand, slightly more than half of 41 patients in whom these two tests were normal before surgery showed increased serum bilirubin after surgery, and slightly less than half of the patients showed an increase in dye retention. In other words, there was no significant difference between the findings in the "normal" and "abnormal" groups. Both groups evidenced approximately the same incidence of postoperative abnormalities in these two liver function tests.

In 1941, Boyce addressed this issue and came to the opposite conclusion, that the hepatic dysfunction following anesthesia and surgery was more severe in patients with preexisting liver disease than in those without. He also concluded that the anesthetic agent played only a minor role in determining the extent of the dysfunction. Although he presented many illustrative cases, Boyce provided no systematic analysis of cases to prove or disprove this claim.

In 1945, Engstrand and Friberg presented a large, well-documented series of cases, but included only seven patients with abnormal liver function preoperatively. These seven patients underwent various operations; four of them had cyclopropane and three had spinal anesthesia combined with nitrous oxide. On the basis of these cases, the authors concluded that cyclopropane was the anesthetic of choice in patients with liver disease.

In 1952, French, *et al.* also studied the question of the effects of anesthetics on the abnormal liver. On the basis of well-controlled series of
cases in numbers sufficient to allow statistical evaluation, the authors
reached two conclusions. First, patients with abnormal liver before anesthesia and surgery showed more severe and more prolonged hepatic
dysfunction following surgery than did normal patients undergoing similar operations with the same anesthetics. Second, when similar operations were performed under different general anesthetics (e.g., ether and
cyclopropane), there was no difference in postoperative liver function
related to the type of anesthesia. They restricted their study, however,
to the effects of inhalation anesthetics. Greene, *et al.* (1954), working in
the same laboratory as French, *et al.*, investigated the effects of spinal
anesthesia on the abnormal liver. Because of the similarity of the methods in the two studies, comparison of the results is possible. In the paper
by Greene, *et al.*, six patients with "mild" liver disease (as defined by
Fairlie, *et al.*, 1951) and seven patients with "moderate" liver disease
underwent major operative procedures performed under spinal anesthesia. These operations consisted of seven vascular shunts for portal
hypertension, four radical excisions of pelvic carcinoma, one lumbodor-
sal sympathectomy, and one exploratory laparotomy. The spinal anesthesia in all of these cases was "hypotensive," in which the arterial blood
pressure was lowered deliberately. If spinal anesthesia in itself has any
specific deleterious effect on liver function, it should be apparent in these
patients. Table 4.4 illustrates the results of bromsulfalein retention tests
for patients undergoing "hypotensive spinal" as reported by Greene, *et
al.* (1954), and for those patients reported by French, *et al.* (1952), who
had operations of similar magnitude under general anesthesia. Although
both groups of authors included patients with "mild" liver disease,
French, *et al.*, did not study patients with "moderate" liver disease.

Table 4.4.
Comparison of the Effect of Anesthetic Agents on Bromsulfalein Retention in
Patients with Liver Disease Undergoing Comparable Operative Procedures

Anesthetic	Degree of Liver Disease	No. Patients	Preoperative	Average Bromsulfalein Retention (%) Postoperative Day				
				1st	3rd	4th	5th	10th
Gas-oxygen-ether[a]	"Mild"	8	6.4	28.8	29.0		23.8	17.8
Cyclopropane[a]	"Mild"	7	4.7	26.5	23.8		19.5	15.0
Spinal[b]	"Mild"	6	6.8	24.2		17.5		10.8
Spinal[b]	"Moderate"	7	22.3	34.6		33.2		20.8

[a] From French, *et al.*, Ann. Surg. *135:* 145, 1952.
[b] From Greene, *et al.*, Ann. Surg. *140:* 641, 1954.

Hence a comparison cannot be made in respect to the effects of anesthetics on "moderate" liver disease. Patients with "moderate" liver disease undergoing spinal anesthesia are included in order to emphasize the importance of the degree of preexisting liver disease to the development of postoperative liver dysfunction. The significance of preexisting liver disease becomes even more apparent when the postoperative bromsulfalein retention in patients with "mild" liver disease is compared with that occurring following similar operations and anesthetics in patients with no liver disease (pp. 237–239 and Table 4.3). Postoperatively, patients with "mild" liver disease show a threefold increase in bromsulfalein retention which remains above normal levels even after the 10th postoperative day (Table 4.4). Study of these patients with "mild" liver disease also shows no significant difference in bromsulfalein retention related to whether gas-oxygen-ether, cyclopropane, or spinal anesthesia was used. These data suggest that any difference which might tend to imply that spinal anesthesia has less deleterious effect on the abnormal liver, is more apparent than real, for there was no statistically significant difference between the three types of anesthesia.

More recently, Zinn, *et al.* (1985) conducted a study comparing the effects of both spinal anesthesia and modern intravenous (narcotic, type unspecified) anesthesia or enflurane anesthesia, both with nitrous oxide and muscle relaxants in 30 patients with preoperative mild alcoholic hepatitis. The diagnosis of alcoholic hepatitis was based on a history of heavy alcohol intake over an extended period of time, plus two or more of the following: hepatomegaly of such an extent that the liver was palpable more than 10 cm below the right costal margin, and increased serum levels of bilirubin, SGOT, SGPT, or lactic dehydrogenase (LDH). Five patients had spinal anesthesia, 12 had intravenous narcotic anesthesia, and 13 had enflurane anesthesia. Blood samples were obtained immediately prior to induction of anesthesia and again on the first and third postoperative days. Operations consisted of superficial procedures on the extremities, the perineum, the chest or the head. Twenty-six of the patients had three of the above-mentioned abnormalities defining alcoholic hepatitis preoperatively, 14 patients had four abnormalities, and 2 patients had five abnormalities. There was no significant difference in the postoperative occurrence of the markers of alcoholic hepatitis in the three groups. Remarkably enough, mean serum enzyme and bilirubin levels were below preoperative levels in all three groups, though the difference was not statistically significant. These data confirm the generalization based on older data that mild preoperative hepatic dysfunction is not worsened following superficial operations performed under either spinal or modern general anesthesia, either inhalational or intravenous.

Although the abnormal liver function that may occur during the latter part of pregnancy probably does not represent hepatic disease in the usual sense, it is interesting to note that this condition is not associated with any special susceptibility to the effects of anesthetics. Smith, *et al.* (1962) found that 80% of 98 healthy women had more than 5% retention of bromsulfalein during labor. In the patients who had bromsulfalein excretion tests performed postoperatively, the rate at which the ability to excrete dye returned to normal was the same among the women who had regional anesthesia (spinal or epidural) for delivery (17 patients), as it was among those who had chloroform (31), cyclopropane (12), or local anesthesia (10).

In summary, there is no evidence to indicate that the particular anesthetic agent or technique is a major consideration in the anesthetic management of patients with mild preexisting liver disease, in terms of worsening the hepatic dysfunction in the postoperative period. This may not be equally true in the presence of severe preoperative liver disease, but even then all currently employed anesthetic agents and techniques would be expected to have similar and equally adverse effects on postoperative hepatic function.

This conclusion is in no way meant to detract from, or to minimize the importance of, meticulous and skillful anesthesia in patients with hepatic disease; for hemorrhagic shock, hypoxia, and other similar conditions can exacerbate the hepatic damage produced by anesthesia and surgery. Patients with severe liver disease need special attention and skillful anesthesia, but the choice of the anesthetic agent itself is of secondary consideration.

Effects of Spinal Anesthesia on Hepatic Blood Flow

In the above discussion on liver function, it was shown that spinal anesthesia when combined with surgery often is associated with varying but usually minor degrees of hepatic dysfunction as measured by usual liver function tests. It is, nevertheless, appropriate to consider the effects of spinal anesthesia on hepatic blood flow to determine, first, if hepatic hypoperfusion can contribute to postoperative hepatic dysfunction described above; and, second, to determine whether spinal anesthesia, by altering liver blood flow, can change the distribution and elimination of perioperatively administered drugs, since their biotransformation by hepatic microsomal enzyme systems determines the magnitude and duration of their effects.

The classic studies of Mueller, *et al.* (1952) and Lynn, *et al.* (1952), working in the same laboratory, were the first to measure hepatic blood flow during spinal anesthesia. These investigators studied five patients during "low" spinal anesthesia (sensory levels of T_7–T_{10}) and five patients during "high" spinal anesthesia (sensory levels of T_2–T_3). None of the patients underwent surgery and none received vasopressors to maintain blood pressure. The patients under "low" spinal anesthesia had a 22% reduction in mean arterial blood pressure (from an average of 110.0 to 85.5 mmHg). At the time the blood pressure had decreased, these five patients showed an 18.5% decrease in estimated hepatic blood flow (from an average of 979 to 798 ml·m^{-2}·min^{-1}), a 10.4% increase in brachial artery–hepatic vein oxygen difference (average 4.78 to 5.34 vol%), a 13.7% decrease in hepatic venous oxygen content (7.12 to 6.04 vol%), a 4.7% decrease in splanchnic oxygen consumption (46.6 to 44.2 ml·m^{-2}·min^{-1}), and a 4.0% decrease in splanchnic vascular resistance (7.4 to 7.1 mmHg·ml^{-1}·sec^{-1}·m^{-2}). With "high" spinal anesthesia the mean arterial blood pressure decreased 28.4% (883 to 632 ml·m^{-2}·min^{-1}), the brachial artery–hepatic vein oxygen difference increased 35.5% (5.09 to 7.90 vol%), the hepatic venous oxygen content decreased 30.3% (11.05 to 7.70 vol%), the splanchnic oxygen consumption increased 8.8% (45 to 49 ml·m^{-2}·min^{-1}), and the splanchnic vascular resistance increased 7.0% (6.6 to 7.1 mmHg·ml^{-1}·sec^{-1}·m^{-2}). The individual variability of the control data (five patients who were not given spinal anesthesia) led the authors to regard changes in hepatic blood flow and in arteriovenous oxygen difference as statistically insignificant in the "low" spinal group. Similarly, they did not consider the changes in splanchnic vascular resistance and splanchnic oxygen consumption to be significant in either group. They noted a "close but not absolute relation" between changes in blood flow and the level of spinal anesthesia and explained the increased extraction of oxygen from splanchnic blood as the result of more prolonged contact of blood in this area with cells "available for extraction." There was, however, a fairly close correlation between the reductions in blood pressure and those in hepatic blood flow. Similar results were also obtained by Papper, *et al.* (1950), as well as by Kennedy, *et al.* (1970). The data of the latter group of investigators are particularly instructive. Kennedy, *et al.* studied 19 nonoperative volunteers with sensory levels of spinal anesthesia to T_5. They found that hepatic blood flow, estimated by the rate of clearance of indocyanine green, decreased 15.6% ± 5.5% (SEM) below preanesthetic control levels immediately following induction of anesthesia. This decrease was statistically significant. A further decrease in hepatic blood flow was seen one half-hour after induction of anesthesia, to 23.5% ± 6.3% below control levels. Thereafter, liver blood flow started to normalize, being 9.9% ± 6.2% below normal at 60 min, and 8.3% ± 6.2% above normal 90 min following induction of anesthesia. Neither of these latter two changes were significantly different from control values. Unlike Mueller, *et al.*, and Lynn, *et al.*, Kennedy, *et al.* found that splanchnic vascular resistance tended to increase, rather than decrease, during spinal anesthesia. It averaged $6.8 \pm 11.1\%$, $13.9\% \pm 10.3\%$, and $11.9\% \pm 9.3\%$ above, and $5.0\% \pm 8.4\%$ below, preanesthetic control levels immediately following, and 30, 60, and 90 min after, induction of anesthesia. None of these changes were statistically significant. The significant decreases in hepatic blood flow were therefore due to decreases in, or to redistribution of, cardiac output, rather than to increases in resistance to liver blood flow. In their subjects, cardiac output did not decrease significantly, however, during spinal anesthesia. This finding suggests that the significant decrease in hepatic blood flow associated with spinal anesthesia may have been due to redistribution of cardiac output and not to changes in output. This conclusion is supported by their observation that the percentage of cardiac output perfusing the liver ($20.6\% \pm 2.1\%$ prior to induction of anesthesia) was $18.3\% \pm 6.7\%$ and $21.5\% \pm 5.9\%$ below control levels immediately following, and 30 min after, induction of anesthesia. Both these changes were statistically significant. By the time hepatic blood flow had returned to its preanesthetic level, the percentage of cardiac output going to the liver also was no longer different during the anesthesia than it was before the anesthesia.

Redistribution of cardiac output as the cause of the decrease in hepatic blood flow during spinal anesthesia was not supported, however, by the data obtained by Sivarajan, et al. (1975), when they measured liver blood flow in Rhesus monkeys using radioactive microsphere techniques. They found that liver blood flow accounted for $19.7\% \pm 1.41\%$ (SEM) (207 ± 20.6 ml$\cdot$100 g$^{-1}\cdot$min^{-1}) of cardiac output prior to T_1 levels of spinal anesthesia. Ten minutes following induction of anesthesia, liver blood flow represented $18.5\% \pm 1.38\%$ (180 ± 16.9 ml$\cdot$100 g$^{-1}\cdot$min^{-1}) of cardiac output. Comparable figures 20, 40, and 80 min after induction of anesthesia were $20\% \pm 1.39\%$, $19.9\% \pm 1.89\%$, and $19.5\% \pm 1.94\%$ of cardiac output, respectively. None of the data on distribution of cardiac output differed significantly from preanesthetic control values. On the other hand, hepatic blood flow decreased significantly below control levels in these animals 20 and 40 min after induction of anesthesia. These decreases in hepatic blood flow during spinal anesthesia suggest that the cause of decreased flow to the liver might be related to decreases in cardiac output rather than redistribution of output. Reasons for the difference in results of these two studies may be related to species differences. Kennedy, et al. (1970) studied normal humans. Sivarajan, et al. (1975) studied Rhesus monkeys. The difference may also be related to the techniques used for measuring blood flow to the liver. The technique used by Sivarajan, et al. also measured blood flow to the gastrointestinal tract, to the mesentery, to the spleen, and to the pancreas. The technique used by Kennedy, et al. measured hepatic flow more directly. Both sets of observations could be reconciled if it were hypothesized that the redistribution of cardiac output which was found by Kennedy, *et al.* to be responsible for the diminution of hepatic blood flow occurred within the splanchnic circulation.

Mather, *et al.* undertook an extensive series of studies of the effects of spinal anesthesia in conscious sheep with chronically implanted catheters that permitted measurement of a variety of cardiovascular, including hepatic vascular functions (Mather, *et al.*, 1982 and 1986; Runciman *et al.*, 1984 a, b, 1985, 1986). The consistency with which they found, in their many studies over the years, that hepatic blood flow remained little affected by spinal anesthesia with sensory levels usually at the T_4 level or higher is indeed notable. When blood flow to the liver did decrease, it was only 8–10% below baseline levels, changes that were not statistically significant. These investigators found that cardiac output and arterial blood pressure were not significantly affected by spinal anesthesia. This was, as these authors emphasize, because intravenous fluids were administered in volumes great enough to avoid significant decreases in blood pressure. This finding stands in contrast to the experimental designs used in the above-mentioned studies of hepatic blood flow during spinal anesthesia in humans and in monkeys, studies in which spinal anesthesia was associated with decreases in arterial blood pressure. Another interesting finding in the studies of Mather, *et al.* was the fact that, although cardiac output, mean arterial pressure, and hepatic blood flow failed to be significantly changed by spinal anesthesia, the percentage of cardiac output perfusing the liver did decrease. In fact, it decreased to levels as much as 86% of preanesthetic baseline values at a time when total hepatic blood flow was within 10% of baseline values. The sheep were awake and breathing spontaneously during the studies. Their arterial oxygen tension levels did not change during spinal anesthesia, nor, equally important, did hepatic venous oxygen tensions. That pulmonary arterial, that is, mixed venous oxygen tension, was also not affected, is not unexpected in view of the absence of significant changes in cardiac output, arterial pressure, and hepatic venous oxygen tension. The significance of these studies by Mather, *et al.*, in terms of the effects of spinal anesthesia on hepatic function as reflected by hepatic extraction of various xenobiotics, the purpose of their research project, is considered on p. 259. It should be noted that in these studies, the minimal effects of spinal anesthesia on hepatic blood flow contrast strikingly with the significant decreases in hepatic blood flow associated with halothane anesthesia in their animals.

It is interesting to note that although spinal anesthesia lasted for 2 hr or longer in the subjects studied by Kennedy, *et al.* (1970), the decreases in blood flow were relatively transient. Hepatic blood flow had returned to normal levels between 30 to 60 min following induction of anesthesia. This suggests the presence of time-dependent compensatory mechanisms which acted to restore hepatic blood flow to normal levels before the anesthesia had worn off. Where such compensatory adjustments take place remains as unclear as whether they do in fact usually exist.

In the presence of arterial hypotension, Mueller, et al. (1952) and Lynn, et al. (1952) observed an increase in the difference between brachial arterial and hepatic venous oxygen content. In the absence of hypotension during spinal anesthesia, Runciman, et al. (1984 b) noted no changes in hepatic venous oxygen tension. When these findings are combined with the decrease in hepatic blood flow that occurs during spinal anesthesia, they suggest that, during levels of hypotension commonly seen clinically during spinal anesthesia, hepatic perfusion may decrease to the point where oxygen supply is no longer adequate to meet hepatic oxygen requirements. This would represent a situation different from that observed during inhalation anesthesia. Potent inhalation anesthetics decrease hepatic blood flow to approximately the same degree as does high spinal anesthesia. Inhalation anesthetics also decrease oxygen consumption. Spinal anesthesia decreases oxygen supply (flow) without decreasing oxygen consumption (Chapter 3; Mueller, et al., 1952; Lynn, et al., 1952; Davis et al., 1956). Thus, spinal anesthesia might appear to set the stage for the development of hepatic hypoxia with subsequent evidence of hepatic dysfunction as evidenced by changes in postoperative liver function tests and serum enzyme levels. This is unlikely. The frequency and magnitude of postoperative hepatic dysfunction are, as discussed above, similar after general anesthesia and after spinal anesthesia when all other factors other than anesthetic technique are kept constant. That changes in hepatic function are the same after general and spinal anesthesia might be explained on the basis that the potential for hepatic hypoxia is as great during general anesthesia as it is during spinal anesthesia because general anesthetics decrease hepatic perfusion more than they decrease hepatic oxygen consumption (Ngai, 1980). This finding would mean that both general and spinal anesthesia may be associated with roughly the same potential for development of hepatic hypoxia. But if the development of hepatic hypoxia were likely during spinal anesthesia as a result of cardiovascular perturbations brought about by the anesthesia, then the more severe the cardiovascular changes, the greater the likelihood of postoperative hepatic dysfunction. In view of the fact that hepatic blood flow varies directly with mean arterial pressure during spinal anesthesia (Papper, et al., 1950; Mueller, et al., 1952; Kennedy, et al., 1970), there should be a relation between the degree of hypotension during spinal anesthesia and both frequency and magnitude of abnormalities of postoperative liver function. Specifically, postoperative hepatic dysfunction should be more evident in patients whose blood pressure has been deliberately decreased by use of spinal anesthesia to decrease surgical blood loss. Levy, et al. (1961) studied the effect of this form of induced hypotension on hepatic plasma flow. In seven subjects, hypotensive spinal anesthesia was associated with a 31% decrease in estimated hepatic plasma flow, the absolute values being 1300 ± 191.7 ml before induction of spinal anesthesia and 899 ± 173.87 ml during spinal anesthesia. The anesthetic technique included endotracheal nitrous oxide-oxygen anesthesia, as well as induction with thiopental. The same decrease in estimated hepatic plasma flow occurred during hypotensive spinal anesthesia combined with thiopental and nitrous oxide as during thiopental–nitrous oxide anesthesia alone. It is not known whether equal decreases in hepatic plasma flow would have been observed had hypotensive spinal anesthesia been administered in the absence of supplemental thiopental and nitrous oxide. It also should be mentioned that the decreases in hepatic plasma flow were essentially the same with general anesthetics alone as with hypotensive spinal anesthesia.

It has been suggested by many investigators that a relationship exists between blood pressure during spinal anesthesia and the magnitude and frequency of postoperative hepatic dysfunction (Schmidt, *et al.*, 1942; Boyce and McFetridge, 1938 b; Johnson, 1949), and this clinical impression remains widespread. There have been, however, few attempts to confirm this by controlled studies. Engstrand and Friberg (1945) analyzed the results of their studies on liver function to see if there was any relationship between hypotension during spinal anesthesia and postoperative liver dysfunction. They believed not only that such a relationship did exist, but also that spinal anesthesia did not induce any reduction in hepatic function as long as blood pressure remained normal. Aside from the problems associated with their reliance on the hippuric acid excretion test, analysis of their data is difficult because of the considerable variation in the types of operation in the normotensive and in the hypotensive groups. There was also such wide individual variation in the postoperative excretion rates, that statistical evaluation becomes difficult, if not impossible. For example, while the blood pressure actually increased in three patients during spinal anesthesia, their average decrease in postoperative hippuric acid excretion amounted to 52%. If the severity of postoperative liver dysfunction were related to the degree of hypotension, patients with increased blood pressure would be expected to do no worse than those with normal blood pressure during anesthesia. In 11 patients whose blood pressure remained normal during spinal anesthesia, the average postoperative hippuric acid excretion decreased by 30%.

Using serum enzyme levels as indices of postoperative hepatic dysfunction, Brohult and Gillquist (1969) came to the same conclusion as did Engstrand and Friberg. These authors studied 26 patients having herniorrhaphies or urologic operations under spinal anesthesia. In 18 patients there was no change in the blood pressure during anesthesia and surgery and no significant change in levels of either SGOT or SGPT. Levels of SOCT remained unchanged compared to preoperative levels on the 1st, 4th, 8th, and 11th days postoperatively. SOCT was significantly elevated above control levels on the seventh postoperative day. In eight patients, arterial pressure decreased 60 mmHg or more for 25 minutes or longer during anesthesia. In these patients, levels of SGOT and SGPT also showed no change following surgery and anesthesia. SOCT levels increased significantly, however, on the first and fourth postoperative days. They were normal on the 7th, 8th, and 11th postoperative days. Whether such subtle changes in SOCT accurately reflect changes in intra-operative hepatic oxygenation in the absence of changes in levels of other enzymes, remains debatable. The significance of these changes in levels in SOCT alone is highlighted by the studies of Greene, *et al.* (1954) who reached a different conclusion in studying the effects on liver function of arterial hypotension deliberately induced by spinal anesthesia. They were unable to detect any greater hepatic dysfunction following "hypo-tensive spinal" than was present after similar operations performed under normotensive conditions. The degrees of hypotension in this study varied from systolic levels of 60 mmHg and under, down to, and including pressures that were unobtainable by sphygmomanometry. In the study by Greene, *et al.*, patients with normal preoperative liver func-tion tests underwent radical surgery performed under hypotensive spinal anesthesia. The operations included seven Wertheim hysterecto-mies, two hemipelvectomies, two resections of the ileum, and two crani-otomies. In this series the average bromsulfalein retention on the first postoperative day was 6.6% and on the fourth postoperative day, 4.9%. These figures compare favorably with the results obtained from the same laboratory (Fairlie, *et al.*, 1951), in a separate study of 10 normal patients given "normotensive" spinal anesthesia of procedures such as vaginal hysterectomy (3 patients), inguinal herniorrhaphy (5), and perineorrha-phy (2). Among these 10 patients, the average bromsulfalein retention on the first postoperative day was 6.2%, on the third day 5.0%, and on the fifth day, 5.0%. If hypotension due to spinal anesthesia were a significant determinant of the degree of postoperative hepatic dysfunc-tion, patients subjected to severe and often prolonged decreases in arte-rial pressure should show more abnormalities of bromsulfalein excretion than did the patients whose pressure was normal during the anesthesia. But this was not the case, despite the fact that all patients in the hypoten-sive group underwent more radical surgery than did any of the normo-tensive patients.

Whereas hypotension due to blood loss is associated with abnormali-ties of liver function lasting beyond the period of hypotension, such has not been the case when hypotension is due to spinal anesthesia. This is not to suggest that hypotension during spinal anesthesia and subsequent changes in hepatic blood flow can never cause liver damage that persists after normal blood pressure and blood flow have been restored. Undoubtedly a point is reached where blood flow is no longer adequate to maintain normal cellular respiration and metabolism, and when the blood flow does return to normal, the hepatic cells cannot resume normal function until regeneration takes place. But no data are available to suggest at what level blood flow becomes too low, a figure which will be especially hard to obtain in the case of the liver because of its dual blood supply. The inference remains that a reduction in hepatic blood flow produced by a moderate degree of hypotension for a moderate period of time during spinal anesthesia does not in itself contribute to postoperative changes in liver function. The reason for this may be due to the dual blood supply of this organ. The portal vein normally supplies about 80% of the blood entering the liver, but only about 62% of the oxygen used by the liver comes from this source. Because of the admixture of portal venous and hepatic arterial blood at the periphery of the lobules, liver cells are normally exposed to lower oxygen tensions than are cells of any other organ. During a decrease in blood pressure due to blood loss, the proportions of hepatic blood flow derived from the portal system and from the hepatic artery are altered by a decrease in splanchnic blood flow. Under such circumstances, the liver gets proportionately more of its oxygen from hepatic arterial blood. At a pressure of 60 mmHg (following hemorrhage) the portal vein supplies only 35.5% of the oxygen used by the liver, instead of the normal 62 percent (McMichael, 1938). Whether this happens during the hypotension of spinal anesthesia is unknown, but it is probable that the relative amounts of blood coming from the hepatic artery and the portal vein are altered after sympathetic denervation by spinal anesthesia.

Changes in liver blood flow during spinal anesthesia are, then, not consequential enough, even in the presence of marked hypotension, to be related to either intra- or postoperative changes in liver function as determined by classic and usual liver function tests. What about the possibility that spinal anesthesia might significantly affect the pharmacokinetics of perioperatively administered drugs that are normally eliminated by uptake into the liver with subsequent biotransformation and, thus, pharmacologic inactivation? This might be particularly important perioperatively when drugs that have high hepatic clearances are administered. This issue was studied extensively in conscious sheep by Mather, et al. They found that spinal anesthesia did not alter hepatic clearance of meperidine, chlormethiazole, or cefoxitin, although clearance of all three drugs was significantly decreased by halothane anesthesia (Mather, et al., 1982 and 1986; Runciman, et al., 1984 a, 1985, 1986). Whelan, et al. (1989) reported similar results when propranolol, a drug with a high hepatic extraction ratio, was infused into awake dogs who had chronically implanted catheters. Mean hepatic plasma flow remained unchanged during spinal anesthesia. Similarly, intrinsic hepatic clearance of propranolol, a reflection of drug metabolizing capacity of hepatic microsomal enzyme systems, was unaffected by spinal anesthesia. Systemic clearance and elimination half-life of propranolol were likewise unaffected.

The above studies suggesting that spinal anesthesia has no effect on hepatic metabolism of xenobiotics stand in contrast to the study by Loft, *et al.* (1985) of the effects of halothane and spinal anesthesia on two indices of hepatic microsomal enzyme activity, antipyrine and aminopyrine metabolism, carried out in healthy patients having arthrotomies. The amount of labeled carbon in exhaled air 2 hr after its oral ingestion was significantly above preoperative levels in patients having had their surgery performed under either anesthetic. The increase after spinal anesthesia was observed only on the 1st postoperative day, not on the 10th or 21st postoperative days. After halothane anesthesia, aminopyrine metabolism was significantly above baseline levels on the 10th but not on the 1st or 21st postoperative days. Antipyrine clearance, measured by the amount of antipyrine in 5 ml saliva 24 hr after oral ingestion of antipyrine, similarly increased significantly above preoperative values when first measured on the 5th postoperative day after both spinal and halothane anesthesia, but had returned to normal levels when again measured on the 10th and 21st postoperative days.

Reasons for the differences between the data of Loft, *et al.* on the one hand, and Mather, *et al.*, and Runciman, *et al.*, on the other hand, are not immediately apparent, nor, given the timing of their publications, were either team of investigators able to comment on the finding of the other team. Certainly the subject warrants further investigation, including studies in patients with and without preexisting disease.

REFERENCES

BECKMAN, V., BROHULT, J., AND REICHARD, H.: Elevations of liver-enzyme activities in serum after halothane, ether and spinal anaesthesias. Acta Anaesthesiol. Scand. *10:* 55, 1966.

BORGSTROM, S.: Prothrombin index after operation. Bull. War Med. *4:* 217, 1943.

BOYCE, F. F.: *The Role of the Liver in Surgery.* Springfield, Ill.: Charles C Thomas, 1941.

BOYCE, F. F., AND MCFETRIDGE, E. M.: Studies of hepatic function by the Quick hippuric acid test. I. Biliary and hepatic disease. Arch. Surg. *37:* 401, 1938 a.

BOYCE, F. F., AND MCFETRIDGE, E. M.: Studies of hepatic function by the Quick hippuric acid test. III. Various surgical states. Arch. Surg. *37:* 443, 1938 b.

BROHULT, J., AND GILLQUIST, J.: Serum ornithine carbamoyl transferase activity in man after halothane anaesthesia and spinal anaesthesia with and without systolic blood pressure fall. Acta Chir. Scand. *135:* 113, 1969.

CANTAROW, A., GARTMAN, E., AND RICCHIUTI, G.: Hepatic function. III. The effect of cholecystectomy on hepatic function. Arch. Surg. *30:* 865, 1935.

COLEMAN, F. P.: The effect of anesthesia on hepatic function. Surgery 3: 87, 1938.

DAVIS, H. C., MORSE, I. S., LARSON, E., AND WYNN, M.: Study of respiratory liver metabolism in surgical patients. J.A.M.A. 162: 561, 1956.

ENGSTRAND, L., AND FRIBERG, O.: On the function of the liver as affected by various operations and anaesthetics. Acta Chir. Scand. 92: (Suppl. 104) 1945.

FAIRLIE, C. W., BARSS, T. P., FRENCH, A. B., JONES, C. M., AND BEECHER, H. K.: Metabolic effects of anesthesia in man. IV. A comparison of the effects of certain anesthetic agents on the normal liver. N. Engl. J. Med. 244: 615, 1951.

FRENCH, A. B., BARSS, T. P., FAIRLIE, C. S., BENGLE, A. L., JONES, C. M., LINTON, R. R., AND BEECHER, H. K.: Metabolic effects of anesthesia in man. V. A comparison of the effects of ether and cyclopropane anesthesia on the abnormal liver. Ann. Surg. 135: 145, 1952.

GRAY, H. K., BUTSCH, W. L., AND McGOWAN, J. M.: Effect of biliary operations on the liver. Their relation to the concentration of bile acids in bile. Arch. Surg. 37: 609, 1938.

GREENE, N. M., BUNKER, J. P., KERR, W. S., VON FELSINGER, J. M., KELLER, J. W., AND BEECHER, H. K.: Hypotensive spinal anesthesia: respiratory, metabolic, hepatic, renal, and cerebral effects. Ann. Surg. 140: 641, 1954.

JOHNSON, F. L.: Liver damage in anaesthesia. Br. J. Anaesth. 21: 164, 1949.

KEETON, R. W., COLE, W. H., CALLOWAY, N., GLICKMAN, N., MITCHELL, H. H., DYNIEWICZ, J., AND HOWES, D.: Convalescence: study in physiological recovery of nitrogen metabolism and liver function. Ann. Intern. Med. 28: 521, 1948.

KENNEDY, W. F., JR., EVERETT, G. B., COBB, L. A., AND ALLEN, G. D.: Simultaneous systemic and hepatic hemodynamic measurements during high spinal anesthesia in normal man. Anesth. Analg. 49: 1016, 1970.

LEVY, M. L., PALAZZI, H. M., NADI, G. L., AND BUNKER, J. P.: Hepatic blood flow variations during surgical anesthesia in man measured by radioactive colloid. Surg. Gynecol. Obstet. 112: 289, 1961.

LOFT, S., BOEL, J., KYST, A., RASMUSSEN, B., HANSEN, S. H., AND DØSSING, M.: Increased hepatic microsomal enzyme activity after surgery under halothane or spinal anesthesia. Anesthesiology 62: 11, 1985.

LYNN, R. B., SANCETTA, S. M., SIMEONE, F. A., AND SCOTT, R. W.: Observations on the circulation in high spinal anesthesia. Surgery 32: 195, 1952.

MATHER, L. E., RUNCIMAN, W. B., AND ILSLEY, A. H.: Anesthesia-induced changes in regional blood flow: implications during drug disposition. Reg. Anesth. (Suppl.) 7: S 24, 1982.

MATHER, L. E., RUNCIMAN, W. B., ILSLEY, A. H., CARAPETIS, R. J., AND UPTON, R. N.: A sheep preparation for studying interactions between blood flow and drug disposition. V: The effects of general and subarachnoid anaesthesia on blood flow and pethidine disposition. Br. J. Anaesth. 58: 888, 1986.

MENDELOFF, A. I.: Some mechanisms involved in testing hepatic excretory function. Bull. N. Engl. Med. Center 11: 163, 1949.

McMICHAEL, J.: The oxygen supply of the liver. Q. J. Exp. Physiol. 27: 73, 1938.

MUELLER, R. P., LYNN, R. B., AND SANCETTA, S. M.: Studies of hemodynamic changes in humans following induction of low and high spinal anesthesia. II. The changes in splanchnic vascular resistance in humans not undergoing surgery. Circulation 6: 894, 1952.

NGAI, S. H.: Effects of anesthetics on various organs. N. Engl. J. Med. 302: 564, 1980.

PAPPER, E. M., HABIF, D. V., AND BRADLEY, S. E.: Studies of renal and hepatic function in normal man during thiopental, cyclopropane and high spinal anesthesia. J. Clin. Invest. 29: 838, 1950.

POHLE, F. J.: Anesthesia and liver function. Wis. Med. J. 47: 476, 1948.

RUNCIMAN, W. B., MATHER, L. E., ILSLEY, A. H., CARAPETIS, R. J., AND McLEAN, C. F.: A sheep preparation for studying interactions between blood flow and drug disposition. II. Experimental applications. Br. J. Anaesth. 56: 1117, 1984 a.

RUNCIMAN, W. B., MATHER, L. E., ILSLEY, A. H., CARAPETIS, R. J., AND UPTON, R. N.: A sheep preparation for studying interactions between blood flow and drug disposition. III. Effects of general and spinal anaesthesia on regional blood flow and oxygen tensions. Br. J. Anaesth. 56: 1247, 1984 b.

RUNCIMAN, W. B., MATHER, L. E., ILSLEY, A. H., AND UPTON, R. N.: A sheep preparation for interactions between blood flow and drug dispositions in general or subarachnoid anaesthesia on blood flow and disposition. Br. J. Anaesth. 58: 1308, 1986.

RUNCIMAN, W. B., MATHER, L. E., ILSLEY, A. H., CARAPETIS, R. J., AND UPTON, R. N.: A sheep preparation for studying interactions between blood flow and drug disposition. IV. The effects of general and spinal anaesthesia on blood flow and cefoxitin disposition. Br. J. Anaesth. 57: 1239, 1985.

SCHMIDT, C. R., UNRUH, R. T., AND CHESKY, V. E.: Clinical studies of liver function. I. Effect of anesthesia and certain surgical procedures. Am. J. Surg. 57: 43, 1942.

SIVARAJAN, M., AMORY, D. W., LINDBLOOM, L. E., AND SCHETTMAN, R. S.: Systemic and regional blood-flow changes during spinal anesthesia in the Rhesus monkey. Anesthesiology 43: 78, 1975.

SMITH, B. E., MOYA, F., AND SHNIDER, S.: The effects of anesthesia on liver function during labor. Anesth. Analg. 41: 24, 1962.

TYLER, F. H., SCHMIDT, C. D., EIK-NES, K., BROWN, H ., AND SAMUELS, L. T.: The role of the liver and the adrenal in producing elevated plasma 17-hydroxycorticosteroid levels in surgery. J. Clin. Invest. 33: 1517, 1954.

WHELAN, E., WOOD, A. J. J., SHAY, S., AND WOOD, M.: Lack of effect of spinal anesthesia on drug metabolism. Anesth. Analg. 69: 307, 1989.

ZAMCHECK, N., CHALMERS, T. C., AND DAVIDSON, C. S.: Pathologic and functional changes in liver following upper abdominal operations. Am. J. Med. 7: 409, 1949.

ZINN, S. E., FAIRLEY, H. B., AND GLENN, J. D.: Liver function in patients with mild alcoholic cirrhosis after enflurane, nitrous oxide-narcotic, and spinal anesthesia. Anesth. Analg. 64: 487, 1985.

CHAPTER 5

Renal Function

Spinal anesthesia has no effect on renal function unless the preganglionic sympathetic block produced by the anesthesia involves sympathetic fibers at the 11th thoracic through the first lumbar spinal segments (White, *et al.*, 1952). If the level of sympathetic blockade reaches this level, spinal anesthesia may then affect renal function in one of two ways or by a combination of both. It may influence renal function purely by interfering with the normal autonomic innervation of the kidney, or it may do so by modifying arterial blood pressure to the extent that renal hemodynamics are altered. Before reviewing the effects of sympathetic denervation and the effects of hypotension on renal function, it is, however, appropriate to consider certain aspects of the mechanisms normally involved in maintenance of renal homeostasis in the absence of anesthesia.

Mechanisms of Renal Homeostasis

Glomerular filtration and selective tubular reabsorption are mechanisms by which the kidneys contribute to the maintenance of the internal milieu of the body as a whole. Three steps are involved in regulation of these functions (Badr and Ichikawa, 1988). First is the existence of intrarenal mechanisms for maintenance of a constant ratio of renal to total systemic vascular resistance that assures delivery to the kidneys of a constant fraction of cardiac output. Second are the intrinsic mechanisms regulating the fraction of the amount of blood delivered to the glomeruli that are filtered to a protein-free ultrafiltrate, the filtration fraction. Third are mechanisms for tubular reabsorption of the majority of the glomerular filtrate with return to the peripheral circulation, thereby regulating blood volume, cardiac output and renal perfusion itself.

Inherent in the above scenario is the presence of vascular autoregulation within the kidney. Similar to but more efficient than the autoregulation seen in several other organs, renal autoregulation involves vascular smooth muscles from renal artery to glomerular arterioles that respond reflexly to changes in intraluminal pressure. Decreases in pressure cause vasodilation, while increases in pressure cause vasoconstriction. Supplementing the myogenic reflex activity is a unique feedback system between renal tubules and glomeruli, whereby a decrease in delivery to macula densa cells produces vasodilation of the adjacent afferent glomerular arteriole with a resulting increase in glomerular perfusion and filtration (Badr and Ichikawa, 1988).

Intrinsic renal control of glomerular filtration fraction (glomerular filtration rate/glomerular plasma flow rate) includes not only a smooth muscle precapillary sphincter on the afferent glomerular arteriole but also a postcapillary sphincter on the efferent glomerular arteriole. A result of this unique arrangement is that even though vascular resistance might increase at the afferent arteriolar level, thereby decreasing glomerular plasma flow, the upstream increase in glomerular capillary pressure tends to increase glomerular filtration. The kidney has a remarkable ability to maintain its main function, filtration, through a wide range of systemic blood pressures and may even contribute to the maintenance of systemic pressure by virtue of its ability to serve as a high vascular resistance organ through which a substantial portion of cardiac output normally flows.

With the preceding information in mind, we can now review the effects of spinal anesthesia on renal function. Since the effects of both sympathetic denervation and arterial hypotension associated with spinal anesthesia could affect renal function, we will consider them separately.

Effects of Sympathetic Denervation

Renal Blood Flow

In the absence of concurrent arterial hypotension, sympathetic denervation of the kidneys produces little or no significant change in renal blood flow. This is true whether the denervation is accomplished surgically (Selkurt, 1946 a; Sartorius and Burlington, 1956), by the administration of ganglionic blocking agents (Miles, et al., 1952; Morris, et al., 1953; Moyer, et al., 1955; Stover, et al., 1956), or by the use of spinal anesthesia (Smith, et al., 1939; Page, et al., 1944; Corcoran, et al., 1948; Mokotoff and Ross, 1948; Papper, et al., 1950; Assali, et al., 1951). Since renal blood flow shows no appreciable change following sympathetic denervation in the presence of a constant blood pressure, renal vascular resistance may be considered to be relatively independent of neurogenic control.

The autonomy of renal vascular resistance could be explained on the basis that sympathetic fibers have little influence on arteries and arterioles within the kidney and that therefore sympathetic denervation produces no significant vasodilation or change in resistance. But the failure of renal vascular resistance to change as the result of sympathetic denervation could also be explained on the basis that renal arteries and arterioles do respond to sympathetic denervation by vasodilation but the vascular resistance remains constant despite changes in arterial and arteriolar size because of the process of "plasma skimming" (Pappenheimer and Kinter, 1956; Kinter and Pappenheimer, 1956). According to the theory of plasma skimming, renal vascular resistance is determined primarily by the viscosity of blood flowing through renal vessels rather than by arterial or arteriolar vasodilation or constriction. Erythrocytes in the renal circulation are normally progressively separated from plasma in the interlobular arteries. Because erythrocytes in the interlobular arteries flow in the center of the vessel in an axial stream with the plasma at the periphery of the vessel, afferent arterioles at the base (i.e., near the site of origin) of the interlobular arteries are supplied primarily with the peripheral layer of plasma while the more distal afferent arterioles are supplied primarily with the central "core" of erythrocytes. Deeper glomeruli which are situated farthest from the cortex are therefore presented with blood containing mainly plasma, while glomeruli nearest the cortex are supplied by blood with a high hematocrit. Since the process of plasma skimming is related to velocity of blood flow, any change in the velocity of blood flow will alter the process of plasma skimming. Because small changes in the degree of plasma skimming taking place in the afferent arterioles at the base of the interlobular arteries produce relatively large changes in the viscosity of the blood reaching the outer arterioles, renal vascular resistance could remain constant despite changes in velocity of blood flow. For example, a 20 percent increase in the hematocrit of blood going to the outer arterioles has been estimated to produce a twofold increase in resistance to flow through these vessels (Pappenheimer and Kinter, 1956). If one hypothesizes that sympathetic denervation does produce renal vasodilation, then the increased intravascular pressures in the smaller arteries and arterioles following such vasodilation could produce increases in the velocity of blood flow with consequent changes in plasma skimming which in themselves could compensate for the decreased resistance produced by the vasodilation. Thus renal vascular resistance would remain unchanged despite vasodilation.

The plasma skimming theory as an explanation for renal vascular autonomy deserves attention. There is no doubt that rheologic changes assumed in such a theory occur in the kidney in response to changes in vascular tone. It is unlikely, however, that rheologic changes play the dominant role in explaining renal vascular autonomy. For example, if rheologic and not myogenic changes were the primary basis for renal vascular autonomy, there is no reason why the same principles of plasma skimming with accompanying rheologic changes could not be applied to various other organs that have autonomous circulations, including the brain. The plasma skimming theory with its corollaries is not nearly as compelling when applied to other organs with autonomous circulations in which there are extensive data quantitating the relationship between vascular tone and perfusing pressure. Also, how can plasma skimming explain the increase in renal vascular pulsations recorded plethysmographically during sympathetic denervation produced by spinal anesthesia (Kusunoki, 1957)?

Renal Function

Although there is evidence that the infusion of adrenergic agonists can affect renal sodium excretion independent of systemic or renal hemodynamic changes (Kim, *et al.*, 1979), studies based on surgical denervation or denervation by spinal anesthesia itself are more relevant to evaluation of the effect of spinal anesthesia on renal function. Thus, for example, it has been shown that *acute* sympathetic denervation in the absence of simultaneous decreases in blood pressure has effects on both glomerular and tubular function. Sartorius and Burlington (1956), for example, studied acute renal denervation in dogs and found that glomerular filtration was greater in a denervated kidney (11 ml/min) than it was in a normally innervated kidney (5 ml/min) when both were exposed to the same mean arterial pressure (105 mmHg). This was true even though the renal plasma flow was slightly less in the denervated than in the intact kidney (59 as compared to 63 ml/min). These authors also found that there was a greater output of urine by the denervated kidney (0.25 ml/min) than there was by the intact kidney (0.10 ml/min). There was also a significant increase in sodium excretion by the denervated kidney although, because of concurrent increases in urinary output, the increase in urinary sodium concentration was relatively slight. Comparable experimental data following acute denervation have also been reported by Blake (1955) as well as by Surtshin and Schmandt (1956). The above studies were carried out in normovolemic animals. In volume-depleted animals, sympathetic denervation produced dilation of the afferent glomerular arteriole with an associated increase in glomerular plasma flow (Kon, *et al.*, 1985).

Unfortunately, reports in humans on the effects of sympathetic denervation on renal function during spinal anesthesia in the absence of arterial blood pressure changes are so scarce that no accurate statement can be made concerning the effect of spinal anesthesia alone. However, Mokotoff and Ross (1948) made the interesting observation that, in patients with congestive heart failure, high spinal anesthesia reversed the previously low renal plasma flow and glomerular filtration rates to normal levels. Similarly, Morales, *et al.* (1957) found, in their patients that were normothermic, that high spinal anesthesia caused relatively little effect on arterial blood pressure, yet reduced glomerular filtration by 12 percent, renal plasma flow by 8 percent, the filtration fraction by 2 percent, and sodium and potassium excretion by 66 percent and 30 percent, respectively. However, all their patients received intravenous thiopental anesthesia, and it is impossible to determine which of the changes in renal function are due to the thiopental and which are due to the spinal anesthesia.

Effects of Arterial Hypotension

Renal Blood Flow

The relationship between arterial blood pressure and renal blood flow under experimental conditions has been the subject of several reports. Noteworthy among these is the paper by Selkurt (1946 a). Altering arterial pressure by applying clamps to the aorta of dogs, Selkurt studied effective arterial pressures up to 110 mmHg but found that increases above approximately 80 mmHg produced relatively little change in renal blood flow. This occurred regardless of whether the kidney was intact or surgically denervated. The similarity of the pressure-flow curves that Selkurt found in the intact and in the denervated kidneys can be observed by comparing the two illustrations in Figure 5.1. Selkurt's findings have since been confirmed several times in other animal investigations (Bounos, et al., 1960). Taylor, et al. (1948), for example, found that although the mean arterial blood pressure of dogs given high spinal anesthesia decreased from 172 to 122 mmHg as a result of the anesthesia, there was little change in renal plasma flow. In fact, in 9 of the 11 dogs there was an increase in renal plasma flow, averaging 10 percent at the time when arterial pressure had decreased an average of 50 mmHg. Utilizing a pump as a method of altering blood pressure, Shipley and Study (1951) studied even greater ranges of blood pressure than did Selkurt. They found that increasing the mean arterial pressure from 80 to approximately 180 mmHg produced relatively little change in renal plasma flow. Their results are summarized in Figure 5.2 where it can be seen that pressures above 80 mmHg do not significantly affect renal blood flow. Pressures below this level, however, result in proportionate decreases in renal plasma flow, with zero flow occurring at about 10 mmHg. Shipley and Study also found, as did Selkurt, that the pressure-flow relationships were essentially the same in both intact and in surgically denervated kidneys. Although the above pressure-flow relationships are altered by hemorrhagic shock (Lauson, et al., 1944; Selkurt, 1946 b), and although other investigators have reported results different somewhat from the above (Brull, et al., 1955; Sartorius and Burlington, 1956), it is now the consensus that the vascular arrangements of the kidney are such that blood flow is relatively independent of blood pressure in the physiologic range (Pappenheimer, 1952). Whether this is due to baroreceptors in the renal vessels which permit them to constrict or

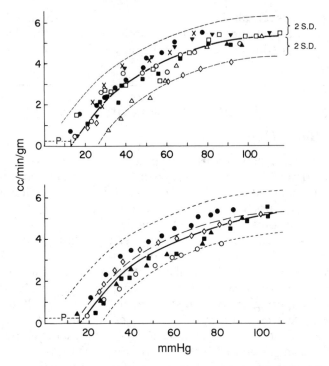

Figure 5.1. Mean curves (±2 SD) of renal blood flow (ml·min^{-1}·g^{-1}) at various effective arterial pressures. Top, with nerves intact; bottom, in denervated kidneys. (Redrawn with permission from Selkurt, Am. J. Physiol. *147:* 537, 1946 a.)

dilate according to the arterial pressure or whether this is due to plasma skimming remains undecided.

A review of the literature indicates that under clinical conditions spinal anesthesia has, in the absence of vasopressors, little effect on renal blood flow when the blood pressure remains in the normal physiologic range. If, however, the blood pressure decreases below a critical level, any further reduction in pressure is associated with a proportional decrease in renal blood flow. Reports indicate that in normal patients the critical level below which normal renal blood flow is no longer maintained during spinal anesthesia is approximately 80–85 mmHg mean arterial pressure (Smith, *et al.*, 1939; Page, *et al.*, 1944; Gregory, *et al.*, 1946; Corcoran, *et al.*, 1948; Mokotoff and Ross, 1948; Papper, *et al.*, 1950; Assali, *et al.*, 1951; Assali and Rosenkrantz, 1951; Bachman, 1953; Morales, *et al.*, 1957). Mean arterial pressures below 80–85 mmHg are, of course, still associated with output of urine and flow of blood through the kidneys, but these are no longer within normal ranges. As already

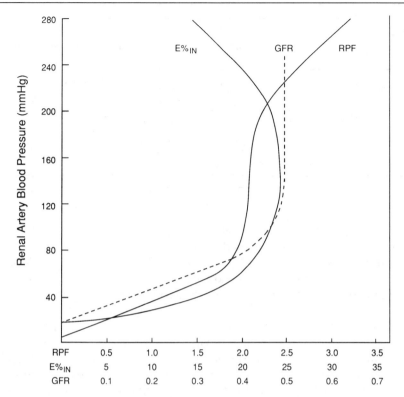

Figure 5.2. Effect of changes in mean arterial pressure on renal function and renal plasma flow. $E\%_{IN}$, extraction percentage of inulin; GFR, glomerular filtration rate in $ml \cdot min^{-1} \cdot g^{-1}$; RPF, renal plasma flow in $ml \cdot min^{-1} \cdot g^{-1}$. (Redrawn with permission from Shipley and Study, Am. J. Physiol. *167:* 676, 1951.)

mentioned, renal blood flow does not cease completely until levels of 10–15 mmHg mean arterial pressure are attained.

The data reported on the effects of spinal anesthesia on renal hemodynamics by Kennedy, *et al.* (1970), are particularly interesting. The authors obtained their data in normal humans in the absence of premedication and surgery. They studied enough subjects (20) to allow statistical analysis of the data. They simultaneously measured a number of relevant cardiovascular functions. All subjects were studied in the supine position before and immediately following induction of spinal anesthesia and again at 15-min intervals for $1\frac{3}{4}$ hr, at which time cutaneous anesthesia had disappeared. Sensory levels of T_5 were obtained initially with hyperbaric lidocaine. No vasopressors were used. Intravenous 5 percent mannitol was administered to produce diuresis necessary for renal function studies. Arterial partial pressure of carbon dioxide ($PaCO_2$), partial pres-

Table 5.1.
Cardiovascular and Renal Hemodynamic Measurements during High Spinal Anesthesia in Man[a,b]

	Mean Arterial Pressure (mmHg)	Cardiac Output (L·min^{-1})	Effective Renal Plasma Flow (mL·min^{-1})	Effective Renal Blood Flow (mL·min^{-1})	Renal Vascular Resistance (mmHg·L^{-1}·min^{-1})	Glomerular Filtration Rate (mL·min^{-1})
Control	104 ± 1.8	6.9 ± 0.37	589 ± 27.0	1041 ± 54.8	105 ± 6	105.0 ± 3.8
¼ hr	−18.7 ± 2.0	+3.7 ± 3.6	−1.8 ± 2.1	−3.5 ± 2.1	−14.8 ± 2.9	−5.7 ± 1.8
¾ hr	−13.8 ± 2.6	−4.4 ± 3.6	−6.6 ± 2.8	−9.6 ± 2.9	−2.9 ± 4.3	−10.5 ± 4.3
1¼ hr	−0.6 ± 2.3	−5.1 ± 2.3	+2.0 ± 3.0	−3.1 ± 2.7	−4.3 ± 4.2	−4.3 ± 2.1
1¾ hr	+2.6 ± 2.7	−4.2 ± 1.5	−8.6 ± 3.3	−11.9 ± 3.3	+16.9 ± 5.2	−8.6 ± 3.0

[a] Adapted with permission from Kennedy, et al., Acta Anaesthesiol. Scand. (Suppl.) 37: 163, 1970
[b] Percent changes from preanesthetic control values; mean ± SD.

sure of oxygen (PaO$_2$) (concentration of oxygen in the inspired air (FIO$_2$) = 0.21), and pH levels remained unchanged. The more important data are summarized in Table 5.1. Significant arterial hypotension developed during the first ¾ hr following induction of anesthesia. Despite the decrease in arterial perfusing pressure, there were only transitory decreases in effective renal plasma and blood flows, negligible at ¼ hour (at which time renal vascular resistance had decreased substantially) but more pronounced at ¾ hr (at which time renal vascular resistance had returned to essentially normal levels). The lack of correlation between renal blood and plasma flows, on the one hand, and mean arterial pressure, on the other hand is striking. Glomerular filtration decreased, but the decrease was relatively slight, roughly the same as the decrease in plasma and blood flows.

Cardiac output did not change significantly during spinal anesthesia in the subjects studied by Kennedy, et al. This might account for the lack of changes in renal hemodynamics in the presence of arterial hypotension. This is supported by the data obtained by Sivarajan, et al. (1975) in their studies of the hemodynamic responses to T$_1$ levels of spinal anesthesia in Rhesus monkeys. In these studies renal blood flow, determined by radioactive microsphere techniques, decreased significantly from control values of 960 ± 73.3 (SEM) ml·100 g^{-1}·min^{-1} to 717 ± 53 and 614 ± 19.9 ml·100 g^{-1}·min^{-1} at times when cardiac output also decreased significantly from control values of 268 ± 25.8 ml·kg^{-1}·min^{-1} to 216 ± 27.1 and 209 ± 23.8 ml·kg^{-1}·min^{-1}. When cardiac output was within normal limits renal blood flow also was normal. The decrease in renal blood flow associated with a decrease in cardiac output was attributable solely to the decrease in output *per se*, not to alterations in the distribution of cardiac output. The percentage of cardiac output perfusing the kidneys remained at 13–15 percent, both when cardiac output was normal and when it was decreased. Decreases in renal blood flow also cannot be ascribed to increases in renal vascular resistance during periods of diminished cardiac output. Renal vascular resistance was the same during decreases in renal flow as it was when renal flow and cardiac output were normal.

Of particular value and interest are the studies performed in sheep by Mather, *et al.* quantitating the effect of spinal anesthesia with sensory levels at T_4 or above on renal function. Not only was renal blood flow measured (by iodohippurate clearance), but also, measurements were simultaneously made of systemic hemodynamics as well as rates of renal clearance of various drugs administered intravenously. For example, although mean cardiac output levels increased to 126 percent of control levels (probably due to assiduous intravenous hydration to avoid hypotension), renal blood flow remained unchanged during spinal anesthesia, as did renal extraction ratios and renal clearance of meperidine (Mather, *et al.*, 1986). In similar studies in which hemodynamic variables did not change more than 10 percent from control levels during spinal anesthesia, renal blood flow as well as renal extraction ratios and clearances of both chlormethiazole (Runciman, *et al.*, 1986) and cefoxitin (Runciman, *et al.*, 1985) were unaffected by anesthesia. In an earlier study in sheep the same group of investigators also found that, in the absence of significant changes in blood pressure and cardiac output, spinal anesthesia had no effect on either renal blood flow or, since flow was unchanged, renal venous oxygen tension (Runciman, *et al.*, 1984). These studies amply demonstrate that renal hemodynamics and excretion of xenobiotics remain unaltered by spinal anesthesia at least as long as cardiac output and blood pressure are maintained within normal limits by adequate intravenous hydration. Similar data on renal elimination of drugs in the presence of normovolemic hypotension produced by spinal anesthesia would be interesting. Data on the effects of general anesthesia on renal blood flow and elimination of drugs gathered in the course of these same studies stand in contrast to the data obtained during spinal anesthesia.

Patients with essential hypertension or parenchymatous renal disease show essentially the same arterial pressure–renal blood flow relationship as normal patients, but patients with organic obliterative disease involving renal arteries or arterioles have a higher critical level of blood pressure below which changes in pressure are associated with changes in renal flow (Weiss, *et al.*, 1933; Page, *et al.*, 1944; Gregory, *et al.*, 1946; Corcoran, *et al.*, 1948; see also Chapter 8 section on toxemia of pregnancy).

Although renal blood flow decreases as mean arterial pressure decreases below about 85 mmHg, and although changes in blood flow alter renal function, such alterations are usually transient in nature. When blood pressure returns to normal after the spinal anesthesia wears off, blood flow usually also returns promptly to preanesthetic levels, and the glomeruli and tubules resume their normal functioning. What is unknown, however, is the level of arterial pressure during spinal anesthesia which, while not enough to allow normal tubular and glomerular function during the hypotension, is nevertheless sufficient to maintain blood flow adequate to maintain normal renal cellular metabolism so that when the blood pressure does return to normal, function is likewise restored. Renal function has been reported as normal following quite severe degrees of hypotension caused by spinal anesthesia (Lynn, et al., 1952), but renal dysfunction after spinal anesthesia has worn off and the blood pressure has returned to normal level, has also been reported frequently enough to cause concern over the adequacy of renal blood flow during extreme degrees of hypotension, especially if the hypotension is prolonged (Hampton and Little, 1953, a, b; Greene, et al., 1954). Exact information is lacking on how low the pressure may decrease during spinal anesthesia before the danger of irreversible changes becomes apparent. However, the pressures within renal capillaries being 13–18 mmHg (Brun, et al., 1956; Gottschalk and Mylle, 1956), it should be assumed for reasons already mentioned (Chapter 2) that *mean* arterial pressures below 35 mmHg during spinal anesthesia will be followed so frequently by renal damage that they should not be permitted. In certain patients, notably those in whom organic changes have reduced the size of their renal vessels, the safe level of mean arterial pressure will be in excess of 35 mmHg.

Renal Function

The rate of glomerular filtration is not linearly related to arterial blood pressure. Much as in the case of renal blood flow, glomerular filtration remains relatively constant through a wide range of arterial pressures. There is, however, a level of arterial pressure as illustrated in Figure 5.2 below which further decreases in pressure result in decreases in glomerular filtration even though increases in pressure above this point fail to produce proportionate increases in glomerular filtration. Experimentally the critical level below which arterial blood pressure and glomerular filtration do show a linear relationship is about 115 mmHg mean arterial pressure, with glomerular filtration ceasing completely at about 35 mmHg mean pressure (Selkurt, 1946 a; Shipley and Study, 1951; Sartorius and Burlington, 1956).

During spinal anesthesia the relationship between arterial blood pressure and glomerular filtration is comparable to that existing under experimental conditions with the exception that the critical level of the mean arterial pressure appears to be approximately 100 mmHg. During spinal anesthesia mean pressures below about 100 mmHg are associated with decreases in glomerular filtration that are proportionate to the degree to which mean blood pressure has fallen below 100 mmHg (Table 5.1; Berglund, *et al.*, 1935; Smith, *et al.*, 1939; Gregory, *et al.*, 1946; Mokotoff and Ross, 1948; Corcoran, *et al.*, 1948; Papper, *et al.*, 1950; Assali and Rosenkrantz, 1951; Assali, *et al.*, 1951; Morales, *et al.*, 1957; Yamada, 1958). Since the filtration fraction remains unchanged during spinal anesthesia even in the presence of arterial hypotension (Gregory, *et al.*, 1946; Assali and Rosenkrantz, 1951; Assali, *et al.*, 1951), the decrease in glomerular filtration is associated with a decrease in urinary output that is roughly proportionate to the degree of decrease in mean arterial pressure below about 100 mmHg. A preanesthetic mean arterial blood pressure of approximately 100 mmHg being a frequent finding, spinal anesthesia is, therefore, so often associated with a decrease in urinary output that a diminished urinary flow may be considered a characteristic of spinal anesthesia. By and large the decrease in urinary output during spinal anesthesia is transient. There is usually a prompt return to normal levels of urinary flow as the anesthesia wears off, and there is no significant rise in blood urea nitrogen level after spinal anesthesia (Saklad, 1931; Boyd, 1936). If, however, hypotension has been severe or prolonged, oliguria or anuria may persist beyond the time when arterial pressure returns to normal. In such cases, organic parenchymal damage has occurred secondary to inadequate renal blood flows during the period of hypotension.

Urinary electrolyte excretion is also reduced by spinal anesthesia. Characteristically the urinary concentration of both sodium and chloride ions is decreased during spinal anesthesia (Papper, *et al.*, 1950; Assali, *et al.*, 1951; Morales, *et al.*, 1957). These lower urinary electrolyte concentrations appear to be related to the development of hypotension and may be the result of slower rates of tubular urine flow with consequently more complete tubular reabsorption (Selkurt, 1951). The urinary concentration of potassium has variously been described as increased (Assali, *et al.*, 1951), decreased (Morales, *et al.*, 1957), or unchanged (Papper, *et al.*, 1950). While the precise role of the sympathetic nervous system in the regulation of tubular reabsorption remains undefined (as does its role in renin production and renal response to antidiuretic hormone), there is general agreement that the more conspicuous of the alterations in renal function produced by sympathetic denervation are not immediate (Mason and Bartter, 1968). The changes in pattern of urinary electrolyte excretion associated with the acute sympathetic denervation of spinal anesthesia differ significantly from those observed following chronic denervation (Pearce and Sonnenberg, 1965).

Plasma levels of aldosterone, though significantly increased by general anesthesia with halothane, methoxyflurane, or ether, remain unchanged during spinal anesthesia and during surgery performed under spinal anesthesia (Oyama, *et al.*, 1979). Under epidural anesthesia, however, the increase in plasma levels of aldosterone is blunted (Kehlet, 1978). Plasma renin activity is also unaffected by either spinal anesthesia or surgery performed during spinal anesthesia (Oyama, et al., 1979).

The effects of spinal anesthesia on renal function in patients with preexisting renal disease have not been studied in detail. Orko, et al. (1986) prospectively compared 20 healthy, control patients and 20 patients with chronic renal failure having lower abdominal surgery performed under spinal anesthesia. There were no conspicuous differences in the two groups peri- or postoperatively with respect to renal function. Similarly, Linke and Merin (1976) found spinal anesthesia satisfactory in 64 patients with severe chronic renal failure having implantation of donor kidneys. Such reports, though bordering on the anecdotal, suggest that, when properly managed, the hypothetical complications such as hematoma formation, exacerbation of preexisting peripheral neuritis, and undue hypotension are not encountered.

In considering the effect of spinal anesthesia on renal function, a note should be included concerning the effect of this type of anesthesia on the rest of the urinary tract, including the bladder. In the bladder there are two main muscles: the detrusor and the muscles about the bladder neck. They constitute a coordinating unit for the storage and voiding of urine. The main innervation of the detrusor muscle is derived from sacral parasympathetic fibers. Sympathetic fibers innervate the base of the bladder and the proximal smooth muscle sphincter; innervation of the more distal, striated muscle sphincter remains to be clearly identified. Detrusor relaxation and closure of the sphincters lead to storage of urine. Detrusor contraction coordinated with sphincter relaxation results in voiding.

Given the innervation of the muscles of the bladder it is essentially inevitable that spinal anesthesia is associated with the inability to void. With urodynamic studies using cystometry in 21 patients, Axelsson, et al. (1985) found that within 1 min of the lumbar intrathecal injection of bupivacaine there was loss of the desire to void when the bladder was overdistended, and within 5 min there was inability to void. It was not until 7–8 hr after subarachnoid injection that detrusor strength had completely returned. Ability to feel a pinprick in sacral dermatomes returned somewhat before, or simultaneously with, return of complete detrusor strength. The authors emphasized that "urine production during spinal anesthesia with routine fluid therapy (ca. 300 ml·hr^{-1}) was so great that if the patient had not been catheterized there would have been a risk of overdistension of the bladder." Neither the incidence of the complication of spinal anesthesia represented by the need for postoperative bladder catheterization, nor its relation to the almost routine overzealous use of intraoperative intravenous fluids in normovolemic patients to maintain "normal" levels of blood pressure are as clinically widely appreciated as they should be. Anesthesiologists should also bear in mind the high risk of iatrogenic lower urinary tract infections associated with even single catheterization of hospitalized patients, limit intravenous fluids, and keep the duration of the spinal anesthesia according to the individual needs of each patient. The risk was recently addressed by Carpiniello, *et al.* (1988), who evaluated the incidence of urinary tract infection, urinary retention, and the need for postoperative urinary catheterization following total joint replacement under spinal anesthesia with tetracaine in elderly females. The incidence of postoperative urinary tract infections was found to be 4 percent–10 percent, despite preoperative negative urine cultures. Straight catheterization of the patients in the recovery room was not beneficial in preventing urinary infection or retention. Based on the findings by Carpiniello, *et al.*, it would not be unreasonable to suspect that male patients may likewise carry a risk of developing postoperative urinary tract infections with at least similar frequency as female patients. The frequency with which bladder catheterization is needed in the postoperative period increases even further, of course, in the presence of obstruction to outflow, particularly by an enlarged median prostatic bar in middle-aged and elderly males.

Distension of the urinary bladder after spinal anesthesia has worn off may cause hypotension. It has also been suggested that distension of the bladder during transurethral prostatic resections may be associated with hypotension as the spinal anesthesia begins to wear off, even though anesthesia is still adequate to block surgical stimuli (Aldrete, 1969). Hypotension can, however, be caused by so many other factors during the latter stages of a transurethral prostatectomy that the role of bladder distension in the presence of surgical levels of spinal anesthesia would be difficult to define. Spinal anesthesia is, however, an excellent means for prevention of mass autonomic discharge and hypertension during distension of the bladder associated with transurethral procedures in paraplegic patients.

Though spinal anesthesia prevents normal penile erection, it is usually of little therapeutic use in management of priapism. The majority of cases of priapism are due to organic obstruction to venous outflow from the penis, most often intravenous obstruction, which is unaffected by sacral parasympathetic blockade.

Spinal anesthesia has no effect on ureteral motility or peristalsis (Andersson and Ulmsted, 1975).

Data available on the effects of spinal anesthesia on plasma renin activity in humans are too fragmentary for interpretation (Robertson and Michelakis, 1972). Though there are reports on plasma aldosterone (pp. 273–274), there are no data on the effects of spinal anesthesia on rates of secretion of aldosterone or antidiuretic hormone or on the effects of spinal anesthesia on the tubular action of these two hormones. It is unlikely that the effects of these hormones on tubular function would be altered by spinal anesthesia. The effects of spinal anesthesia on their secretion deserve investigation, however.

REFERENCES

ALDRETE, J. A.: Transurethral resection with subarachnoid block. Complication of late hypotension. J. A. M. A. *208:* 1012, 1969.

ANDERSSON, K. E., AND ULMSTED, U.: Effects of spinal anesthesia, lidocaine, and morphine on the motility of the human ureter in vivo. Scand. J. Urol. Nephrol. *9:* 236, 1975.

ASSALI, N. S., KAPLAN, S. A., FOMON, S. J., DOUGLASS, R. A., AND TADA, Y.: The effects of high spinal anesthesia on the renal hemodynamics and the excretion of electrolytes during osmotic diuresis in the hydropenic normal pregnant woman. J. Clin. Invest. *30:* 916, 1951.

ASSALI, N. S., AND ROSENKRANTZ, J. G.: Studies on autonomic blockade. V. Inhibition of water diuresis in pregnant women by high spinal anesthesia. Surg. Gynecol. Obstet. *93:* 468, 1951.

AXELSSON, K., MÖLLEFORS, OLSSON, G., LINGÅRDH, G., AND WIDMAN, B.: Bladder function in spinal anaesthesia. Acta Anaesthesiol. Scand. *29:* 315, 1985.

BACHMAN, L.: Renal circulation: relation to some anesthetic problems. Anesth. Analg. *32:* 136, 1953.

BADR, K. F., AND ICHIKAWA, I.: Prerenal failure: a deleterious shift from renal compensation to decompensation. N. Engl. J. Med. *319:* 623, 1988.

BERGLUND, H., MEDES, G., BENSON, T. Q., AND BLUMSTEIN, A.: Effects of spinal anaesthesia on glomerular function in hypertension. Acta Med. Scand. *86:* 292, 1935.

BLAKE, W. D.: Pathways of adrenaline action on renal function with observations on a blood pressure reflex regulating water and electrolyte excretion. Am. J. Physiol. *181:* 399, 1955.

BOUNOS, G., ONNIS, M., AND SHUMACKER, H. B.: Renal autoregulation. Surg. Gynecol. Obstet. *111:* 540, 1960.

BOYD, E. A.: Investigations into the urea nitrogen content of blood following anaesthesia. Br. J. Anaesth. *13:* 56, 1936.

BRULL, L., LOUIS-BAR, D., AND LYBECK, H.: The action of chronic denervation and of the use of a ganglioplegic or a sympatholytic agent on the baresthetic device of the renal arteries. Acta Physiol. Scand. *34:* 175, 1955.

BRUN, C., CRONE, C., DAVIDSEN, H. G., FABRICUS, J., HANSEN, A. T., LASSEN, N. A., AND MUNCK, O.: Renal interstitial pressure in normal and in anuric man based on wedged renal vein pressure. Proc. Soc. Exp. Biol. Med. *91:* 199, 1956.

CARPINIELLO, V. L., CENDRON, M., ALTMAN, H. G., MALLOY, T. R., AND BOOTH, R.: Treatment of urinary complications after total joint replacement in elderly females. Urology 32(3): 186, 1988.

CORCORAN, A. C., TAYLOR, R. D., AND PAGE, I. H.: Circulatory responses to spinal and caudal anesthesia in hypertension: relation to the effect of sympathectomy. II. Effect on renal function. Am. Heart J. *36:* 226, 1948.

GOTTSCHALK, C. W., AND MYLLE, M.: Micropuncture study of pressures in proximal tubules and peritubular capillaries of the rat kidney and their relation to ureteral and renal venous pressures. Am. J. Physiol. *185:* 430, 1956.

GREENE, N. M., BUNKER, J. P., KERR, W. S., VON FELSINGER, J. M., KELLER, J. W., AND BEECHER, H. K.: Hypotensive spinal anesthesia: respiratory, metabolic, hepatic, renal, and cerebral effects. Ann. Surg. *140:* 641, 1954.

GREGORY, R., LEVIN, W. C., ROSS, G. T., AND BENNETT, A.: Studies on hypertension. VI. Effect of lowering the blood pressures of hypertensive patients by high spinal anesthesia on the renal function as measured by inulin and diodrast clearances. Arch. Intern. Med. 77: 385, 1946.

HAMPTON, L. J., AND LITTLE, D. M.: Results of a questionnaire concerning controlled hypotension in anaesthesia. Lancet 264: 1299, 1953 a.

HAMPTON, L. J., AND LITTLE, D. M.: Complications associated with the use of "controlled hypotension" in anesthesia. Arch. Surg. 67: 549, 1953 b.

KEHLET, H.: Influence of epidural analgesia on the endocrine-metabolic response to surgery. Acta Anaesthesiol. Scand. (Suppl.) 70: 39, 1978.

KENNEDY, W. F., JR., SAWYER, T. K., GERBERSHAGEN, H. J., EVERETT, G. B., CUTLER, R. E., AND BONICA, J. J.: Simultaneous systemic cardiovascular and renal hemodynamic measurements during high spinal anaesthesia in man. Acta Anaesthesiol. Scand. (Suppl.) 37: 163, 1970.

KIM, J. K., LINAS, S. L., AND SCHRIER, R. W.: Catecholamines and sodium transport in the kidney. Pharmacol. Rev. 31(3): 169, 1979.

KINTER, W. B., AND PAPPENHEIMER, J. R.: Renal extraction of PAH and of diodrase-I^{131} as a function of arterial red cell concentration. Am. J. Physiol. 185: 391, 1956.

KON, V., YARED, A., AND ICHIKAWA, I.: Role of renal sympathetic nerves in mediating hypoperfusion of renal cortical microcirculation in experimental congestive heart failure and acute extracellular fluid volume depletion. J. Clin. Invest. 76: 1913, 1985.

KUSUNOKI, Y.: Changes in renal volume during spinal anesthesia. J. Jpn. Obstet. Gynecol. Soc. 4: 150, 1957.

LAUSON, H. D., BRADLEY, S. E., AND COURNAND, A.: The renal circulation in shock. J. Clin. Invest. 23: 381, 1944.

LINKE, C. L., AND MERIN, R. G.: A regional anesthetic approach for renal transplantation. Anesth. Analg. 55: 69, 1976.

LYNN, R. B., SANCETTA, S. M., SIMEONE, F. A., AND SCOTT, R. W.: Observations on the circulation in high spinal anesthesia. Surgery 32: 195, 1952.

MASON, D. T., AND BARTTER, F. C.: Autonomic regulation of blood volume. Anesthesiology 29: 681, 1968.

MATHER, L. E., RUNCIMAN, W. B., ILSLEY, A. H., CARAPETIS, R. J., AND UPTON, R. N.: A sheep preparation for studying interactions between blood flow and drug disposition. V. The effects of general and subarachnoid anaesthesia on blood flow and pethidine disposition. Br. J. Anaesth. 58: 888, 1986.

MILES, B. E., DE WARDENER, H. E., CHURCHILL-DAVIDSON, H. C., AND WYLIE, W. D.: The effect on the renal circulation of pentamethonium bromide during anesthesia. Clin. Sci. 11: 73, 1952.

MOKOTOFF, R., AND ROSS, G.: Effect of spinal anesthesia on the renal ischemia in congestive heart failure. J. Clin. Invest. 27: 335, 1948.

MORALES, P., CARBERY, W., MORELLO, A., AND MORALES, G.: Alterations in renal function during hypothermia in man. Ann. Surg. 145: 488, 1957.

MORRIS, G. C., JR., MOYER, J. H., SNYDER, H. B., AND HAYNES, B. W., JR.: Vascular dynamics in controlled hypotension: study of cerebral and renal hemodynamics and blood volume changes. Ann. Surg. 138: 706, 1953.

MOYER, J. H., MORRIS, G. C., JR., AND SEIBERT, R. A.: Renal function during controlled hypotension with hexamethonium and following norepinephrine. Surg. Gynecol. Obstet. 100: 27, 1955.

ORKO, R., PITKÄNEN, M., AND ROSENBERG, P. H.: Subarachnoid anaesthesia with 0.75% bupivacaine in patients with chronic renal failure. Br. J. Anaesth. 58: 605, 1986.

OYAMA, T., TANIGUCHI, K., JIM, T., SATONE, T., AND KUDO, T.: Effects of anaesthesia and surgery on plasma aldosterone concentration and renin activity in man. Br. J. Anaesth. 51: 747, 1979.

PAGE, I. H., TAYLOR, R. D., CORCORAN, A. C., AND MUELLER, L.: Correlation of clinical types with renal function in arterial hypertension. II. The effect of spinal anesthesia. J. A. M. A. 124: 736, 1944.

PAPPENHEIMER, J. R.: Peripheral circulation. Annu. Rev. Physiol. 14: 259, 1952.

PAPPENHEIMER, J. R., AND KINTER, W. B.: Hematocrit ratio of blood within mammalian kidney and its significance for renal hemodynamics. Am. J. Physiol. 185: 377, 1956.

PAPPER, E. M., HABIF, D. V., AND BRADLEY, S. E.: Studies of renal and hepatic function in normal man during thiopental, cyclopropane, and high spinal anesthesia. J. Clin. Invest. 29: 838, 1950.

PEARCE, J. W., AND SONNENBERG, H.: Effects of spinal section and renal denervation on the renal response to blood volume expansion. Can. J. Physiol. Pharmacol. 43: 211, 1965.

PFLUG, A. E., AASHEIM, G. M., AND FOSTER, C.: Sequence of return of neurological function and criteria for safe ambulation following subarachnoid block (spinal anaesthetic). Can. Anaesth. Soc. J. 25: 133, 1978.

ROBERTSON, D., AND MICHELAKIS, A. M.: Effects of anesthesia and surgery on plasma renin activity in man. J. Clin. Endocrinol. 34: 831, 1972.

RUNCIMAN, W. B., MATHER, L. E., ILSLEY, A. H., CARAPETIS, R. J., AND UPTON, R. N.: A sheep preparation for studying interactions between blood flow and drug disposition. III. Effects of general and spinal anaesthesia on regional blood flow and oxygen tensions. Br. J. Anaesth. 56: 1247, 1984.

RUNCIMAN, W. B., MATHER, L. E., ILSLEY, A. H., CARAPETIS, R. J., AND UPTON, R. N.: A sheep preparation for studying interactions between blood flow and drug disposition. IV. The effects of general and spinal anaesthesia on blood flow and cefoxitin disposition. Br. J. Anaesth. 57: 1239, 1985.

RUNCIMAN, W. B., MATHER, L. E., ILSLEY, A. H., CARAPETIS, R. J., AND UPTON, R. N.: A sheep preparation for studying interactions between blood flow and drug disposition. VI. Effects of general or subarachnoid anaesthesia on blood flow and chlormethiazole disposition. Br. J. Anaesth. 58: 1308, 1986.

SAKLAD, M.: Studies in spinal anesthesia. Am. J. Surg. 11: 452, 1931.

SARTORIUS, O. W., AND BURLINGTON, H.: Acute effects of denervation on kidney function in the dog. Am. J. Physiol. 185: 407, 1956.

SELKURT, E. E.: The relation of renal blood flow to effective arterial pressure in the intact kidney of the dog. Am. J. Physiol. 147: 537, 1946 a.

SELKURT, E. E.: Renal blood flow and renal clearance during hemorrhagic shock. Am. J. Physiol. 147: 699, 1946 b.

SELKURT, E. E.: Effect of pulse pressure and mean arterial blood pressure modification on renal function. Fed. Proc. 10: 124, 1951.

SHIPLEY, R. E., AND STUDY, R. S.: Changes in renal blood flow, extraction of inulin, glomerular filtration rate, tissue pressure and urine flow with acute alterations of renal artery pressure. Am. J. Physiol. 167: 676, 1951.

SIVARAJAN, M., AMORY, D. W., LINDBLOOM, L. E., AND SCHWETTMAN, R. S.: Systemic and regional blood-flow changes during spinal anesthesia in the Rhesus monkey. Anesthesiology 43: 78, 1975.

SMITH, H. W., ROVENSTINE, E. A., GOLDRING, W., CHASIS, H., AND RANGES, H. A.: The effects of spinal anesthesia on the circulation in normal, unoperated man with reference to the autonomy of the arterioles and especially those of the renal circulation. J. Clin. Invest. 18: 319, 1939.

STOVER, J. W., GRIFFIN, R. W., AND FORD, R. V.: The effects of chronic pentapyrrolidinium-induced hypotension on renal hemodynamics and on the excretion of water and electrolytes in hypertension. Ann. Intern. Med. 44: 893, 1956.

SURTSHIN, A., AND SCHMANDT, W. P.: Comparison of continuously collected urines from the two normal kidneys and some effects of unilateral denervation. Am. J. Physiol. 185: 418, 1956.

TAYLOR, R. D., CORCORAN, A. C., AND PAGE, I. H.: Effects of denervation of experimental renal hypertension. Fed. Proc. 7: 123, 1949.

WEISS, S., PARKER, F., JR., AND ROBB, G. P.: A correlation of the hemodynamics, function, and histologic structure of the kidney in malignant arterial hypertension with malignant nephrosclerosis. Ann. Intern. Med. 6: 1599, 1933.

WHITE, J. C., SMITHWICK, R. H., AND SIMEONE, F. A.: *The Autonomic Nervous System.* Third Edition. New York: The Macmillan Company, 1952.

YAMADA, M.: Spinal anesthesia and renal functions. I. Changes in renal circulation in spinal anesthesia (as determined by renal clearance test). Acta Med. Biol. 5: 235, 1958.

CHAPTER 6
Endocrine Function

Spinal anesthesia itself has no effect on endocrine function. Spinal anesthesia plays, nevertheless, a critical role in determining the frequency, magnitude, and type of endocrine responses to the stress of surgery. It plays this role because the major cause of changes in endocrine function is bombardment of the central nervous system by nociceptive stimuli arising from the operative field, stimuli that are blocked by spinal anesthesia. The multiplicity of responses generated by such stimuli causes a condition often referred to as stress. Spinal anesthesia, therefore, blocks stress responses to surgery.

Exactly what constitutes surgical stress defies precise definition. The term covers everything from cardiovascular to metabolic to endocrine responses, and much in between. Not only that, many responses making up surgical stress are so intertwined as to make difficult, if not impossible, to define and separate cause from effect. Hormonal responses may contribute to, or even cause some of, the cardiovascular responses and vice versa. Especially close is the integration of hormonal and metabolic manifestations of stress, although certain aspects of metabolic stress responses are independent of concurrent endocrine responses and vice versa.

The purpose of this chapter is not to define surgical stress but, rather, to isolate certain components of endocrine responses that most people would agree are involved in surgical stress, and to examine how spinal anesthesia affects these responses. Included in this overall view are studies of the effects on the adrenal cortex, catecholamines, pituitary neuroendocrines, immunocompetence, and thyroid. Evaluation of the effect of spinal anesthesia on insulin activity during surgery is delayed until the effect of spinal anesthesia on carbohydrate metabolism is considered in Chapter 7.

The reader is offered a caveat at this point: contrary to the almost, but not quite (Longnecker, 1984) universal belief that blocking of metabolic and endocrine responses to surgical stress is beneficial and desirable, no attempt is made to judge what are purely phenomenologic events or nonevents. There are no data to prove that prevention of surgically induced changes in blood levels of hormones by spinal anesthesia is either beneficial or detrimental based on prospective statistically valid studies of outcome.

Adrenal Cortex

One method for evaluating the response of an organism to stress is to measure output of hormones by the adrenal cortex, especially the glucocorticoids. This is most conveniently accomplished by measuring blood levels of glucocorticoids. Since adrenocorticosteroids are not stored in the adrenals, the rate of biosynthesis and the rate of secretion are essentially the same. Blood levels therefore represent the balance between biosynthesis and secretion on the one hand, and uptake and biodegradation, on the other. A high blood level can indicate either an increase in production or a decrease in rate of elimination from the vascular space. The following discussion uses the single term, corticosteroids, to cover all glucocorticoids whose blood levels have been reported in studies of spinal anesthesia, regardless of terminology used in the cited original communication. Perhaps this approach is an oversimplification from the purist's point of view, but semantics in this field have changed over the decades, and in many instances there is uncertainty in the older literature about which corticoids and their metabolites were originally measured. The effect of spinal anesthesia on blood levels of the main adrenal mineralocorticoid, aldosterone, during surgery is presented separately on p. 285.

Spinal anesthesia in the absence of surgery is unassociated with significant changes in plasma levels of corticosteroids (Sandberg, et al., 1954; Virtue, et al., 1957; Oyama and Matsuki, 1970; Matsuki and Oyama, 1972). This is not surprising, since neither output of corticosteroids by the adrenal cortex nor their rate of utilization would be expected to be altered appreciably by sympathetic or somatic denervation in resting man.

After the start of an operation, there is usually a significant increase in plasma levels of corticosteroids during general anesthesia. It is associated with afferent impulses from the operative site which, when transmitted to the central nervous system, cause an increase in output of adrenocorticotropic hormone from the pituitary (Oyama, et al., 1979). Comparable increases in plasma levels of corticosteroids are not observed during surgery performed under spinal anesthesia. Sandberg, et al. (1954) found in seven patients that after 2 hr of surgery performed under general anesthesia, the average plasma level of corticosteroids had increased from a preanesthetic control level of 19 μg/100 ml plasma (after anesthesia but before surgery) to an average level of 33.8 μg/100 ml plasma, an increase of 14.8 μg/100 ml blood. The average increase in four patients having operations under spinal anesthesia was less—from control levels of 17.0 up to 25.7 μg/100 ml plasma during surgery, an increase of only

8.7 µg/100 ml. Virtue, et al. (1957) found that the increase in plasma corticosteroids after the start of surgery under general anesthesia ranged from 8.4 to 12.0 µg/100 ml plasma, depending on the type of general anesthesia used. Comparable procedures performed under spinal anesthesia were, however, associated with insignificant (average 1.4 µg/100 ml) increases in plasma levels of corticosteroids. These findings have also been confirmed by Hammond, et al. (1956, 1958), who found no increase in circulating levels of corticosteroids in seven patients during spinal anesthesia either before the start of surgery or during operation. Oyama and Matsuki (1970) also found slight increases in plasma levels of corticosteroids during surgery performed under spinal anesthesia. Their results are particularly noteworthy because the number of patients they studied was large enough to permit statistical analyses not possible with the restricted number of patients reported by earlier investigators. Oyama and Matsuki studied 40 patients, 20 with lidocaine spinals, 20 with dibucaine spinals. The type of local anesthetic had no effect on the results. Peripheral venous plasma levels of corticosteroids averaged 13.8 µg/100 ml after induction of spinal anesthesia but before the start of surgery. Fifteen minutes after surgery had started plasma levels of corticosteroids averaged 18.4 µg/100 ml, a slight but statistically significant increase of 4.6 µg/100 ml. The same authors (Matsuki and Oyama, 1972) found comparable increases (5.0 µg/100 ml) in plasma corticosteroid levels in an additional 10 patients having lower abdominal or lower extremity operations under spinal anesthesia. They also found that increases in plasma levels of corticosteroids were greater (average increase of 9.8 µg/100 ml) in eight patients having cesarean sections under spinal anesthesia than they were in surgical patients. The difference between the obstetrical patients and the surgical patients appears retrospectively to border on being statistically significant. The point deserves further study.

More recently, Blunnie, et al. (1983) found that the intraoperative increase in plasma corticosteroid levels observed in patients having abdominal hysterectomies during intravenous Althesin infusion was attenuated by spinal anesthesia to at least the T_{10} level, but was completely abolished by anesthesia with infusion of both fentanyl and Althesin. Their findings confirm that spinal anesthesia does not necessarily block intraoperative increases in plasma levels of corticosteroids, even though the sensory level of denervation may be adequate for intra-abdominal procedures. The report of Blunnie, et al. also demonstrates that it is possible for intravenous anesthesia to be more effective in blocking endocrine responses to surgery than are inadequate levels of spinal anesthesia, if the doses of intravenous anesthetics are large enough.

The level of spinal anesthesia which is considered adequate to block corticosteroid responses to surgery depends upon site and type of operation. Davis, et al. (1987), found that primarily unilateral levels of spinal anesthesia below T_{10} in patients having hip arthroplasties completely blocked the increases in plasma corticosteroid levels seen in patients having the same operation performed under general anesthesia (intravenous morphine and thiopental for induction and halothane-nitrous oxide for maintenance of anesthesia).

Spinal anesthesia may only attenuate, not completely eliminate the increase in blood corticosteroid levels associated with surgery, even in the presence of adequate clinical anesthesia at the operative site, which suggests the existence of afferent input of nonnociceptive impulses along sympathetic or sensory fibers (Kehlet, 1989). These afferent impulses enter the spinal cord at a level above the level made anesthetic to painful stimuli (Chapter 1). Perhaps intraoperative apprehension causes the increase in corticosteroid levels. Such increases in plasma corticosteroid levels, as occur during surgery performed under spinal anesthesia, might be attributable to increased output of steroids from the adrenal cortex rather than to decreased utilization. If so, the mechanism causing the slight and significant increase in output of adrenocortical steroids is unclear. Plasma levels of adrenocorticotropic hormone increase slightly during spinal anesthesia before surgery starts (Oyama, et al., 1979), but the increase is not statistically significant. There is also no significant increase in plasma levels of adrenocorticotropic hormone during spinal anesthesia after surgery has started (Oyama, et al., 1979).

The slight increases in plasma levels of corticosteroids during surgery performed under spinal anesthesia are inadequate to produce the eosinopenia observed during surgery performed under general anesthesia (Roche, et al., 1950).

Although operations performed under spinal anesthesia are associated with only slight changes in plasma corticosteroid levels, the blood concentrations of these substances rise rapidly in the postoperative period and soon attain levels comparable to those seen following surgery performed under general anesthesia. Two hours after the completion of surgery under spinal anesthesia, the blood levels of corticosteroids have been reported as averaging (10 patients) 26.6 μg/100 ml of plasma (Sandberg, et al., 1954), while 2 hr following surgery performed under general anesthesia, the average plasma level (17 patients) was 32.0 μg/100 ml. Four hours postoperatively comparable figures were 34.3 μg/100 ml plasma for spinal, and 34.6 μg/100 ml plasma for general anesthesia. Six hours after surgery the levels were 36.2 and 37.7 μg/100 ml plasma, respectively. Similar findings have also been reported in the immediate postoperative period by Tyler, et al., (1954). After reaching their peak between 4 and 12 hr postoperatively, plasma levels of corticosteroids usually decline gradually and return to preoperative levels between the first and the third postoperative days. A similar postoperative elevation of blood steroid levels when spinal anesthesia wears off was observed by Hammond, *et al.*, (1958). Oyama and Matsuki (1970) and Matsuki and Oyama (1972), on the other hand, failed to detect an increase in plasma levels of corticosteroids in their surgical patients after the spinal anesthesia wore off. In 40 patients, plasma levels of corticosteroids averaged 16.5 μg/100 ml 3½ hr after the anesthesia had worn off. During surgery plasma levels had averaged 18.2 μg/100 ml (Oyama and Matsuki, 1970). In an additional 10 patients, corticosteroid levels averaged 16.4 μg/100 ml during surgery, and 10.1 μg/ml 3½ hr after the start of surgery. Similar results were also obtained in patients having cesarean sections under spinal anesthesia: 28.8 μg/ml during surgery and 26.8 μg/ml 3½ hr later. Plasma levels of corticosteroids reported in the immediate postoperative period by these investigators were not significantly lower than they were intraoperatively, but they did not increase postoperatively to the extent reported in other studies. The reason for this remains unclear. Perhaps in the cases reported by Oyama and Matsuki plasma levels of corticosteroids increased intraoperatively to the levels equal to those expected if surgery had been performed with general, instead of with spinal anesthesia. This appears unlikely, but the authors did not study patients having comparable operations under general anesthesia. Perhaps liberal use of narcotics in the postoperative period was so effective in relieving pain that corticosteroid levels remained unaltered. Although complete data that permit a final conclusion are lacking, studies to date suggest that the rate at which plasma steroid levels return to normal postoperatively is not related to the anesthetic agent or technique, and is the same for spinal as for general anesthesia (Le Femine, *et al.*, 1957). The fact that postoperative blood steroid levels are unrelated to the type of anesthesia is confirmed by the fact that the decrease in circulating eosinophils averages 95–100 percent 4 hr postoperatively, regardless of the type of anesthesia employed (Järvinen, *et al.*, 1959).

Aldosterone, an adrenal mineralocorticoid, has as its primary stimulus for release increased plasma concentrations of angiotensin II (Shizgal, 1989). The level of stimulation of the renin-angiotensin system, with resultant increases in plasma levels of angiotensin II during surgery, is greater with general than with spinal anesthesia. It is not surprising that plasma levels of aldosterone increase substantially during operations performed under general anesthesia and remain essentially unchanged when surgery is performed under spinal anesthesia (Oyama, *et al.*, 1979).

Adrenal Medulla

The adrenal medulla is innervated by preganglionic sympathetic fibers arising from T_{11}, T_{12}, and L_1 spinal segments with, possibly, additional fibers from T_{10} and L_2 in some instances (White, *et al.*, 1952). These preganglionic sympathetic fibers pass uninterruptedly through extrinsic ganglia and terminate around the chromaffin cells of the adrenal medulla. Therefore, spinal anesthesia might be expected to decrease the amount of circulating epinephrine, by blocking efferent impulses to the adrenal medulla. Since relatively little norepinephrine is normally secreted by the adrenal medulla, block of preganglionic fibers to the gland would have little influence on circulating levels of norepinephrine, most of which is released at effector organ sites throughout the body.

One of the first reports of plasma levels of epinephrine and norepinephrine during spinal anesthesia in humans was that by Hamelberg, *et al.* (1960 a, b). Peripheral venous (antecubital) blood samples were obtained before and during spinal anesthesia, the latter being obtained at the time surgery was in progress. Epinephrine levels averaged 0.35 $\mu g \cdot L^{-1}$ before anesthesia and 0.41 $\mu g \cdot L^{-1}$ during anesthesia and surgery. Corresponding values for norepinephrine were 1.37 and 1.46 $\mu g \cdot L^{-1}$. Shimosato and Etsten (1969) similarly found no significant change in plasma levels of epinephrine or norepinephrine in 15 unpremedicated volunteers following induction of continuous (catheter) spinal anesthesia with sensory levels of T_{4-7}.

Pflug and Halter (1981), on the other hand, using radioenzymatic techniques, reported that intraoperative plasma levels of norepinephrine increased significantly above baseline levels during surgery performed on the lower half of the body under spinal anesthesia. In their study, plasma levels of epinephrine were not statistically significantly different from preoperative levels during surgery performed under either general or spinal anesthesia. This suggests that release of epinephrine from the adrenal medulla remains unchanged or it is changed minimally intraoperatively with both spinal and general anesthesia; it is the release of norepinephrine from postganglionic sympathetic nerve endings that is blocked by spinal anesthesia. There was a statistically significant relationship between the dermatomal level of spinal anesthesia and intraoperative changes in plasma levels of both epinephrine and norepinephrine. Vasopressors were not used in this study. The changes in catecholamine levels observed intraoperatively were transient; within 2½–3 hr of intraoperative blood sampling, the differences had essentially disappeared in blood samples obtained when the effects of both the spinal and the general anesthesia had worn off.

The absence of significant changes in blood catecholamine levels during surgery performed under spinal anesthesia is in contrast to the elevations usually observed during surgery performed under general anesthesia. The changes indicate that with adequate levels of spinal anesthesia the autonomic nervous system is denervated to the extent that neither surgery, apprehension, nor pain result in a reflex increase in sympathetic nervous system with release of norepinephrine from nerve endings and epinephrine from the adrenal medullae (at least in amounts greater than can be instantly metabolized and redistributed to keep circulating blood levels constant).

Actually, paralysis of preganglionic fibers to the adrenal medulla by spinal anesthesia would be expected to prevent reflex increases in blood epinephrine levels rather than to decrease these levels below those found in normal subjects at rest. One situation in which reflex release of epinephrine can prove especially dangerous is in patients with pheochromocytomas. Here, spinal anesthesia might appear to be especially useful, for although such an anesthetic would not decrease the paroxysms of hypertension due to release of epinephrine during surgical manipulation of the tumor, it would tend to prevent reflex increases in blood epinephrine levels. Very few authors however, have advocated the use of spinal anesthesia in the management of pheochromocytomas. Some have advised spinal anesthesia because of the profound muscular relaxation (Bauer and Belt, 1947), but use of spinal anesthesia as a method of functionally denervating pheochromocytomas (Tuohy, 1952) is infrequently mentioned in the literature. Most authors specifically condemn the use of spinal anesthesia in patients with pheochromocytomas because of the arterial hypotension associated with levels of anesthesia high enough to allow excision of the tumors (Wells and Boman, 1937; McCullagh and Engel, 1942; Esperson and Dahl-Iversen, 1946; Apgar and Papper, 1951). The present authors feel that in the absence of some definite contraindication, spinal anesthesia high enough to denervate the adrenal glands is useful in patients with a known or suspected pheochromocytoma who are having surgery below the diaphragm for purposes other than removal of the pheochromocytoma. One of the authors (NMG) has in the past advocated and used high (hypotensive) spinal anesthesia as the primary anesthetic for excision of pheochromocytoma. Spinal anesthesia has the advantage of blocking reflex release of epinephrine during the surgical approach to the adrenal gland. It also has the disadvantage of failing to prevent hypertensive crises during manipulation of the tumor. The availability of today's alpha- and beta-adrenergic blocking agents makes well administered general anesthesia preferable to the use of high spinal anesthesia for excision of pheochromocytomas.

An infrequent situation in which spinal anesthesia might also prove useful because of its block of sympathetic fibers to the adrenal medulla is in patients with adrenal cortical hypofunction, whether of iatrogenic (i.e., post-steroid therapy) or of morphological origin. Adrenal cortical hypofunction has been shown to be associated with an abnormally great sensitivity to the effects of epinephrine and norepinephrine (Ramey and Goldstein, 1957), and spinal anesthesia has experimentally been shown to be of benefit in such a situation (Kleinberg, *et al.*, 1942).

Pituitary

Factors involved in release of hormones from the pituitary are as numerous as the myriad of pituitary hormones that have been identified. Spinal anesthesia has little or no effect on release and, therefore, little or no effect on function of, or intraoperative blood levels of, pituitary hormones except for those hormones whose release from the pituitary is governed at least in part by neuraxial bombardment from peripherally originating noxious stimuli.

Because of the close neuroanatomic and functional interrelationship between anterior and posterior portions of the pituitary, data are reviewed on the effects of spinal anesthesia on intraoperative blood levels of hormones derived from both sources, that is, the effect of spinal anesthesia on neuroendocrine function. Included are data on blood levels of adrenal corticotropin, aldosterone, growth hormone, prolactin, antidiuretic hormone, and oxytocin. Thyrotropin is included below in the section on the thyroid. Because immunocompetence is also related to neuroendocrine function, a brief comment on spinal anesthesia and immunocompetence is also offered (pp. 292–293).

Adrenal Corticotropin

The increased plasma levels of corticosteroids during surgery described above are due to afferent nerve impulses arising from the operative site. These impulses, acting on the neurosecretory center in the ventral hypothalamus which controls the release of adrenocorticotropic hormone from the anterior pituitary, cause an increased output of adrenocorticotropic hormone, and therefore an increased level of circulating corticosteroids. Since nerve impulses from the operative area are responsible for eliciting this response, it is evident that spinal anesthesia can prevent the normal response by blocking afferent fibers from the injured area. Adrenal corticotropin blood levels have not been reported during surgery. There is no evidence, however, that spinal anesthesia prevents release of adrenal corticotropin from the pituitary if normally effective neural stimuli reach the pituitary. Nor is there evidence that corticosteroid blood levels that remain constant during surgery performed under spinal anesthesia are the result of impairment by spinal anesthesia of the ability of the adrenal cortex to release corticosteroids when stimulated by corticotropin released from the pituitary. When spinal anesthesia wears off postoperatively, afferent impulses from the operative site are no longer blocked, adrenal corticotropin is released from the pituitary, the adrenal cortex responds, and blood levels of corticosteroids increase to levels comparable to those generally found in patients undergoing general anesthesia. The value of the transient intraoperative relief provided by spinal anesthesia from surgical stress, as reflected by corticosteroid blood levels, remains to be quantitated.

Growth Hormone

Plasma levels of growth hormone were measured by Blunnie, *et al.* (1983) in three groups of middle-aged females undergoing abdominal hysterectomy surgery. Their anesthesia consisted of either induction and maintenance with intravenous Althesin, or spinal anesthesia to at least T_{10} levels combined with either general anesthesia (intravenous Althesin), or fentanyl induction of anesthesia with intravenous Althesin for maintenance of anesthesia. Peripheral venous blood samples were obtained at skin incision and $\frac{1}{2}$, 1, $1\frac{1}{2}$, 2, 3, 4, 24, and 48 hr later. Although there was considerable intrapatient variability, mean levels of plasma growth hormone did not change significantly during spinal anesthesia but did increase significantly during general anesthesia. The differences in plasma levels of growth hormone achieved statistical significance at $1\frac{1}{2}$, 2, 3, and 4 hr. The duration of these differences cannot be determined since data beyond 4 hr were not reported.

Release of growth hormone, normally episodic with a pronounced circadian rhythm, is governed by two hypothalamic hormones: growth hormone–releasing hormone and growth hormone release–inhibiting hormone. Production of these two hormones appears, in turn, to be increased by peripheral trauma, decreases in blood glucose levels and hypovolemia (Shizgal, 1989). Spinal anesthesia has no effect on blood volume (Chapter 2) or blood glucose levels (pp. 300–304) and blocks peripherally generated noxious afferent stimuli from reaching the hypothalamus. It is perhaps not surprising that plasma levels of growth hormone remain unchanged during surgery performed under spinal anesthesia, while increasing during surgery performed under general anesthesia. The increase in plasma growth hormone concentrations during general anesthesia reported by Blunnie, *et al.* suggests that either output of growth hormone release–inhibiting hormone decreases or that output of growth hormone–releasing hormone increases. The latter seems more likely. The pattern seems to be for pituitary hormonal output to increase during surgery performed under general anesthesia.

Plasma levels of growth hormone during spinal and during general anesthesia may contribute to changes in carbohydrate metabolism described in Chapter 7.

Prolactin

The study cited above (Blunnie, *et al.*, 1983) also reported changes in plasma levels of prolactin. With all three anesthetic techniques there was an increase in plasma concentrations of prolactin that achieved statistical significance at 30 min and decreased thereafter. Why the levels increased is unclear. That they increased equally with all three anesthetic techniques suggests that afferent noxious stimuli from the periphery are not major determinants of pituitary release of prolactin.

Gonadotropin

Goyadotropin plasma levels have not been reported during spinal anesthesia.

Antidiuretic Hormone

Antidiuretic hormone (vasopressin) increases reabsorption of free water by renal tubules. It also exerts a vasopressor effect by acting directly on arteriolar smooth muscle. Antidiuretic hormone is stored in the posterior pituitary, and the principal stimulus for its release from the pituitary is an increase in plasma osmolality acting on hypothalamic osmoreceptors. The increase in reabsorption of water increases vascular volume and reduces vascular osmolality at the cost of decreased output of more highly concentrated urine (Philbin, 1989). Decreases in blood volume, when associated with increases in osmolality, also increase output of antidiuretic hormone. Though not as powerful a stimulus for release of antidiuretic hormone as increases in plasma osmolality, afferent neural stimuli from peripheral trauma also can increase release of this hormone from the pituitary (Shizgal, 1989).

Spinal anesthesia is singularly devoid of changes in plasma osmolality. Spinal anesthesia also blocks afferent stimuli from the operative site that might release antidiuretic hormone from the pituitary. Spinal anesthesia is, therefore, not accompanied by changes in output of antidiuretic hormone and associated changes in fluid and electrolyte balance.

Iatrogenically induced changes in osmolality and vascular volume during spinal anesthesia are, however, not uncommon in clinical practice. Most frequent are decreases in plasma osmolality and increases in vascular volume associated with overly enthusiastic intravenous hydration for maintenance of arterial blood pressure during spinal anesthesia. In a normovolemic patient rendered hypervolemic (and hypo-osmolar) by overly generous intravenous infusions, the decrease in antidiuretic hormone release contributes to an intraoperative and postoperative increase in urinary output. This increase in urinary output occurs at a time when the muscles of micturition are still anesthetized, thus leading to overdistension of the urinary bladder.

Thyroid

There are few studies of the effects of anesthesia, spinal or regional, on thyroid function. Early studies reported that general anesthesia and surgery are usually accompanied by increased plasma levels of thyroxine (Goldenberg, *et al.*, 1956) and with increased rates of utilization of thyroxine (Goldenberg, *et al.*, 1957).

In all probability, the elevation of plasma thyroxine levels are, as Goldenberg, *et al.*, suggested, the result of increased production of thyrotropic hormone by the pituitary gland. The cause of the increased production of thyrotropic hormone remains, however, unclear. It may be related to increased activity of the neurosecretory center in the hypothalamus. If so, spinal anesthesia might prevent stimulation of the neurosecretory center that regulates output of thyrotropic hormone during surgery. This is similar to the intraoperative deafferentation by spinal anesthesia of the neurosecretory center governing release of adrenocorticotropic hormone. Blood levels of thyroid hormone would then be expected to become elevated during surgery performed under general anesthesia in the same way corticosteroids levels are (p. 283), while during spinal anesthesia blood levels of thyroid hormone would not increase. This was, however, not found to be the case by Greene and Goldenberg (1959). These authors studied 5 patients during spinal and 13 patients during general anesthesia. Thyroid activity was evaluated using a conversion ratio based on the ratio between protein-bound ^{131}I and free [131]I. Thyroid activity increased in venous blood during surgery in all patients regardless of the type of anesthesia. This suggests that the neurosecretory center regulating output of thyrotropic hormone from the pituitary does not respond to afferent stimuli during operation. More direct and more accurate evaluation of thyroid activity during surgery performed under spinal anesthesia (by measurement of serum thyroxine levels) suggests, however, that spinal anesthesia may be associated with only slight decreases in thyroid activity. Oyama and Matsuki (1971) measured plasma thyroxine levels in 40 patients before and during spinal anesthesia and surgery. Preanesthetic plasma levels of thyroxine averaged 9.4 µg/100 ml. Ten minutes after induction of spinal anesthesia but before the start of surgery, plasma thyroxine levels averaged 8.9 µg/100 ml. Fifteen minutes after commencement of surgery the levels averaged 8.8 µg/100 ml. Three and one-half hours after induction of anesthesia, at a time when the anesthesia had worn off, plasma levels of thyroxine averaged 9.0 µg/100 ml. None of the changes were statistically significant. The same authors subsequently reported comparable findings in 8 patients having cesarean sections and in 10 additional patients having surgery under spinal anesthesia (Matsuki and Oyama, 1972). These findings during spinal anesthesia stand in contrast to the increase in plasma thyroxine levels observed by Oyama, *et al.* during general anesthesia (Oyama, *et al.*, 1969 a, b). Plasma thyroxine levels increased during general anesthesia even before surgery started. These elevations therefore apparently represent an effect of the anesthetic, not the effect of surgical trauma. The reason for the increased plasma levels of thyroxine during general anesthesia lies neither with increased spontaneous release of hormone from the thyroid gland, nor with its increased release mediated by thyroid stimulating hormone from the pituitary (Fore, *et al.*, 1966). The reason apparently lies with anesthetically induced release of thyroxine from the liver (Harland, *et al.*, 1974). Clearly a difference exists between the effects of spinal and general anesthesia on circulating levels of thyroxine.

Spinal anesthesia is advantageous in the anesthetic and surgical management of patients with uncontrolled or incompletely controlled hyperthyroidism at the time operation is needed (Rea, 1944; Knight, 1945; Tuohy, 1952). Its value in such cases is probably twofold. First, spinal anesthesia is unassociated with increased plasma levels of thyroxine. Second, and perhaps more important, spinal anesthesia alters the normal relationship between adrenal medullary activity and thyroid hormone activity. The metabolic and cardiovascular effects of increased concentrations of thyroid hormones are rapidly and totally eliminated by total preganglionic sympathetic block (Brewster, *et al.*, 1956) or by adrenergic blocking agents. In view of the fact that sympathetic block prevents the reflex release of epinephrine and norepinephrine and also abolishes the physiologic effects of increased blood levels of thyroid hormones, spinal anesthesia may be the anesthetic technique of choice in the management of those rare patients whose hyperthyroidism cannot be controlled preoperatively.

Immunocompetence

The 1980s saw a marked increase in study of the possible effects of anesthesia on immunologic responses associated with surgery. In part, this was due to the increase in numbers of patients with acquired immunodeficiency syndrome. In part it was also due to the increase in iatrogenically induced immunodeficiency associated with increasing numbers of patients having organ transplantations. The relatively few data on this subject, reviewed by Stevenson, *et al.* in 1990, are conspicuous for the paucity of studies on the effect of spinal anesthesia on immunologic responses. There are data on how epidural anesthesia affects immunologic responses, but it is difficult to apply them to spinal anesthesia for reasons stated in Chapter 10. Of particular concern is the possibility that blood levels of local anesthetics, high enough to produce systemic pharmacologic responses as can be seen with epidural anesthesia, may influence immunocompetency in a way that spinal anesthesia, with its low blood levels of local anesthetics, does not.

There are only two studies of spinal anesthesia and immunologic responses to surgery. In one of these, Whelan and Morris (1982) studied 15 patients undergoing transurethral resection of the prostate randomly assigned to have either general ($N = 8$) anesthesia (thiopental induction; maintenance with nitrous oxide and halothane or trichloroethylene) or spinal anesthesia ($N = 7$). Blood samples taken 2 hr before premedication, at the conclusion of the procedure, and 24 hr, 5 days, and 6 wk postoperatively were used for measurement of various indices of immune responses. In patients having general anesthesia, the changes were restricted to a statistically significant decrease in the numbers of both T and B lymphocytes 24 hr postoperatively. Decreases in total lymphocyte and B lymphocyte counts were seen immediately postoperatively in patients having spinal anesthesia, but not thereafter. Responses of lymphocytes to the purified protein derivative (PPD) and pokeweed mitogen (PWM) mitogens, as well as to histocompatibility antigens in mixed lymphocyte cultures, were seen following general anesthesia, and were considered indicative of immunodepression. These responses were not observed after spinal anesthesia. These authors concluded that postoperative immunodepression does occur and that it is due to general anesthesia, not to surgery. It is also possible, of course, that immunodepression was, in fact, due to surgery, but that spinal anesthesia blocked afferent stimuli causing the immunodepression, while general anesthesia did not.

In the other study of the effects of spinal anesthesia on immunologic responses to surgery, Cullen and van Belle (1975) studied 42 patients having regional anesthesia (spinal anesthesia in 16) and in 35 patients having general (inhalation) anesthesia for a wide variety of surgical procedures. They found that the decrease in lymphocytic transformation averaged 7 percent after spinal anesthesia and 261 percent after general anesthesia. This statistically significant difference disappeared, however, when the results were adjusted to the same mean duration of anesthesia and the same mean level of operative trauma.

The present data are inadequate to define exactly what effect, if any, spinal anesthesia has on immunologic responses associated with surgery. The subject deserves further study.

REFERENCES

APGAR, V., AND PAPPER, E. M.: Pheochromocytoma: anesthetic management during surgical treatment. Arch. Surg. 62: 634, 1951.

BAUER, J., AND BELT, E.: Paroxysmal hypertension with concomitant swelling of thyroid due to pheochromocytoma of right adrenal gland: cure by surgical removal of pheochromocytoma. J. Clin. Endocrinol. 7: 30, 1947.

BLUNNIE, W. P., MCILROY, P. D. A., MERRETT, J. D., AND DUNDEE, J. W.: Cardiovascular and biochemical evidence of stress during major surgery associated with different techniques of anaesthesia. Br. J. Anaesth. 55: 611, 1983.

BREWSTER, W. R., JR., ISAACS, J. P., OSGOOD, P. F., AND KING, T. L.: The hemodynamic and metabolic interrelationships in the activity of epinephrine, norepinephrine and the thyroid hormones. Circulation 13: 1, 1956.

CULLEN, B. F., AND VAN BELLE, G.: Lymphocytic transformation and changes in leukocyte count: effects of anesthesia and operation. Anesthesiology 43: 563, 1975.

DAVIS, F. M., LAURENSON, V. G., LEWIS, J., WELLS, J. E., AND GILLESPIE, W. J.: Metabolic response to total hip arthroplasty under hypobaric subarachnoid or general anaesthesia. Br. J. Anaesth. 59: 725, 1987.

ESPERSON, T., AND DAHL-IVERSEN, E.: Clinical picture and treatment of phaeochromocytomas of suprarenal origin: two own cases, one with paroxysmal hypertension improved by treatment with methylthiouracil and cured by surgical intervention. Acta Chir. Scand. 4: 271, 1946.

FORE, W., KOHLER, P., AND WYNN, J.: Rapid redistribution of serum thyroxine during ether anesthesia. J. Clin. Endocrinol. 26: 821, 1966.

GOLDENBERG, I. S., LUTWAK, L., ROSENBAUM, P. J., AND HAYES, M. A.: Thyroid activity during surgery. Surg. Gynecol. Obstet. 102: 109, 1956.

GOLDENBERG, I. S., ROSENBAUM, P. J., WHITE, C., AND HAYES, M. A.: The effect of operative trauma on utilization of thyroid hormone. Surg. Gynecol. Obstet. 104: 295, 1957.

GREENE, N. M., AND GOLDENBERG, I. S.: The effect of anesthesia on thyroid activity in humans. Anesthesiology 20: 125, 1959.

HAMELBERG, W., SPROUSE, J. H., MAHAFFEY, J. E., AND RICHARDSON, J. A.: Catecholamine levels during light and deep anesthesia. Anesthesiology 21: 297, 1960 a.

HAMELBERG, W., SPROUSE, J. H., MAHAFFEY, J. E., AND RICHARDSON, J. A.: Plasma level of epinephrine and norepinephrine: anesthetic significance. J. A. M. A. 172: 1596, 1960 b.

HAMMOND, W. G., ARONOW, L., AND MOORE, F. D.: Studies in surgical endocrinology. III. Plasma concentrations of epinephrine and norepinephrine in anesthesia, trauma, and surgery, as measured by a modification of the method of Weilmalherbe and Bone. Ann. Surg. 144: 715, 1956.

HAMMOND, W. G., VANDAM, L. D., DAVIS, J. C., CARTER, R. D., BALL, M. R., AND MOORE, F. D.: Studies in surgical endocrinology. IV. Anesthetic agents as stimuli to change in corticosteroids and metabolism. Ann. Surg. 148: 199, 1958.

HARLAND, W. A., HORTON, P. W., STRANG, R., FITZGERALD, B., RICHARDS, J. R., AND HOL-LOWAY, K. B.: Release of thyroxine from the liver during anaesthesia and surgery. Br. J. Anaesth. 46: 818, 1974.

JÄRVINEN, P. A., KIVALO, I., AND VARA, P.: Effect of different anesthesia methods on eosino-penic response to surgical stress. Acta Anaesthesiol. Scand. 3: 75, 1959.

KEHLET, H.: Surgical stress: The role of pain and analgesia. Br. J. Anaesth. 63: 189, 1989.

KLEINBERG, W., REMINGTON, J. W., DRILL, V. A., AND SWINGLE, W. W.: The nervous factor in the circulatory failure induced in adrenalectomized dogs by intestinal stripping and a single stage bilateral adrenalectomy. Am. J. Physiol. 137: 362, 1942.

KNIGHT, R. A.: The use of spinal anesthesia to control sympathetic overactivity in hyperthy-roidism. Anesthesiology 6: 225, 1945.

LE FEMINE, A. A., MARKS, L. J., TETER, J. G., LEFTIN, J. H., LEONARD, M. P., AND BAKER, D. V.: The adrenocortical response in surgical patients. Ann. Surg. 146: 25, 1957.

LONGNECKER, D. E.: Stress free: to be or not to be? Anesthesiology 61: 643, 1984.

MCCULLAGH, E. P., AND ENGEL, W. J.: Pheochromocytoma with hypermetabolism: report of two cases. Ann. Surg. 116: 61, 1942.

MATSUKI, A., AND OYAMA, T.: Thyroid-adrenocortical relationship during caesarean section and minor surgery under spinal anaesthesia. Anaesthesist 21: 122, 1972.

OYAMA, T., AND MATSUKI, A.: Plasma levels of cortisol in man during spinal anaesthesia and surgery. Can. Anaesth. Soc. J. *17:* 243, 1970.

OYAMA, T., AND MATSUKI, A.: Serum levels of thyroxine in man during spinal anesthesia and surgery. Anesth. Analg. *50:* 309, 1971.

OYAMA, T., SHIBATA, S., MATSUKI, A., AND KUDO, T.: Thyroxine distribution during halothane anesthesia in man. Anesth. Analg. *48:* 715, 1969 a.

OYAMA, T., SHIBATA, S., MATSUKI, A., AND KUDO, T.: Serum endogenous thyroxine levels in man during anaesthesia and surgery. Br. J. Anaesth. *41:* 103, 1969 b.

OYAMA, T., TANIGUCHI, K., JIN, T., SATONE, T., AND KUDO, T.: Effects of anaesthesia and surgery on plasma aldosterone concentration and renin activity in man. Br. J. Anaesth. *51:* 747, 1979.

PFLUG, A. E., AND HALTER, J. B.: Effect of spinal anesthesia on adrenergic tone and the neuroendocrine responses to surgical stress in humans. Anesthesiology *55:* 120, 1981.

PHILBIN, D. M.: Antidiuretic hormone and surgery, in Bevan, D. R., *Ballières Clinical Anaesthesiology,* Vol. 3, No. 2, September: Metabolic response to surgery. Philadelphia: 1989.

RAMEY, E. R., AND GOLDSTEIN, M. S.: The adrenal cortex and the sympathetic nervous system. Physiol. Rev. *37:* 155, 1957.

REA, C. E.: A new plan in the operative treatment of patients with severe hyperthyroidism. The use of spinal anesthesia as an adjunct to their preoperative care. Surgery *16:* 731, 1944.

ROCHE, M., THORN, G. W., AND HILLS, A. G.: The levels of circulating eosinophils and their response to ACTH in surgery. N. Engl. J. Med. *242:* 307, 1950.

SANDBERG, A. A., EIK-NES, K., SAMUELS, L. T., AND TYLER, F. H.: The effects of surgery on the blood levels and metabolism of 17-hydroxycorticosteroids in man. J. Clin. Invest. *33:* 1509, 1954.

SHIMOSATO, S., AND ETSTEN, B.: The role of the venous system in cardiocirculatory dynamics during spinal and epidural anesthesia in man. Anesthesiology *30:* 619, 1969.

SHIZGAL, H. M.: Metabolic response to surgery: Essentials, in Bevan, D. R., *Ballières Clinical Anaesthesiology,* Vol. 3, No. 2, September: Metabolic response to surgery. Philadelphia: 1989.

STEVENSON, G. W., HALL, S. C., RUDNICK, S., SELENY, F. L., AND STEVENSON, H. C.: The effect of anesthetic agents on the human immune response. Anesthesiology *72:* 542, 1990.

TUOHY, E. G.: The adaptations of continuous spinal anesthesia. Anesth. Analg. *31:* 372, 1952.

TYLER, F. H., SCHMIDT, C. D., EIK-NES, K., BROWN, H., AND SAMUELS, L. T.: The role of the liver and the adrenal in producing elevated plasma 17-hydroxycorticosteroid levels in surgery. J. Clin. Invest. *33:* 1517, 1954.

VIRTUE, R. W., HELMREICH, M. L., AND GAINZA, E.: The adrenal cortical response to surgery. I. The effect of anesthesia on plasma 17-hydroxycorticosteroid levels. Surgery *41:* 549, 1957.

WELLS, A. H., AND BOMAN, P. G.: The clinical and pathologic identity of pheochromocytoma. J. A. M. A. *109:* 1176, 1937.

WHELAN, P., AND MORRIS, P. J.: Immunological responsiveness after transurethral resection of the prostate: general *versus* spinal anesthesia. Clin. Exp. Immunol. *48:* 611, 1982.

WHITE, J. C., SMITHWICK, R. H., AND SIMEONE, F. A.: *The Autonomic Nervous System.* Third Edition. New York: The Macmillan Company, 1952.

CHAPTER 7

Metabolism and Acid-Base Balance

Oxygen Consumption

Only one author (Bühler, 1933) has reported an increase in total body oxygen consumption during spinal anesthesia. Several have observed no significant change (Burch and Harrison, 1930; Schuberth, 1936; Pugh and Wyndham, 1950; Tardieu, *et al.*, 1957). The majority, however, have reported that spinal anesthesia is associated with slight decreases in oxygen consumption. Johnson (1951) found a decrease in oxygen consumption averaging 14 percent among six patients under spinal anesthesia but without supplemental intravenous barbiturates. These patients had been given ephedrine. Lynn, *et al.*, (1952) found in 10 operative patients under intravenous barbiturate anesthesia plus high spinal anesthesia that oxygen consumption decreased from an average control level of 188 ml of oxygen/min to 124 ml of oxygen/min (a 33 percent decrease). In six patients who had no intravenous barbiturates, the same authors found only a 10 percent decrease in oxygen consumption (182 to 164 ml of oxygen/min). Similar reductions in oxygen consumption have also been reported by others (Sancetta, *et al.*, 1952, 1953; Nakayama, *et al.*, 1956). Egbert, *et al.* (1961) found that oxygen uptake in 20 normal males averaged 361 ± 92 ml·min^{-1} in the preanesthetic control period, but that it decreased to 276 ± 85 ml·min^{-1} after sedation with a barbiturate and a narcotic and further decreased to 267 ± 77 after induction of spinal anesthesia with sensory levels of T_{2-6}. The decrease in oxygen consumption associated with premedication was statistically significant. The decrease associated with the anesthesia was not. The subjects studied by Egbert, *et al.* all received ephedrine; perhaps the observed changes in oxygen consumption would have been greater if this vasopressor with recognized metabolic effects had not been administered. The data of Egbert, *et al.* nonetheless emphasize the necessity for differentiating changes in oxygen consumption brought about by premedicants from those brought about by the anesthesia itself. The data furthermore suggest that in patients who are in a truly basal, resting state, spinal anesthesia diminishes total body oxygen consumption to only a minor extent. Thus, the statistically significant decrease in oxygen consumption (from

130.0 ± 15.6 to 118.1 ± 9.9 ml·min^{-1}) observed in nine unpremedicated patients during mid- or high thoracic levels of spinal anesthesia by Paskin, *et al.* (1969) might have been due to the fact that the patients were not in a completely basal state when preanesthetic control measurements of oxygen consumption were made.

On the basis of the above reports it appears that spinal anesthesia is usually accompanied by slight but consistent decreases in total body oxygen consumption. The consistency with which they are reported is perhaps even more impressive than the fact that in any given study the decrease produced by premedication in the presence of basal conditions, is not statistically significant. Since there is no change in oxygen consumption by the splanchnic organs during spinal anesthesia (Mueller, *et al.*, 1952), such minor decreases in oxygen consumption suggest that oxygen utilization may be decreased in the central nervous system, in the myocardium, in skeletal muscles, or in all three. Theoretically, a widespread sensory and motor blockade with concurrent decrease in central nervous system activity might lead to reduction in oxygen consumption by the brain. This possibility has not been examined by studies of cerebral oxygen consumption during operative spinal anesthesia. Kety, *et al.* (1950) found, however, no change in oxygen uptake by the brain in humans during total preganglionic sympathetic block produced by differential spinal anesthesia. Paralysis of skeletal muscles during spinal anesthesia would not be expected to decrease muscle oxygen consumption appreciably, if at all, below the level of muscle oxygen consumption in a truly resting basal state. On the other hand, myocardial work (Chapter 2) is decreased during spinal anesthesia, especially during high spinal anesthesia with extensive sympathetic denervation. Though not measured in man during clinical spinal anesthesia, myocardial oxygen consumption would be expected to decrease proportionately. The modest but slight decrease in total body oxygen consumption observed during spinal anesthesia is probably due in part to a decrease in myocardial oxygen consumption.

The effects of spinal anesthesia on oxygen consumption were combined with simultaneous measurements of carbon dioxide production by Paskin, *et al.* (1969). They found that when oxygen consumption had decreased from 130.0 ± 15.6 ml·min^{-1} before anesthesia to 118.1 ± 9.9 ml·min^{-1} during anesthesia there was a simultaneous decrease in carbon dioxide production from 114.3 ± 42.2 to 99.3 ± 28.7 ml·min^{-1}, a statistically significant decrease. Since carbon dioxide production decreased more than oxygen consumption, the respiratory quotient decreased. It averaged 0.91 ± 0.17 before anesthesia, and 0.83 ± 0.19 during anesthesia, again a statistically significant decrease. The reason for this decrease in respiratory quotient remains unclear, especially in view of reports discussed below which indicate that spinal anesthesia is not associated with demonstrable changes in carbohydrate, protein, or fat metabolism. Perhaps the decrease in respiratory quotient reported by Paskin, et al., may be related to the fact that their unpremedicated patients were not in the same basal metabolic state preanesthetically as they were during spinal anesthesia. Perhaps the respiratory quotient would not decrease if measurements of carbon dioxide output and oxygen uptake were made in the truly resting state before induction of spinal anesthesia. Apprehension and anxiety would, however, make this a difficult state to achieve in even the most cooperative and informed patients in the absence of premedication.

It should be emphasized that the reduction in oxygen consumption associated with spinal anesthesia occurs at a time when heat dissipation is increasing as a result of cutaneous vasodilation (Brill and Lawrence, 1930; Felder, et al., 1951). An increase in surface temperature at a time when oxygen consumption has decreased means that during spinal anesthesia the usual direct linear relationship between metabolic rate and skin temperature no longer exists. For this reason the animal whose sympathetic outflow has been blocked becomes less capable of maintaining a constant body temperature. On this basis spinal anesthesia has been used as an adjunct to the induction of deliberate hypothermia (Morales, et al., 1957). Under clinical conditions skeletal muscle and rectal temperatures usually decrease somewhat during spinal anesthesia (von Brandis, 1938; Smith, 1962; Roe and Cohn, 1972). Roe and Cohn found in five patients with unstated levels of sensory anesthesia that rectal temperatures started to decrease within minutes following induction of spinal anesthesia and reached their lowest points, 0.6–2.6°C below preanesthetic levels, within 2 hr. Shivering occurred in these patients, as core temperature decreased to a critical level. When shivering was "mild," rectal temperature had decreased an average of 1°C. When shivering was "severe," it had decreased 1.4°C. Roe and Cohn noted that the onset of shivering occurred in unanesthetized, unclothed humans within minutes following exposure to cold at a time when core temperature had not yet decreased. Their subjects did not shiver until after core temperatures had decreased (the level of motor paralysis in their patients prevented shivering only in the lower extremities). Roe and Cohn therefore suggested that the sensitivity of central thermoregulatory mechanisms is impaired by spinal anesthesia. Since spinal anesthesia does not directly affect hypothalamic temperature sensors, Roe and Cohn hypothesized that the observed disruption of normal temperature control is mediated during spinal anesthesia through changes in cutaneous thermosensory mechanisms. Certainly the onset of thermocompensatory shivering is governed by different factors in normal unanesthetized humans than it is during spinal anesthesia. In the absence of spinal anesthesia the gradient between surface temperature and core temperature is a major determinant of when shivering starts. During spinal anesthesia core temperature appears to play a greater role than does the surface-core temperature gradient.

Metabolism

Carbohydrate metabolism is influenced very little by spinal anesthesia. The metabolic effect of increased blood levels of metabolically active hormones, such as growth hormone and adrenal corticosteroids associated with many types of general anesthesia, are not seen during spinal anesthesia.

Although assimilation of glucose by the body as a whole is unaffected by spinal anesthesia (Pareira and Probstein, 1949), the only organ in which glucose consumption has been specifically studied during spinal anesthesia is the central nervous system. In six normal subjects, Kleinerman, et al. (1959) found that cerebral glucose utilization averaged 4.4 mg·100 g^{-1}·min^{-1} before anesthesia, and 3.9 mg·100 g^{-1}·min^{-1} during spinal anesthesia with levels high enough to produce sympathetic denervation of the upper extremities. The difference was not statistically significant and was not associated with a change in the arterio-venous glucose difference across the brain. In an exhaustive study, Cole, et al. (1990) measured glucose consumption in 29 different regions on both sides of the brain in awake rats without peripheral stimulation and in rats anesthetized with either halothane or spinal anesthesia and subjected to unilateral stimulation of the sciatic nerve. Glucose consumption increased significantly in many areas on both sides of the brain following sciatic stimulation during halothane anesthesia. Glucose consumption following sciatic nerve stimulation in rats given spinal anesthesia, however, remained similar, on both sides of the brain, to glucose consumption in awake, unstimulated rats. The results confirm the direct relation between cerebral metabolism and afferent stimulation. They also confirm that spinal anesthesia attenuates transmission of peripheral stimuli to the brain so completely that few cerebral responses are evoked (Chapter 1).

In the same study, Cole, et al. found, in 16 different areas on both sides of the cord, that glucose metabolism decreased during sciatic stimulation in rats given spinal anesthesia. The metabolism was decreased to levels below those observed in unstimulated awake rats only in two lumbar gray matter areas at the site of drug injection.

Blood levels of glucose, an indirect indication of glucose metabolism, have long been known to remain unchanged during spinal anesthesia with or without concurrent surgery (Saklad, 1931; Neff and Stiles, 1936; Johnson, 1949; Kleinerman, et al., 1959). Oyama and Matsuki (1970), however, found that while blood glucose levels remained within the normal range in 24 patients during lower abdominal surgery performed under spinal anesthesia, there was a slight but statistically significant increase over preanesthetic control levels. Similarly, Møller, et al. (1984) found in patients having abdominal hysterectomies under spinal anesthesia to at least the T_4 level that there was a slight but significant increase in plasma glucose levels that occurred 1 hr after skin incision. The change in glucose levels mirrored similar changes in plasma cortisol levels. Both changes were significantly less during spinal anesthesia than in patients in the same study having neuroleptanesthesia for hysterectomy. Why plasma glucose and cortisol levels increased after an hour is not clear. Davis, et al. (1987) also observed similar changes in patients having unilateral low (L_1–T_6) spinal anesthesia for hip arthroplasties: a slight but transient increase in plasma glucose shortly after induction of anesthesia. Plasma levels of glucose in patients in the same study having general (nitrous oxide-halothane) anesthesia for their arthroplasties increased early, too, but stayed elevated.

The effect of spinal anesthesia on release of glucagon from *alpha* pancreatic cells was studied by Halter and Pflug (1980). They found that the increase in plasma glucagon in response to the intravenous infusion of arginine was 26 ± 4 percent greater during T_5 levels of anesthesia than it was prior to induction of spinal anesthesia. This finding suggests the possibility that adrenergic tone may be involved in maintenance of pancreatic cell function and that removal of this adrenergic tone by the sympathetic blockade associated with spinal anesthesia may influence release of metabolically active enzymes from the pancreas. This possibility was strengthened by studies of the same investigators (Halter and Pflug, 1980) on the effect of spinal anesthesia on response of plasma levels of glucose and immunoreactive insulin to the intravenous infusion of glucose. In six patients with low (T_9–T_{12}) levels of spinal anesthesia, plasma levels of insulin and glucose were not statistically significantly different when glucose was infused intravenously before and after induction of anesthesia. In the presence of T_{2-6} levels of anesthesia ($N = 5$), the acute response of plasma levels of insulin to the intravenous infusion of glucose was inhibited by an average of 56 ± 6 percent. These data agree with the finding of Oyama and Matsuki (1970) that plasma levels of insulin did not change despite slight increases in blood glucose levels.

The findings of Halter and Pflug that high levels of spinal anesthesia decrease responses of both plasma levels of insulin to the intravenous infusion of glucose, and plasma levels of glucagon to the intravenous infusion of arginine, suggest that normal sympathetic tone is needed to assure normal secretory responses of pancreatic *alpha* and *beta* islet cells. These findings were not, however, confirmed by Ishihara, et al. (1981).

These investigators found that T_1-C_4 levels of spinal anesthesia in dogs were associated with plasma levels of immunoreactive insulin induced by intravenous infusion of glucose that were statistically significantly greater after induction of spinal anesthesia than they were before induction. Insulinogenic indices (area above basal plasma insulin curve divided by area above basal plasma glucose curve) were also significantly greater over time with spinal than they were in control studies. These authors also obtained similar data in animals anesthetized with halothane, enflurane, thiopental, or Innovar (fentanyl/droperidol). Thiopental stimulated the insulin response to hyperglycemia to the same degree as spinal anesthesia; conversely, enflurane and halothane depressed the response.

Reasons for the diametrically opposed results of the effects of spinal anesthesia on the response of insulin to a loading dose of intravenous glucose are not clear. Nor is the clinical significance of these data. Even with extreme hypotension during high levels of spinal anesthesia there is no biochemical evidence of abnormal carbohydrate metabolism. If anaerobic carbohydrate metabolism were taking place, one would expect to find increased blood levels of lactic and pyruvic acids with an increase in the lactate/pyruvate ratio, i.e., "excess lactate." The fact that blood lactate and pyruvate levels and the ratio between lactate and pyruvate are not significantly altered even during deliberate hypotension induced by spinal anesthesia (Greene, et al., 1954) indicates that in such circumstances peripheral blood flow is sufficient to maintain aerobic carbohydrate metabolism. Those cases in which an increase in lactate and pyruvate have been observed during spinal anesthesia (Kleinerman, et al., 1958) have also shown a parallel increase in both lactate and pyruvate with the result that lactate/pyruvate ratio remained unaltered.

Although spinal anesthesia has no significant direct effect on carbohydrate metabolism, it significantly alters the response of carbohydrate metabolism to other types of anesthesia. Annamunthodo, et al. (1958) found that the decrease in liver glycogen and the increase in blood glucose levels were less in patients who had gastrectomies performed under spinal anesthesia combined with nitrous oxide, oxygen, and ether than in patients who had the same operation performed under nitrous oxide, oxygen, and ether alone. Similarly, the hyperglycemia seen with intravenous infusion of Althesin is lessened when the Althesin is infused in combination with spinal anesthesia (Blunnie, et al., 1983).

The absence of changes in carbohydrate metabolism during spinal anesthesia is reflected by the absence of changes in serum inorganic phosphate levels (Foldes, et al., 1950), an index of carbohydrate-linked high-energy phosphate production.

Despite the above conflicting data on the effect of spinal anesthesia on responses of insulin release to changes in blood glucose levels, spinal anesthesia has been and still is often preferred over general anesthesia in patients with diabetes mellitus, especially when surgery can be carried out with low levels of anesthesia. There may be advantages to use of spinal anesthesia in diabetic patients. Inadvertent hypoglycemia due to overzealous insulin replacement will be more readily recognized in awake, conscious patients during spinal anesthesia than in patients under general anesthesia if the hypoglycemia is severe enough to affect cerebral function. Patients may also be able to resume their normal diets more rapidly after spinal anesthesia than after general anesthesia and thus allow better control of the diabetes postoperatively. There are, however, no data to prove that spinal anesthesia is preferable to general anesthesia in diabetic patients. There are not even any data to prove what effect, if any, spinal anesthesia may have on insulin requirements or carbohydrate metabolism in diabetic patients. Much less are there data from appropriately controlled and statistically valid series of cases to prove whether or not carbohydrate metabolism is more adversely affected by general anesthesia than by spinal anesthesia in diabetic patients. Intuitively it might be reasonable to expect spinal anesthesia to have less effect on carbohydrate metabolism than general anesthetics in patients unable to metabolize glucose normally, but biochemically acceptable data are simply not available to prove this. Certainly blood levels of glucose alone are insufficient to prove the superiority of one type of anesthesia over another in diabetic patients. The fact that certain general anesthetics are associated with elevation of blood glucose levels in both normal and diabetic patients, whereas spinal anesthesia is not, proves little about carbohydrate metabolism at the cellular level. Blood glucose levels are a product of the rate of glucose production (and release into blood) on the one hand and the rate of glucose removal from blood on the other hand. The rate of removal of glucose from blood is, in turn, a function of tissue uptake of glucose and tissue metabolism of glucose. The former may not be synonymous with the latter. There are also no adequately controlled data to prove that blood levels of the products of deranged carbohydrate metabolism are related to the type of anesthesia in diabetic patients. Blood levels and urinary output of ketones and fixed acids have not been demonstrated to be significantly different in diabetic patients during spinal anesthesia than they are during general anesthesia. Indeed, the best controlled study of this point suggests no difference exists. In 15 well-controlled diabetic females having elective cesarean sections under spinal anesthesia, Datta and Brown (1977) found that acid-base balance intra- and postoperatively was no different than that in 15 equally well-controlled diabetic females having elective cesarean sections performed with general anesthesia (thiopental-nitrous oxide-oxygen with succinylcholine). The difference in the condition of the infants in the two groups of patients at the time of delivery was due to abnormalities of uteroplacental circulation associated with diabetes (Chapter 8), not to differences in carbohydrate metabolism in the mothers or in the infants.

Protein metabolism during spinal anesthesia has not been extensively studied. The negative nitrogen balance normally associated with surgery has been reported as being shorter in duration following spinal anesthesia than it is following comparable types of surgery performed using general anesthesia (Manku, 1970), but this deserves to be more closely quantitated. Blood levels of amino acid nitrogen remain unaffected by spinal anesthesia (Greene, *et al.*, 1954).

The effect of spinal anesthesia on fat metabolism has not been studied except for measurements of levels of plasma free fatty acids. These were found to be unchanged by Oyama and Matsuki (1970) and slightly elevated, though not as much as by general anesthesia, by Blunnie, *et al.* (1983). Given the paucity of sympathetic innervation of white fat, spinal anesthesia would be expected to have little if any effect on regulation of metabolism in this type of fat. Brown fat, on the other hand, has a rich sympathetic innervation that is involved in regulation of thermogenesis (Himms-Hagen, 1984), but the effect of spinal anesthesia on metabolism of brown fat has not been reported.

In regard to thermogenesis, the abnormal metabolic state represented by malignant hyperthermia might be expected to be influenced by spinal anesthesia in view of data suggesting that the sympathetic nervous system plays a role in this syndrome. Phentolamine (but not propranolol) as well as reserpine increase survival of susceptible pigs following challenge with succinylcholine (Lister, *et al.*, 1976). Epidural anesthesia has also been reported to prevent porcine malignant hyperthermia (Kerr, *et al.*, 1975). Gronert, *et al.* (1977), however, found that total spinal anesthesia in susceptible pigs failed to prevent or attenuate malignant hyperthermia after exposure to halothane or to halothane plus succinylcholine. In support of this is a possible but less than probable case of malignant hyperthermia associated with spinal anesthesia reported by Malz, *et al.* (1982) and a somewhat more strongly suggestive case reported by Katz and Krich (1976). On the other hand, vaginal deliveries in patients demonstrably susceptible to malignant hyperthermia have been successfully managed both by spinal (Wadhwa, 1977) and by epidural (Willatts, 1979) anesthesia.

Acid-Base Balance

Acid-base balance is little influenced by spinal anesthesia. As mentioned in Chapter 3 , there is no evidence that either respiratory alkalosis or acidosis is associated with conventional spinal anesthesia. Nor has metabolic acidosis or alkalosis been reported. The blood pH remains essentially constant (Kety, *et al.*, 1950; Greene, *et al.*, 1954; Kleinerman, *et al.*, 1959; Linderholm and Norlander, 1958; Shimosato and Etsten, 1969; Samii, *et al.*, 1979). Release of an arterial tourniquet applied for 75 min to a lower extremity during spinal anesthesia is associated with an average decrease of 2.3 mmole·L^{-1} in arterial base excess for 20 min (Hassan, *et al.*, 1978), but a similar response following restoration of circulation to an ischemic extremity is also observed during general anesthesia.

Although some authors have observed an increase in serum carbon dioxide content during spinal anesthesia (Antonin, 1930; Seevers and Waters, 1932), it is the concensus that neither preganglionic sympathetic block nor spinal anesthesia has any significant effect on carbon dioxide content or capacity of either arterial or venous blood (Nowak and Downing, 1938; Latterell and Lundy, 1949; Greene, *et al.*, 1954; Kleinerman, *et al.*, 1959; Linderholm and Norlander, 1958). Similarly, as already mentioned, spinal anesthesia has no significant effect on blood levels of fixed acids. Nor does it significantly change serum concentrations of electrolytes such as sodium, chloride, and potassium (Greene, *et al.*, 1954; Morales, *et al.*, 1957).

Although urinary excretion of electrolytes may be reduced during spinal anesthesia, their concentrations in serum are unchanged. This could be accounted for by the fact that excretion of water is simultaneously depressed or by possible changes in intracellular ion concentrations. Unfortunately data on the effect of spinal anesthesia on intracellular ion concentrations are sparse. The only report dealing with this subject is that by Barnes, *et al.* (1957) who studied such concentrations in skeletal muscle in 10 operative patients, 4 of whom had specimens of muscle removed during gas-oxygen-ether anesthesia, the other 6 during spinal anesthesia. It was not the purpose of their study to correlate ionic concentrations with types of anesthesia, but analysis of their data shows that during spinal anesthesia there was, per 100 g of wet fat-free muscle, an average of 5.18 mEq of sodium, 8.91 mEq of potassium, 1.66 mEq of magnesium, 5.36 mmol of phosphorus, 2.63 mEq of chloride, and 80.94 g of water. Comparable figures for muscle removed during gas-oxygen-ether anesthesia were 2.89 mEq of sodium, 9.41 mEq of potassium, 1.57 mEq of magnesium, 5.38 mmol of phosphorus, 1.82 mEq of chlorine, and 79.31 g of water. Statistically the intracellular concentrations of sodium and chlorine were significantly greater with spinal than with gas-oxygen-ether anesthesia. This is also seen in these authors' calculations of ionic concentrations in terms of mEq/kg of intracellular water. During spinal anesthesia there was an average of 32.24 mEq of sodium/kg of intracellular water, while during gas-oxygen-ether the corresponding value for sodium was 16.80 mEq. There was no difference in the concentrations of potassium, magnesium, or phosphorus in the two groups when these substances were calculated in terms of the amount of intracellular water present (chloride concentration was not calculated in this fashion). Interesting as these findings may be, however, it is impossible to say whether the differences in levels of intracellular sodium and chloride were related to the form of anesthesia or whether they could be accounted for by the fact that all muscle specimens taken during spinal anesthesia were obtained from the thigh while those taken during gas-oxygen-ether anesthesia were obtained from the chest or neck. Again, the differences might have been due to the patients' diseases. Patients under spinal anesthesia had peripheral obliterative arterial disease involving the toes, while those having gas-oxygen-ether had carcinoma. The question as to whether spinal anesthesia alters intracellular ionic concentrations awaits further investigation.

Data are lacking on the effect of spinal anesthesia on either ionized or total serum calcium. It is doubtful if it has any significant effect. Carpopedal spasm relieved by calcium gluconate injections has been reported (always in females) following spinal anesthesia (Barnes and Ordorica, 1957). Such spasms are more likely due to an hysterical type of hyperventilation than they are to changes in serum calcium levels produced by the anesthesia.

REFERENCES

ANNAMUNTHODO, H., KEATING, V. J., AND PATRICK, S. J.: Liver glycogen alterations in anaesthesia and surgery. Anaesthesia 13: 429, 1958.

ANTONIN, V.: Einfluss der Lokal- und Lumbalanästhesie auf den acido-basischen Hauschalt in der postoperative Zeit und die Bedeutung der Vorbereitung des Kranken auf diese Verhältnisse. Acta Chir. Scand. 66: 79, 1930.

BARNES, B. A., GORDON, E. B., AND COPE, O.: Skeletal muscle analyses in health and in certain metabolic disorders. I. The method of analysis and the values in normal muscle. J. Clin. Invest. 36: 1239, 1957.

BARNES, F. E., JR., AND ORDORICA, E. J.: Tetany in women following spinal analgesia. North Carolina Med. J. 18: 114, 1957.

BLUNNIE, W. P., MCILROY, P. D. A., MERRETT, J. D., AND DUNDEE, J. W.: Cardiovascular and biochemical evidence of stress during major surgery associated with different techniques of anaesthesia. Br. J. Anaesth. 55: 611, 1983.

BRILL, S., AND LAWRENCE, L. B.: Changes in temperature of the lower extremities following the induction of spinal anesthesia. Proc. Soc. Exp. Biol. Med. 27: 728, 1930.

BÜHLER, K.: Experimentelle Untersuchungen über die Wirkung verschiedener Betäubungsmittel auf den respiratorischen Gasstoffwechsel. Arch. Klin. Chir. 172: 657, 1933.

BURCH, J. C., AND HARRISON, T. R.: The effect of spinal anesthesia on the cardiac output. Arch. Surg. 21: 330, 1930.

COLE, D. J., LIN, D. M., DRUMMOND, J. D., AND SHAPIRO, H. M.: Spinal tetracaine decreases central nervous system metabolism during somatosensory stimulation in the rat. Can. J. Anaesth. 37: 231, 1990.

DATTA, S., AND BROWN, W. U., JR.: Acid-base status in diabetic mothers and their infants following general or spinal anesthesia for cesarean section. Anesthesiology 47: 272, 1977.

DAVIS, F. M., LAURENSON, V. G., LEWIS, J., WELLS, J. E., AND GILLESPIE, W. J.: Metabolic response to total hip arthroplasty under hypobaric or general anaesthesia. Br. J. Anaesth. 59: 725, 1987.

EGBERT, L. D., TAMERSOY, K., AND DEAS, T. C.: Pulmonary function during spinal anesthesia: the mechanism of cough depression. Anesthesiology 22: 882, 1961.

FELDER, D. A., LINTON, R. R., TODD, D. P., AND BANKS, C.: Changes in the sympathectomized extremity with anesthesia. Surgery 29: 803, 1951.

FOLDES, F. F., MURPHY, A. J., AND WILSON, B. C.: The effect of various anesthetic agents on inorganic serum phosphate levels. J. Pharmacol. Exp. Ther. 100: 14, 1950.

GREENE, N. M., BUNKER, J. P., KERR, W. S., VON FELSINGER, J. M., KELLER, J. W., AND BEECHER, H. K.: Hypotensive spinal anesthesia: respiratory, metabolic, hepatic, renal, and cerebral effects. Ann. Surg. 140: 641, 1954.

GRONERT, G. A., MILDE, J. H., AND THEYE, R. A.: Role of sympathetic activity in porcine malignant hyperthermia. Anesthesiology 47: 411, 1977.

HALTER, J. B., AND PFLUG, A. E.: Effect of sympathetic block by spinal anesthesia on pancreatic islet function in man. Am. J. Physiol. 239: (Endocrinol. Metab. 2): E150, 1980.

HASSAN, H., GJESSING, J., AND TOMLIN, P. I.: Blood-gas changes following tourniquet release during spinal anaesthesia. Br. J. Anaesth. 50: 76, 1978.

HIMMS-HAGEN, J.: Thermogenesis in brown adipose tissue as an energy buffer. N. Engl. J. Med. 311: 1549, 1984.

ISHIHARA, H., KALLUS, F. T., AND GIESECKE, A. H., JR.: Intravenous glucose tolerance test during anaesthesia in dogs: insulin response and glucose clearance. Can. Anaesth. Soc. J. 28: 381, 1981.

JOHNSON, S. R.: The mechanism of hyperglycemia during anesthesia: an experimental study. Anesthesiology 10: 379, 1949.

JOHNSON, S. R.: The effect of some anaesthetic agents on the circulation in man. Acta Chir. Scand. (Suppl.) 158, 1951.

KATZ, J. D., AND KRICH, L. B.: Acute febrile reaction complicating spinal anaesthesia in a survivor of malignant hyperthermia. Can. Anaesth. Soc. J. 23: 285, 1976.

KERR, D. D., WINGARD, D. W., AND GATZ, E. E.: Prevention of porcine malignant hyperthermia by epidural block. Anesthesiology 42: 307, 1975.

KETY, S. S., KING, B. D., HORVATH, S. M., JEFFERS, W. A., AND HAFKENSCHIEL, J. H.: The effects of an acute reduction in blood pressure by means of differential spinal sympathetic block on the cerebral circulation of hypertensive patients. J. Clin. Invest. 29: 402, 1950.

KLEINERMAN, J., SANCETTA, S. M., AND HACKEL, D. B.: Effects of high spinal anesthesia on cerebral circulation and metabolism in man. J. Clin. Invest. 37: 285, 1959.

LATTERELL, K. E., AND LUNDY, J. S.: Oxygen and carbon dioxide content of arterial blood before and during spinal analgesia. Anesthesiology 10: 677, 1949.

LINDERHOLM, H., AND NORLANDER, O.: Carbon dioxide tension and bicarbonate content of arterial blood in relation to anaesthesia and surgery. Acta Anaesthesiol. Scand. 2: 1, 1958.

LISTER, D., HALL, G. M., AND LUCKE, J. N.: Porcine malignant hyperthermia. III. Adrenergic blockade. Br. J. Anaesth. 48: 831, 1976.

LYNN, R. B. SANCETTA, S. M., SIMEONE, F. A., AND SCOTT, R. W.: Observations on the circulation in high spinal anesthesia. Surgery 32: 195, 1952.

MALZ, H., GULLOTTA, F., KLEIN, H., AND AEBERT, K.: "Maligne hyperthermie" nach NLA und Spinalanaesthesie. Anaesthesist 31: 248, 1982.

MANKU, R. S.: Effect of anesthesia on protein metabolism in patients undergoing hernioplasty. Anesth. Analg. 49: 446, 1970.

MØLLER, I. W., HJORTSØ, E., KRANTZ, T., WANDALL, E., AND KEHLET, H.: The modifying effect of spinal anaesthesia on intra- and postoperative adrenocortical and hyperglycemic response to surgery. Acta Anaesthesiol. Scand. 28: 266, 1984.

MORALES, P., CARBERY, W., MORELLO, A., AND MORALES, G.: Alterations in renal function during hypothermia in man. Ann. Surg. *145:* 488, 1957.

MORALES, G., AND MORELLO, A.: High spinal anesthesia as an adjunct to hypothermia in man. Fed Proc. *15:* 461, 1956.

MUELLER, R. P., LYNN, R. B., AND SANCETTA, S. M.: Studies of hemodynamic changes in humans following induction of low and high spinal anesthesia. II. The changes in splanchnic blood flow, oxygen extraction and consumption, and splanchnic vascular resistance in humans not undergoing surgery. Circulation *6:* 694, 1952.

NAKAYAMA, E., NOGUCHI, T., KARUBE, Y., BABA, I., AND HARAGUCHI, M.: Circulation and respiration in anesthesia. I. Circulation and respiration during spinal anesthesia. J. Jpn. Obstet. Soc. (Engl. ed.) *3:* 159, 1956.

NEFF, W. B., AND STILES, J. A.: Some experiences with cyclopropane as an anaesthetic, with special reference to the diabetic patient. Can. Med. Assoc. J. *35:* 56, 1936.

NOWAK, S. J. G., AND DOWNING, V.: Oxygen and carbon dioxide changes in arterial and venous blood in experimental spinal anesthesia. J. Pharmacol. Exp. Ther. *64:* 271, 1938.

OYAMA, T., AND MATSUKI, A.: Effects of spinal anaesthesia and surgery on carbohydrate and fat metabolism in man. Br. J. Anaesth. *42:* 723, 1970.

PAREIRA, M. D., AND PROBSTEIN, J. B.: Glucose assimilation during anesthesia and surgery. Ann. Surg. *129:* 463, 1949.

PASKIN, S., RODMAN, T., AND SMITH, T. C.: Effect of spinal anesthesia on the pulmonary function of patients with chronic obstructive pulmonary disease. Ann. Surg. *169:* 35, 1960.

PUGH, L. G. C., AND WYNDHAM, C. L.: The circulatory effects of high spinal anesthesia in hypertensive and control patients. Clin. Sci. *9:* 189, 1950.

ROE, C. F., AND COHN, F. L.: The causes of hypothermia during spinal anesthesia. Surg. Gynecol. Obstet. *135:* 577, 1972.

SAKLAD, M.: Studies in spinal anesthesia. Am. J. Surg. *11:* 452, 1931.

SAMII, K., ELMELIK, E., MOURTADA, M. B., DEBEYRE, J., AND RAPIN, M.: Intraoperative hemodynamic changes during total knee replacement. Anesthesiology *50:* 239, 1970.

SANCETTA, S. M., LYNN, R. B., AND SIMEONE, F. A.: Studies of hemodynamic changes in humans following induction of spinal anesthesia. IV. Observations in low spinal anesthesia during surgery. Surg. Gynecol. Obstet. *97:* 597, 1953.

SANCETTA, S. M., LYNN, R. B., SIMEONE, F. A., AND SCOTT, R. W.: Studies of hemodynamic changes in humans following induction of low and high spinal anesthesia. I. General considerations of the problem. The changes in cardiac output, brachial arterial pressure, peripheral and pulmonary oxygen contents and peripheral blood flows induced by spinal anesthesia in humans not undergoing surgery. Circulation *6:* 559, 1952.

SCHUBERTH, O. O.: On the disturbance of the circulation in spinal anaesthesia. Acta Chir. Scand. *78* (Suppl. 43): 1936.

SEEVERS, M. H., AND WATERS, R. M.: Circulatory changes during spinal anesthesia. Anesth. Analg. *11:* 85, 1932.

SHIMOSATO, S., AND ETSTEN, B.: The role of the venous system in cardiocirculatory dynamics during spinal and epidural anesthesia in man. Anesthesiology *30:* 619, 1969.

SMITH, N. T.: Subcutaneous, muscle, and body temperatures in anesthetized man. J. Appl. Physiol. *17:* 306, 1962.

TARDIEU, G., TARDIEU, C., AND POCIDALO, J. J.: Anesthésie médullaire totale. Etude hémodynamique. Premiers résultats. J. Physiol. (Paris) *49:* 390, 1957.

VON BRANDIS, H. J.: Über die Beziehungen zwischen Wärmehaushalt und chirurgischem eingriff beim Menschen. Arch. Klin. Chir. *192:* 245, 1938.

WADHWA, R. K.: Obstetric anesthesia for a patient with malignant hyperthermia susceptibility. Anesthesiology *46:* 63, 1977.

WILLATTS, S. M.: Malignant hyperthermia susceptibility: management during pregnancy and labour. Anaesthesia *34:* 41, 1979.

CHAPTER 8

Obstetric Physiology

The use of spinal anesthesia in obstetrics warrants specific consideration for two reasons. First, because certain physiologic changes occur
during pregnancy that modify the patient's reaction to spinal anesthesia.
Second, the fact that two patients (mother and child) are involved. The
particular effects of spinal anesthesia in obstetric patients will now be
considered; for complete understanding, however, the reader should
relate the following material to that presented in other chapters.

Physiologic Changes During Pregnancy

It is unnecessary and impractical to review all the physiologic changes
occurring during pregnancy. Certain of these changes, however, deserve
special mention, as they are highly important in relation to spinal anesthesia. Of primary importance are the cardiovascular changes associated
with pregnancy (Table 8.1). Cardiac output increases gradually throughout pregnancy by 30 percent or more with a concurrent 20 percent increase in oxygen consumption. Although maternal blood volume increases have been reported to range from 10 to 15 percent (Pritchard,
1965) to over 40 percent (Campbell, et al., 1972; Cheek and Gutsche,
1987), there is a relative anemia due to a proportionately greater increase
in plasma than in red cell volume. Because arterial blood pressure decreases slightly as pregnancy progresses, relative hypotension may be
present at term. These changes are additive to those occurring in peripheral blood distribution secondary to intrauterine fetal development. As
the placenta and fetus grow, the uterus enlarges until it contains approximately one sixth of the mother's total blood volume at term (Ralston and
Shnider, 1978). The higher peripheral blood volume during pregnancy
increases the potential for hypotension in the parturient at term during
major regional anesthesia such as spinal or epidural anesthesia.

The gravid uterus affects the maternal circulation, not only because
of the blood it contains, but also by its sheer size and weight. By pressing
on the iliac veins, the gravid uterus obstructs venous return from the
legs, causing femoral venous pressure to increase from an average normal level of 11.4 cm H_2O to approximately 24 cm H_2O at term (McLennan, 1943). This is most pronounced when the patient is in the supine

Table 8.1.
Cardiovascular and Respiratory Parameter Changes Induced by Pregnancy

Parameter	Average Change (%)
Cardiovascular system	
Blood volume	+35
Plasma volume	+45
Red blood cell volume	+20
Cardiac output	+40
Stroke volume	+30
Heart rate	+15
Total peripheral resistance	−15
Mean arterial blood pressure	−10
Central venous pressure	0
Respiratory system	
Respiratory rate	+15
Tidal volume	+40
Minute ventilation	+50
Arterial pO_2	+10
Oxygen consumption	+20
Inspiratory capacity	+ 5
Vital capacity	0
Airway resistance	−35
Residual volume	−20
Functional residual capacity	−20
Arterial pCO_2	−25
Total lung capacity	0–5

[a] Adapted from Shnider and Levinson, *Anesthesia for Obstetrics.* Second Edition. Baltimore: Williams & Wilkins, 1987.

position with the full weight of uterus and fetus pressing on the intrapelvic veins. The result is the long and well-recognized syndrome of supine hypotension (Ahltorp, 1935; Brigden, *et al.*, 1950; Holmes, 1960; Eckstein and Marx, 1974). Decreases in maternal blood pressure in the supine position in parturients are the result of decreases in venous return to the heart, and thus to decreases in cardiac output. The resulting hypotension may be further aggravated insofar as placental blood flow is concerned by compression of the aorta by the gravid uterus in the supine position. Aortic compression further decreases the perfusion pressure in uterine arteries (Eckstein and Marx, 1974) and decreases placental blood flow. Displacing the uterus to the left (by manual or mechanical means), by tilting the delivery table to the left, or by elevating the right hip, restores maternal pressure to normal levels in up to 90 percent of patients (Kennedy, *et al.*, 1959). Supine hypotension is somewhat less likely at term after the fetal head descends into the pelvis (Holmes, 1960) than before the head becomes engaged. When supine hypotension occurs during spinal anesthesia, the degree of hypotension bears no relation to the level of anesthesia (Ueland, *et al.*, 1968).

Within the uterus, the developing fetus is exposed to oxygen tensions considerably lower than those found in maternal arterial blood; whereas oxygen tension is 90–100 mmHg in the latter, fetal arterial levels (i.e., umbilical vein) usually average 32–35 mmHg, while umbilical artery oxygen tension is approximately 27 mmHg (Brett, 1989). This is somewhat compensated for by the higher hemoglobin concentration of fetal blood (15 g·100 ml^{-1}) as compared to maternal blood (12 g·100 ml^{-1}) and by the fact that the oxygen dissociation curve for fetal blood is shifted to the left of that found in adult blood. Thus, with an oxygen tension of only 18 mmHg, fetal arterial blood is approximately 50 percent saturated with oxygen (Oski and Delivoria-Papadoupoulos, 1970), but because of the shift of the dissociation curve to the left, this oxygen is given up less readily to the tissues (Fig. 8.1).

Because the oxygen content of fetal blood is normally low, any interference with placental blood flow may have immediate and adverse effects on fetal oxygenation. It has been estimated that uterine contractions normally result in intrauterine pressures of 25–95 mmHg, depending on their severity, while between contractions, the pressure is approximately

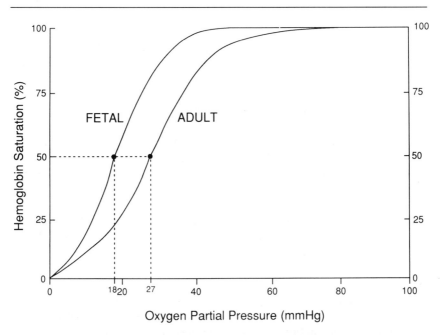

Figure 8.1. Oxygen dissociation curves for fetal and adult hemoglobin. In the adult, the oxygen partial pressure at which hemoglobin is 50% saturated (P_{50}) is 27 mmHg. In the neonate, the P_{50} is approximately 18 mmHg, and increases to 30 mmHg by 8 mo of age.

5 mmHg. It has also been noted that uterine blood flow usually stops when intrauterine pressures during contractions are between 60 and 70 mmHg. Consequently, during strong contractions of normal labor, maternal blood flow to the placenta may cease temporarily. The normal systolic blood pressure of 69 mmHg present in full-term infants is also insufficient during these strong contractions to return fetal blood to the placenta. Thus, during strong labor contractions, there will be periods when placental gas exchange ceases almost completely. The resulting fetal hypoxemia is manifested clinically by brief periods of fetal bradycardia which may occur during labor. The periods of diminished uterine blood flow during contractions may be prolonged by several factors, the most important being maternal arterial hypotension. Any significant lowering of maternal blood pressure lengthens the period of time when intrauterine pressure exceeds maternal arterial pressure, thereby extending the period of fetal hypoxemia. Although the degree of maternal hypotension which may lead to fetal distress varies (Hon, et al., 1960), generally, the lower the maternal arterial pressure, the greater the incidence of fetal bradycardia. The critical level of maternal systolic blood pressure appears to be approximately 70 mmHg. As Ebner, et al. (1960) demonstrated in a study of 29 patients scheduled for elective cesarean section, the potential for fetal bradycardia was greater if the mother's systolic pressure decreased below 70 mmHg than if it remained above this level during spinal anesthesia. The incidence of fetal bradycardia was 20 percent when the maternal systolic pressure was 60–69 mmHg, but was 38 percent when the pressure was 50–59 mmHg and 67 percent when the pressure decreased below 50 mmHg. Thus, the relationship between uterine perfusion pressure and uterine blood flow is linear with no evidence of autoregulation of uterine blood flow (Greiss, 1966). A linear relationship between maternal blood pressure and the incidence of fetal bradycardia therefore exists only when maternal systolic pressure is below approximately 70 mmHg. At a given level of hypotension during anesthesia the incidence of fetal bradycardia increases, however, as the duration of hypotension increases. None of the infants studied by Ebner, et al. (1960), developed fetal bradycardia when the duration of maternal hypotension (systolic pressure below 80 mmHg) was under 4 min. However, when the hypotension lasted 4–6 min, the fetus was bradycardic 33 percent of the time. With hypotension that persisted more than 6 minutes, the incidence of fetal bradycardia increased to 44 percent. Thus, when the maternal systolic blood pressure is 70 mmHg or less, fetal oxygenation is likely to diminish even when the uterus is not contracting. During labor, contractions and ensuing periods of uterine hypoperfusion may exacerbate this hypoxemia and bradycardia.

Changes in mechanics of pulmonary ventilation are less during pregnancy than are the relatively major changes occurring in the cardiovascular system (Table 8.1). Lung volumes do not change significantly. The reduction in functional residual capacity during the last trimester is compensated for by an increased inspiratory capacity, leaving vital capacity and total lung capacity unchanged (Prowse and Gaensler, 1965). The dyspnea so common in pregnancy, apparently unrelated to altered respiratory mechanics, probably represents altered threshold or sensitivity of the respiratory center to carbon dioxide.

Obstetric Neuroanatomy

Almost 60 years ago Cleland (1933) reported that paravertebral nerve blocks at T_{11} and T_{12} relieved the pain of uterine contractions during the first stage of labor without affecting the pain associated with stretching of the birth canal. The latter pain, it was hypothesized, involved sacral nerve roots. On this basis the concept developed that labor pain is transmitted by two anatomically separate groups of nerve fibers: one group of fibers enters the cord at T_{11} and T_{12}, transmitting pain from the body of the uterus, the other group enters the cord at S_{2-4}, transmitting pain from the cervix and the birth canal (Fig. 8.2). Therefore, it was held that labor pain could be relieved by blockade of T_{11} and T_{12} during the first stage of labor and blockade of sacral roots during the second stage. How-

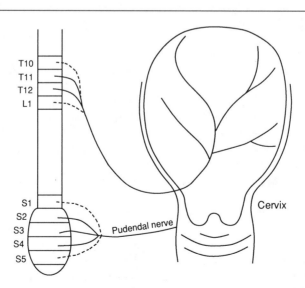

Figure 8.2. Diagram of the sensory innervation of the uterus and cervix. (Redrawn with permission from Moir, Br. J. Anaesth. *58:* 747, 1986.)

ever, it has since been shown that the situation is more complex. Bonica, for example, has demonstrated by a series of meticulous observations made over a period of many years that pain associated with the first stage of labor has two components (Bonica, 1979), one involving the pain of contraction and distension of the uterus, and the other involving the pain associated with dilation of the cervix. Both types of pain are transmitted to the spinal cord by afferent A-delta and C fibers that travel with sympathetic pathways and enter the cord at the levels of T_{10}, T_{11}, T_{12}, and L_1. Thus, sensory innervations of both the cervix and the body of the uterus are the same. While block of T_{11} and T_{12} relieves the pain of uterine contractions during early labor, it is necessary to block T_{10} and L_1 to relieve the pain caused by more intense contractions and cervical dilation as the first stage of labor progresses. During the second stage of labor, it is necessary to block S_1–S_5 as well as T_{10}–L_1 to relieve pain from stretching of the perineum and pelvic structures.

Labor pain can be blocked without interfering with uterine contractions. This may be due in part to the fact that A-delta and C fibers transmitting pain impulses during labor are highly sensitive to the effects of local anesthetics (Chapter 1). More important, however, is the fact that once labor is established, uterine contraction is independent of central neuronal control. Even high sensory levels of spinal anesthesia have little effect on uterine contraction. As Vasicka and Kretchmer (1961) have demonstrated, uterine denervation produced by spinal anesthesia with sensory levels as high as C_6 affects neither the frequency nor the intensity of contractions. Vasicka and Kretchmer did observe, however, that both the frequency and intensity of uterine contractions decreased significantly when spinal anesthesia was accompanied by arterial hypotension. Similar observations by others (Vasicka, *et al.*, 1964; Johnson, *et al.*, 1972; DeVore and Eisler, 1987) attest to the fact that an intact extrinsic nerve supply to the uterus is not a prerequisite for maintenance of normal uterine contractions once labor is established. Whether or not induction of spinal anesthesia before the onset of labor delays onset remains controversial. It if does delay onset, it does so only briefly and would not prevent labor from starting. Even paraplegic females start labor at about the same time as parturients with an intact spinal cord, and furthermore, they also have normal uterine contractions. Spinal anesthesia may, however, prolong the duration of the second stage of labor. This occurs because the muscles of the pelvic outlet are relaxed, thereby delaying rotation of the fetal head during its descent through the birth canal. Additionally, prolongation of the second stage of labor may occur if spinal anesthesia is administered in such a way that relaxation of the abdominal muscles prevents effective "bearing down" by the mother during uterine contractions. It may be for these reasons that a higher incidence of mid-forceps delivery may, in some reports, accompany spinal anesthesia.

Special Aspects of Spinal Anesthesia in Obstetrics

It is widely recognized that small doses of spinal anesthetics produce considerably higher levels of anesthesia in pregnant than in nonpregnant females. To obtain spinal anesthesia high enough for abdominal surgery using hyperbaric solutions in nonpregnant patients, it may be necessary to use the head-down position. However, if this is done in obstetric patients, anesthesia usually extends dangerously high to the upper thoracic spinal segments. This was demonstrated most strikingly by Assali and Prystowsky (1950 a). These authors used a continuous spinal technique with 0.2 percent procaine and found that 5–20 ml were required to obtain anesthesia to pinprick at the level of the fourth cervical dermatome in 10 pregnant females at term. In the same 10 females, 36–48 hr after delivery, three to four times the amount of procaine solution was required to obtain the same level of anesthesia.

Because of the lower requirement for local anesthetics, the amount of anesthetic agent used for spinal anesthesia in obstetrics should be rigidly restricted. For vaginal deliveries, not more than 50 mg of lidocaine or procaine or 5 mg of tetracaine should be used; for cesarean sections, 100 mg of lidocaine or procaine, or 8–10 mg of tetracaine or bupivacaine are sufficient in the majority of cases, although up to 15 mg of isobaric bupivacaine has been used without complications (Russell, 1984, 1987; Bader, et al., 1990).

The reason such high levels of anesthesia are achieved in pregnant women at term when using even small doses of anesthetic agents is not because of changes in cerebrospinal fluid (CSF) protein, and consequently, in binding of local anesthetic within the subarachnoid space (Marx and Orkin, 1965). Neither is it due to any hypothetical increase in CSF pressure during uterine contractions, spreading the anesthetic agent throughout the subarachnoid space (Franken, 1934). Marx, et al. (1962) demonstrated that increases in CSF pressure during labor are a result of skeletal motor activity and not of uterine contractions. They found that spinal anesthesia decreased CSF pressure during labor only insofar as it relieves pain and prevents "bearing down." On the other hand, Hopkins, et al. (1965), found no relation between pain and changes in CSF pressure. Instead, they found the transient increases in CSF pressure during uterine contractions under spinal anesthesia to be related to brief elevations of maternal blood pressure associated with the contractions. Furthermore, Hopkins, *et al.* found the sensory level of spinal anesthesia to be unrelated to whether the local anesthetic was injected into the subarachnoid space during or between uterine contractions. This finding is in agreement with the observation that coughing during induction of spinal anesthesia has no effect on the level of anesthesia achieved (Dubelman and Forbes, 1979) (p. 317). It also agrees with the observation that equally high levels of spinal anesthesia occur in pregnant females who are not in labor.

The propensity for females at term to develop unusually high levels of sensory denervation during spinal anesthesia is probably best explained by at least three factors. The first factor rests on the hypothesis that the volume of CSF in the spinal subarachnoid space of women at term is considerably less than in nonpregnant females. Although there are no studies providing actual measurements of spinal fluid volumes in the spinal subarachnoid during pregnancy, this is the best explanation for Assali and Prystowsky's results. Differences in the rate at which the local anesthetic was absorbed from the subarachnoid space were essentially eliminated by the technique used by these authors. Thus, the differences in dosage required to produce a certain level of anesthesia must be related to differences in the volume of spinal fluid in which the local anesthetic can mix. In other words, there must be differences in the volume of the spinal subarachnoid space in pregnant and nonpregnant females. This reduction in CSF volume is due to venous engorgement in the epidural and subarachnoid spaces because normal venous drainage is obstructed by the weight of the gravid uterus. Such venous obstruction is evidenced in the lower extremities by increased femoral venous pressures, and in the pelvis by frequent development of hemorrhoids at, or near term. The lumbar veins that accommodate the greater part of the venous outflow from the lower portion of the spinal subarachnoid space can also be partially obstructed by the gravid uterus. How venous engorgement influences the spread of local anesthetics for spinal anesthesia in pregnant patients is particularly well demonstrated in the study by Barclay, *et al.* (1968). They studied three groups of patients. An average sensory level of anesthesia of T_{11} was obtained when 4 mg of tetracaine was injected into the subarachnoid space of 20 nonpregnant women of child-bearing age ($N = 20$). The same amount of tetracaine (4 mg) administered in the same manner produced an average sensory level of anesthesia of T_8 in a group of pregnant females at term ($N = 15$) scheduled for elective cesarean section. The third group consisted of nonpregnant women of child-bearing age ($N = 15$). These patients were given 4 mg tetracaine, injected through a subarachnoid catheter after inflating a rubber bladder that was secured over the abdomen by an abdominal binder. Inflation of the bladder increased inferior vena caval pressure to

250 mm H_2O (the catheter that transduced the blood pressure had been placed in the inferior vena cava via the femoral vein). In this third group, the average sensory level of spinal anesthesia was T_7.

The above-mentioned data demonstrate that venous obstruction (induced by the acute increase in intraabdominal pressure) may be the second cause of the high levels of anesthesia seen in pregnant patients given spinal anesthetics. This is supported by data obtained most recently. In a study by Russell (1983), the authors used 0.5 percent plain bupivacaine, and found that the spread of the block with the patient in the lateral position was similar to that in nonpregnant patients. However, there was a marked cephalad extension of the block in pregnant patients following resumption of the supine position. These observations were used to propose that the increase in the vena caval pressure caused by the gravid uterus in the supine position resulted in cephalad displacement of the local anesthetic within the subarachnoid space. Although plain 0.5 percent bupivacaine is slightly hypobaric, the influence of the "head-down" position in the lateral decubitus due to the greater width of the hips than shoulders in females (Greene, 1985) is probably minimal. The data also suggest that similarly increased levels of anesthesia would be observed in any patient, pregnant or not, with increased inferior vena caval pressure, regardless of the reason. The only argument against this theory is the observation (Marx, et al., 1961) that CSF pressure is the same before and immediately after delivery, which should not be the case if venous engorgement within the subarachnoid space were suddenly relieved by delivery of the infant.

The third factor responsible for the reduced local anesthetic requirements to produce spinal anesthesia during pregnancy is that proposed by Datta, et al. (1986). The authors demonstrated that CSF (as well as plasma) concentrations of progesterone increase during pregnancy, and that there is a correlation between the increasing CSF concentration of progesterone and the decreasing dose of lidocaine required to produce equivalent segmental levels of spinal anesthesia (Datta, et al., 1986). Recently, it was demonstrated (Datta, et al., 1983; Flanagan, et al., 1987; and Butterworth, et al., 1990) that the sensitivity of nerve fibers to local anesthetics increased during pregnancy. Although it would be tempting to ascribe the decreased local anesthetic requirements during pregnancy to this increased sensitivity of nerve fibers, this theory does not explain why somatic motor fibers themselves are also not more sensitive to local anesthetic blockade during pregnancy. Also, it is likely that the increased nerve sensitivity would decrease the amount of local anesthetic needed to provide total block of nerve fibers to a given dermatomal level only, while affecting little, if at all, the total dermatomal extent of sensory denervation. These findings, in the context of the decreased CSF volume associated with pregnancy, may nevertheless provide at least a partial explanation for the lesser dose requirements of local anesthetics during spinal anesthesia. Although other factors, such as the lordosis of pregnancy, may contribute to the higher levels of spinal anesthesia seen in pregnant women, reductions in capacity of the subarachnoid space, leading to changes in spinal fluid volume, increased inferior vena caval pressure, and increased nerve sensitivity to local anesthetics probably constitute the most important factors.

Effects of Spinal Anesthesia on Maternal Physiology

Cardiovascular System

Hypotension

One of the most striking characteristics of spinal anesthesia in obstetrics is the high incidence and severity of maternal arterial hypotension following induction of anesthesia. This also represents the greatest risk of spinal anesthesia in obstetric patients. One reason for the high incidence of arterial hypotension is the already mentioned fact that a given amount of spinal anesthetic produces a higher level of anesthesia in pregnant females at term than in nonpregnant females. However, the same level of anesthesia is usually associated with a greater decrease in blood pressure in pregnant than in nonpregnant females. The relationship between pregnancy and the decline in blood pressure during spinal anesthesia has been studied and commented on by many. Especially valuable are the carefully controlled investigations of Assali and Prystowsky (1950 a). These authors found a "negligible" decrease in mean pressure (7 percent) in five normotensive nonpregnant females during total sympathetic block produced by continuous differential spinal anesthesia. However, in 12 normotensive females at term, this same technique produced "dramatic" reductions in blood pressure, averaging a 43 percent decrease in systolic pressure, and 53 percent decrease in diastolic pressure. Ten of the females studied at term were again studied within 36 to 48 hr after delivery, and the results approached normal nonpregnant controls, with an average decrease in systolic pressure of only 12 percent during total sympathetic block.

Decreases in arterial pressure during spinal anesthesia result from the same factors for both pregnant and nonpregnant patients (Chapter 2; also Assali and Prystowsky, 1950 b). Spinal anesthesia decreases cardiac output in obstetric patients (Stenger, et al., 1964) as in nonpregnant females. However, pregnancy involves certain additional factors that may accentuate the cardiovascular response to sympathetic denervation. One such factor is the large amount of blood present in the gravid uterus. In women at term, approximately one sixth of the total blood volume is contained within the uterus. Consequently, a proportionately greater percentage of circulating blood volume is trapped in the peripheral vascular bed during sympathetic blockade. This results in a correspondingly greater decrease in venous return to the heart and reduction in cardiac output and blood pressure. The weight of the uterus also contributes to decreases in cardiac output because it impairs venous return from the lower extremities during spinal anesthesia, especially in the supine position. This is important because immediately after delivery, a sudden, significant increase in arterial blood pressure (Roman and Adriani, 1948; Assali and Prystowsky, 1950 b), as well as a 52 percent increase in cardiac output (Ueland, et al., 1968), often occur at this time. These changes coincide with the removal of obstruction to venous flow in the pelvic veins. Finally, although uterine contractions do not directly influence venous pressures, the "bearing down" of the patient (i.e., Valsalva maneuver) causes contraction of abdominal muscles, which further decreases venous return to the heart by increasing intrathoracic pressure. This is reflected by an increase in femoral venous pressure during "bearing-down" (Runge, 1924). The foregoing three factors, alone or in combination, render pregnant females more likely to experience obstruction of the venous return to the heart than nonpregnant females, even when not undergoing spinal anesthesia. The hemodynamic effects of spinal anesthesia, added to those of pregnancy itself, are such that even a relatively low level of spinal denervation may cause a significant decrease in blood pressure.

Because of the increased incidence of hemodynamic instability, pregnant females should never be placed in the reverse Trendelenburg position during high spinal anesthesia. While this might be dangerous enough in a nonpregnant female, it will be even more so in a parturient, because of development of severe arterial hypotension. Initially, the head-up or the sitting position can control the height of anesthesia when hyperbaric solutions are being used. But should the patient develop hypotension or abnormally high levels of anesthesia while either sitting or in the supine position, the patient must be repositioned immediately and without hesitation, with the head placed slightly lower than the feet (Chapters 1 and 2) and left uterine displacement should be continued.

Correct positioning of the pregnant female is but one means of preventing and managing maternal hypotension during spinal anesthesia. Others include left uterine displacement, intravenous fluid administration, supplemental oxygen administration, and use of vasopressors (Wright and Shnider, 1987; Wright, 1983). Clark, et al. (1976) compared the efficacy of administering intravenous fluids with or without left uterine displacement for the prevention of hypotension associated with spinal anesthesia in 247 patients having cesarean sections. Hypotension

Table 8.2.
Prevention of Arterial Hypotension During Spinal Anesthesia for Cesarean Section[a]

	Patients Not in Labor			Patients in Early Labor		
	No Prevention	Intravenous Fluids	Intravenous Fluids Plus Uterine Displacement	No Prevention	Intravenous Fluids	Intravenous Fluids Plus Uterine Displacement
No. patients	27	76	53	18	39	34
Incidence of hypotension (%)	92	57	53	50	46	15
Ephedrine[b] (%)	52	74	82	44	72	100

[a] Adapted with permission from Clark, *et al.*, Anesthesiology 45: 670, 1976.
[b] Percent of patients who were given intravenous ephedrine for treatment of hypotension.

was defined as a systolic blood pressure of less than 100 mmHg. Left uterine displacement was sustained mechanically. Intravenous fluids consisted of 1000 ml of 5 percent dextrose in lactated Ringer's solution 30 min prior to induction of anesthesia. Intravenous ephedrine was employed if hypotension developed. In the absence of any special preventive measures, 92 percent of term patients not in labor developed hypotension (Table 8.2). On the other hand, only 50 percent of untreated patients in early labor became hypotensive. The reason for this difference is not apparent. Ephedrine was given to correct hypotension almost as often to patients in labor as to those not in labor: 52 percent and 44 percent, respectively. Prophylactic intravenous fluids 30 min prior to induction of anesthesia significantly reduced the occurrence of hypotension among patients not in labor, but had no effect on the incidence of hypotension among those in early labor. This is probably because the frequency of hypotension was already low in patients in labor even without preventive measures. The incidence of hypotension was not decreased in the absence of labor when left uterine displacement was employed along with prophylactic fluid administration. This combination did, however, significantly decrease the incidence of hypotension among patients in early labor. The percentage of hypotensive patients requiring intravenous ephedrine was approximately the same for all groups (the 100 percent of patients in early labor who needed ephedrine after both uterine displacement and fluids represents only five patients). Gutsche (1976), like Clark, *et al.*, did not find intravenous fluids to be consistent in preventing arterial hypotension in pregnant patients. Indeed, Gutsche found that intravenous fluids with uterine displacement served only to decrease, but not to eliminate the incidence of hypotension. Gutsche found a combination of prophylactic ephedrine plus intravenous fluids more reliable than either measure alone in preventing maternal hypotension during spinal anesthesia. Despite generous prehydration with 1500–2000 ml of crystalloid, Norris (1987) also reported that 74 percent of patients having spinal anesthesia for cesarean section became hypotensive (defined as systolic blood pressure less than 100 mmHg or less than 70 percent of baseline).

Wollman and Marx (1968) found, in contrast, that intravenous infusion of a liter of 5 percent dextrose in lactated Ringer's solution prior to induction of spinal anesthesia for either cesarean section or vaginal delivery was effective in preventing hypotension. In fact, Wollman and Marx found that none of the patients given prophylactic fluids intravenously developed hypotension during T_{2-6} levels of spinal anesthesia, in contrast to the findings of Clark, et al., and those of Norris. Wollman and Marx also noted that infusion of the same volume of fluid after induction of anesthesia was not as effective in preventing hypotension as it was when given before induction of spinal anesthesia. They further observed that use of these fluid volumes represented no hazard to the obstetric patient, as central venous pressure did not increase.

Other studies have shown that fluid preloading prior to induction of spinal anesthesia is effective in preventing maternal hypotension (Corke, et al., 1982; Marx, et al., 1969; Mathru, et al., 1980; Caritis, et al., 1980), especially if 1 L or more was used (Caritis, et al., 1980; Bader, et al., 1990). Some studies have employed colloids such as 5 percent albumin, and have found it very effective (Mathru, et al., 1980). Dextran has been used for fluid preloading prior to epidural anesthesia, and it also has been found effective (Wennberg, et al., 1990). Nevertheless, concerns about colloids (whether albumin or dextran) remain, especially regarding cost and the possibility of anaphylactoid reactions (Munoz, 1987; Messmer, 1987).

The preceding discussion regarding the effectiveness of intravenous fluid preloading in preventing maternal hypotension is not meant to imply that blood pressure maintenance is in, and of, itself a measure of adequacy of peripheral perfusion or tissue oxygenation. Certainly maintenance of blood pressure, whether measured in an artery peripherally with a sphygmomanometer or even centrally via a central venous or pulmonary artery catheter, will give but little information on actual oxygen delivery to tissues. As mentioned previously (Chapter 2), the beneficial effects of intravenous fluid preloading must be viewed in the context of the hemodilution, decreased oxygen carrying capacity, and increased coagulability it produces.

The vasopressor used most often in the above-mentioned clinical studies was ephedrine. Although other vasopressors are equally effective in restoring maternal blood pressure during obstetrical spinal anesthesia, most are not used. This is because they may induce uterine vasoconstriction, and thus decrease uterine blood flow, a response especially evident with alpha-adrenergic agonists (Shnider, 1983). Methoxamine (Eng, *et al.*, 1971; Shnider, *et al.*, 1970; Ralston, *et al.*, 1974), phenylephrine (Greiss and Crandell, 1965), norepinephrine (Greiss and Crandell, 1965) and dopamine (Rolbin, *et al.*, 1979) either further accentuate uterine hypoperfusion during maternal hypotension produced by spinal anesthesia, or fail to improve uterine hypoperfusion, even though each of the vasopressors effectively restores maternal blood pressure. Methoxamine, phenylephrine, dopamine, and norepinephrine affect uterine and placental blood flow adversely, and are therefore often associated with development of fetal acidosis. While vasopressors such as metaraminol and mephentermine produce less uterine vasoconstriction than methoxamine, phenylephrine, and norepinephrine, they produce more uterine vasoconstriction than ephedrine (Ralson, *et al.*, 1974). Vasopressors should be given during obstetric anesthesia to maintain adequate placental perfusion, not to restore maternal blood pressure. The two are not synonymous. Ephedrine, especially when administered as an intravenous infusion (Kang, *et al.*, 1982; Lindblad, *et al.*, 1988) is preferable over currently available vasopressors for maintaining both placental blood flow and maternal blood pressure during spinal anesthesia (Eng, *et al.*, 1971, 1973; Gutsche, 1976; Shnider, *et al.*, 1968; Ralston, *et al.*, 1974; Norris, 1987; Kang, *et al.*, 1982; Shnider, 1983; Bader, *et al.*, 1990). Recently, phenylephrine and ephedrine were compared with respect to their ability to prevent development of maternal hypotension for cesarean section (Moran, *et al.*, 1991). Sixty healthy patients were randomly assigned to receive either intravenous bolus injections of 10 mg ephedrine, or 80-μg bolus injections of phenylephrine to maintain systolic blood pressure above 100 mmHg. In both groups, umbilical artery pH, partial pressure of carbon dioxide (pCO_2), and base deficit were normal, and there were no significant differences regarding neonatal Apgar scores, neurobehavioral scores, or frequency of maternal nausea and vomiting. These results suggest that when given in small (80-μg) bolus injections, phenylephrine is effective in treating maternal hypotension and that it has no adverse maternal or neonatal effects (Moran, *et al.*, 1991). Although these results are encouraging, confirmation of the safety of phenylephrine use in obstetric anesthesia is needed.

Despite conflicts in the above data regarding the effectiveness of fluid preloading or of different vasoactive drugs to prevent hypotension during clinical spinal anesthesia, one can conclude that: (a) without prophylactic measures, there is a high incidence of maternal hypotension during spinal anesthesia in obstetric patients at term; (b) the incidence of hypotension can be decreased and existing hypotension can be treated by either prophylactic ephedrine, left uterine displacement, or prophylactic administration of intravenous fluids preferably prior to induction of spinal anesthesia; (c) no one method is by itself totally successful; (d) a combination of all three methods is probably most effective both as prophylaxis and treatment; and (e) the goal in restoring maternal hemodynamic parameters (blood pressure, heart rate) to normal levels is to maximize placental perfusion and tissue oxygenation.

Pregnancy-Induced Hypertension

In recent years, the term "toxemia of pregnancy" has been replaced by the more appropriate term, "pregnancy-induced hypertension" (PIH), as there has been no evidence for the presence of a "toxin." Currently, the hypertensive disorders encountered during pregnancy are classified into four categories:

1. Preeclampsia, or pregnancy-induced hypertension, which consists of the triad of hypertension, proteinuria, and generalized edema. These changes, usually developing after the 20th week of gestation, can be mild or severe. If seizures develop, preeclampsia becomes eclampsia.
2. Chronic hypertension denotes presence of hypertension both prior to pregnancy (or prior to the 20th week of gestation) and following delivery.
3. Superimposed preeclampsia denotes development of the findings triad in a chronic hypertensive patient.
4. Transient gestational hypertension, in which the findings triad in list item (1) do not develop during pregnancy, with return to normotension following delivery (usually within the first 10 postpartum days).

Recent studies (Easterling, et al., 1990) suggest that the development of hypertension during pregnancy is preceded by a hyperdynamic state characterized by increased cardiac output and normal peripheral resistance. Newer investigations have implicated thromboxane A_2 in the pathogenesis of PIH (Fitzgerald, et al., 1990). Because of the relatively high frequency with which it occurs (7 percent of all pregnancies), affecting over 250,000 parturients (Gutsche and Cheek, 1987), the physiologic responses of preeclamptic patients to spinal anesthesia deserve special consideration (Wright, 1983).

The effects of spinal anesthesia on maternal blood pressure, along with the older reports of the value of spinal anesthesia in the management of certain types of oliguria, resulted in the recommendation that spinal anesthesia be used in the management of preeclampsia. Spinal anesthesia was even considered the anesthetic method of choice for delivery of preeclamptic patients (Hingson, 1947; Whitacre, et al., 1948; Lull and Hingson, 1948; McElrath, et al., 1949; Lund, 1951, 1952; Tuohy, 1952; Mylks, et al., 1960). Sympathetic blockade lowers blood pressure in eclamptic and preeclamptic patients and may, as a result, have a beneficial effect on the patient's ocular and central nervous system symptoms.

However, decrease in blood pressure is abrupt and uncontrolled, going from hypertensive to hypotensive levels. This has prompted a feeling among obstetricians that preeclamptic and especially eclamptic patients are hypersensitive to the cardiovascular effects of spinal anesthesia and therefore contraindicated in such patients. Whether or not eclamptic patients are in fact more "sensitive" to spinal anesthesia is open to question. Assali and Prystowsky (1950 a) examined this point in a controlled study by comparing the vascular response to total sympathetic block produced by differential spinal anesthesia. The study involved 15 preeclamptic patients and 12 normotensive patients at term. Before the sympathetic block the average blood pressure in the hypertensive patients was 164/112 mmHg. During the block, the blood pressure averaged 135/94 mmHg, a 17 percent decrease in systolic and a 16 percent decrease in diastolic pressure. This compared to an average decrease of 43 percent in systolic pressure and 53 percent in diastolic pressure in normotensive females at term during an equally extensive sympathetic block. These results were later confirmed by Kaplan and Assali (1953) and by Smith, *et al.* (1966). It appears, therefore, that the decrease in blood pressure during spinal anesthesia in preeclamptic patients may be greater on an absolute scale than in normal patients, but is less on a percentile basis (Moya and Smith, 1962). Preeclamptic or eclamptic patients, therefore, may hardly be considered "hypersensitive" to spinal anesthesia. Indeed, the current consensus is that major regional anesthesia, including spinal anesthesia, is effective and safe when used properly in eclamptic and preeclamptic patients (Rogers, *et al.*, 1969; Gutsche and Cheek, 1987). Spinal anesthesia is particularly useful for preventing hypertension during labor in such patients. Spinal (and epidural) anesthesia are of little or no value, however, in the treatment of hypertension in preeclampsia. Good obstetric management in conjunction with the use of the newer antihypertensive drugs is both more effective and safer in controlling hypertension than spinal anesthesia. On the other hand, spinal anesthesia can be given safely for either vaginal or cesarean delivery of preeclamptic patients, and in itself, the presence of PIH should not contraindicate the use of spinal anesthesia (Gutsche and Cheek, 1987). Whether spinal anesthesia is actually contraindicated or not depends on the obstetric situation and on the skill and training of the person administering the anesthetic; although the method can be used in preeclamptic patients, it should be performed only by those with extensive experience and who possess a thorough understanding of the physiologic disturbances involved (Lechner and Chadwick, 1990).

Those who have advocated spinal anesthesia for the treatment of PIH also believe that renal function is improved by spinal anesthesia, since oliguria is replaced by a normal urinary output, if not by diuresis. Clinical reports on the effects of spinal anesthesia on renal function in preeclamptic patients are, however, extremely difficult to evaluate. There have been no controlled studies in which patients were given a spinal anesthetic alternating with other anesthetic methods. Examination of the published protocols suggesting increased urinary output after induction of spinal anesthesia reveals that spinal anesthesia is usually administered at the same time as the institution of bed rest, heavy sedation, administration of antihypertensive drugs, intravenous fluid administration, and even delivery, any one of which might explain the beneficial effects ascribed to anesthesia. It is impossible, therefore, on the basis of published reports, to evaluate the beneficial effect, if any, of spinal anesthesia on the oliguria of PIH. Even the theoretical basis for its value in this respect is based on four doubtful assumptions: that the oliguria is due to renal arteriolar vasoconstriction; that such vasoconstriction is under neurogenic control of sympathetic nerves; that relief of vasoconstriction results in an increase in renal blood flow; and, finally, that increased blood flow produces greater urinary output. Certainly renal arterioles in both pregnant and nonpregnant women exhibit an inherent vascular tone that is relatively independent of neurogenic impulses (Chapter 5; Assali and Rosenkrantz, 1951; Assali, et al., 1951). Measurements of renal blood flow and urinary output in PIH patients indicate that the same is true in preeclampsia. Turner and Houck (1950) studied renal hemodynamics in nine preeclamptic patients before and during continuous caudal or continuous spinal anesthesia to the sixth thoracic segment. They found that glomerular filtration was reduced below normal in seven of nine patients before anesthesia (average 88.8 ml/min), and was further decreased during anesthesia in seven of the nine patients (average during block 68.3 ml/min). This coincided with the fact that the effect of the block on renal plasma flow was not consistent. Before spinal anesthesia, renal plasma flow was normal in five of the nine patients, above normal in one, slightly below normal in two, and considerably below normal in one. During anesthesia, renal plasma flow did not change in three patients, decreased in four, and increased in two. Similarly, there was no consistent effect on either tubular secretion or filtration fraction. Similar results have been obtained by other investigators. Assali and Rosenkrantz (1951) and Kaplan and Assali (1953) found that in addition to having no affect on renal vascular resistance, high spinal anesthesia usually resulted in decreased urinary output in both normal and preeclamptic females at term. It appears unlikely, therefore, that sympathetic blockade provides any special benefit in the management of oliguria due to preeclampsia.

Respiratory System

Females in labor often complain of breathlessness or of being unable to breathe during spinal anesthesia. This is particularly the case with the higher levels of anesthesia required for cesarean section. While this also can occur in nonobstetric patients, it appears to be more frequent in pregnant females. While spinal anesthesia certainly can cause inadequate ventilation (Stenger, *et al.*, 1964), the subjective sensation of breathlessness is usually not associated with objective evidence of impaired respiration. In fact, in the absence of excessively high levels of motor block, spinal anesthesia in parturient females is not usually accompanied by hypoxia or carbon dioxide retention, but may be associated with emotionally induced hyperventilation (Moya and Smith, 1962). In three of the seven patients studied by Ueland, *et al.* (1968), for example, maternal arterial pCO_2 decreased during spinal anesthesia. None of the four patients studied by de Jong (1965) showed increases in arterial pCO_2 during spinal anesthesia for cesarean section, and one hyperventilated to an arterial pCO_2 of 20 mmHg, a level of alkalosis sufficient to produce seizures (Dumitru, *et al.*, 1962). The etiology of such respiratory distress so often observed in pregnant females during spinal anesthesia is unexplained. It occurs more frequently during high levels of spinal anesthesia, especially during cesarean section, than during lower levels. Perhaps loss of proprioception in the anterior abdominal and thoracic wall contributes to the sense of breathlessness despite adequate or even excessive ventilation. This may render the patient unable to appreciate the fact that the muscles of respiration are functioning normally. If this is the explanation, one must also determine why obstetric patients are more prone to developing this type of breathlessness than are nonobstetric patients.

Effects on Other Organ Systems

The abnormal liver function that may be observed in normal females at term is not associated with increased susceptibility to the hepatic effects of spinal or general anesthesia (Smith, *et al.*, 1962). The increased bromsulfalein retention present at the time of delivery returns to normal by the fourth postpartum day, regardless of the type of anesthesia. The same also holds true for toxemic patients whose hepatic dysfunction at the time of delivery is more pronounced. Here, spinal anesthesia provides no significant advantage from the hepatic point of view compared to general anesthesia (Smith, *et al.*, 1962).

The amount of maternal blood loss during normal vaginal deliveries is unaffected by the type of anesthesia (Bosomworth, *et al.*, 1960). Neither is there evidence to support the hypothesis (Crawford and Murphy, 1960) that spinal anesthesia may predispose to, or even cause, premature separation of the placenta. The effect of spinal anesthesia on the permeability of the human placental barrier is as yet undetermined. It appears, however, that under normal conditions, spinal anesthesia has little effect on the permeability to at least one substance, namely, sodium. Flexner, *et al.* (1948) found in a study dealing with normal labor that the concentration of radioactive sodium in the newborn infant following its intravenous administration to the mother was the same regardless of whether spinal, ether, or thiopental anesthesia was used for delivery. On the other hand, with abnormal labor the situation is reportedly different. Johnson and Clayton (1955) found that the placental transfer of radioactive sodium was increased by continuous caudal anesthesia when placental ischemia was present during labor. Johnson and Clayton found that in nine patients with prolonged labor who were sedated only, "placental function" as measured by sodium transfer was 66 percent of normal, while it was 80 percent of normal in 11 patients given continuous caudal anesthesia. This increase (also expected after spinal anesthesia) is probably the result of vasodilation of decidual vessels.

Effects of Spinal Anesthesia on the Fetus and Neonate

Spinal anesthesia may affect the fetus and neonate in either, or both, of two ways. The local anesthetic used to produce anesthesia for labor and delivery could directly affect the fetus following its absorption into the maternal circulation and subsequent diffusion across the placenta into the fetal circulation. Alternatively, spinal anesthesia could affect the fetus indirectly by altering placental blood flow and the course of labor through the denervation it produces.

Until recently, it was assumed that spinal anesthesia resulted in low or even undetectable maternal plasma levels of local anesthetics. In 1979, Giasi, *et al.* demonstrated that the subarachnoid or epidural administration of 75 mg of lidocaine in 20 nonpregnant patients resulted in measurable plasma concentrations (pp. 1 and 364–371). Their initial findings have since been confirmed for both lidocaine (75 mg) and bupivacaine (15 mg) (Axelsson and Widman, 1981; Burm, *et al.*, 1983). In all of these studies, blood (or plasma) concentrations for lidocaine have been reported to range between 0.300 and 0.444 $\mu g \cdot ml^{-1}$, while for bupivacaine, they were 0.063 $\mu g \cdot ml^{-1}$. These very low plasma concentrations would not be expected to cause any systemic effects (Burm, *et al.*, 1983). Since clinical spinal anesthesia in obstetrics would require local anesthetic dosages that would be at most equal to, though most likely less than, the dosages employed by Burm, *et al.* and by Axelsson and Widman, it is unlikely that plasma local anesthetic concentrations in the parturient would be significantly higher than the levels reported in nonpregnant patients. In light of the possible decrease in CSF in parturients, however, which may in turn result in higher concentrations of local anesthetics, more studies are clearly needed for confirmation, as are studies proving that systemic effects from local anesthetic absorption would likewise be unlikely.

Neonatal blood levels of local anesthetics have also been reported. Tronick, et al. (1976) found umbilical plasma levels of lidocaine to average $0.10 \ \mu g \cdot ml^{-1}$ in four infants whose mothers were given lidocaine spinal anesthesia for delivery. Twenty-four hours after delivery plasma levels of lidocaine in heel-stick blood averaged $0.04 \ \mu g \cdot ml^{-1}$. Similar results were reported by Datta, et al. (1980), who found that 55–65 mg of lidocaine injected intrathecally resulted in maternal venous plasma levels of $0.63 \pm 0.14 \ \mu g \cdot ml^{-1}$, while the umbilical vein and umbilical artery concentrations were 0.17 ± 0.02 and $0.11 \pm 0.02 \ \mu g \cdot ml^{-1}$, respectively. Kuhnert, et al., (1986) confirmed these results following spinal administration of 60–100 mg hyperbaric lidocaine for cesarean section. In their study, maternal plasma levels, umbilical vein and umbilical artery concentrations were 0.65 ± 0.52, 0.20 ± 0.12, and $0.08 \pm 0.06 \ \mu g \cdot ml^{-1}$, respectively; these values were significantly lower than the plasma concentration achieved during epidural anesthesia (Fig. 8.3). The levels reported in the above-mentioned studies are below those associated with either intrauterine toxicity or altered neonatal behavior (Ralston and Shnider, 1978). It is thus unlikely that local anesthetics used for obstetrical spinal anesthesia have any direct effect on the fetus or the neonate.

Spinal anesthesia may, however, affect the fetus and neonate indirectly by causing changes in placental blood flow or in the progression of labor. This may in turn change fetal heart rate or neonatal oxygenation and neonatal acidosis may become evident. Fetal bradycardia does not usually occur when maternal systolic blood pressure is maintained above 100 mmHg in normal parturients. However, with maternal systolic blood pressures below 70 mmHg, fetal bradycardia becomes the rule during active labor (p. 312). The incidence of fetal bradycardia (indicative of placental hypoperfusion) becomes so great when maternal systolic blood pressure decreases below 100 mmHg, that even in normal patients during active labor, corrective measures should be initiated immediately. For patients with preeclampsia, eclampsia, or other obstetric complications, active measures to avoid maternal hypotension should be undertaken even earlier.

Fetal oxygenation, like fetal heart rate, is adversely affected by spinal anesthesia only when maternal hypotension develops and impairs placental blood flow (Lucas, et al., 1966). The level of maternal systolic blood pressure requisite for normal oxygenation at the time of delivery is the same as that necessary to prevent fetal bradycardia. It should be noted, however, that in the absence of maternal hypotension, fetal oxygenation at birth is the same with spinal anesthesia as with general anesthesia or other forms of regional anesthesia (Haselhorst and Stromberger, 1932;

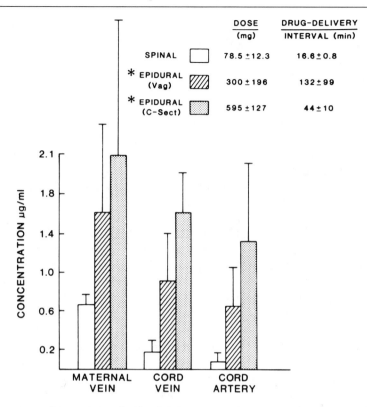

Figure 8.3. Comparison of plasma lidocaine levels at time of delivery following spinal or epidural anesthesia. (Reproduced with permission from Kuhnert, *et al.*, Anesth. Analg. *65:* 139, 1986).

Taylor, *et al.*, 1951 a, b; Henderson, *et al.*, 1957; Quilligan, *et al.*, 1964; Abboud, *et al.*, 1985; Caritis, *et al.*, 1980; Marx, *et al.*, 1984; Bader, *et al.*, 1990). However, the type of anesthesia used for delivery may affect the ability of the neonate to initiate spontaneous respirations, and thus, neonatal oxygenation may be affected. For example, while potent general anesthetics may delay the onset of neonatal respiration, spinal anesthesia does not. General anesthetics, accordingly, may be associated with a greater incidence of neonatal hypoxemia than spinal anesthesia 2 or 3 min following delivery. In the absence of maternal hypotension, depressed neonatal oxygenation 2 or 3 min following delivery under spinal anesthesia usually occurs because the mother received narcotics or other depressants during labor and delivery. Thus, although fetal oxygen measurements taken as close as possible to the time of delivery show no difference related to the type of anesthesia, infants delivered under general anesthesia more often require resuscitation than when delivered under regional (including spinal) anesthesia. The studies of Taylor, et al. (1951 a) provide but one example of the relative ease with which infants delivered under regional anesthesia initiate and then maintain respiration. These authors found that none of 20 neonates delivered under regional (including spinal) anesthesia required resuscitation, while 38 percent of those delivered with ether, 30 percent of those delivered with nitrous oxide, and 54 percent of those delivered with cyclopropane needed resuscitation before breathing spontaneously. Similar data were also obtained by Phillips (1959). Babies born to mothers undergoing general anesthesia or regional anesthesia with heavy premedication show lower oxygen saturations for 30 min to an hour after delivery than do babies born under spinal or other forms of conduction anesthesia alone (Taylor, et al., 1951 a; Shields and Taylor, 1957). These differences are especially marked in premature infants, for whom the attainment of normal oxygen saturation is more difficult than for the full-term neonates, even under the best of circumstances (Taylor, et al., 1951 b). Similar observations were also made by Apgar, et al. (1957). These investigators found that infants born vaginally were more depressed when delivered under general anesthesia than when delivered under regional (including spinal) anesthesia. The onset of sustained respiration following full-term delivery under general anesthesia was delayed three times more often than following regional anesthesia. This was also reflected by different Apgar scores. Approximately 5 percent of full-term infants delivered vaginally under conduction anesthesia had Apgar scores of 0–4, while 95 percent had scores of 5–10. After general anesthesia, 10 percent of the infants had Apgar scores of 0–4, and 90 percent had scores of 5–10. These differences were even more evident following elective cesarean section; 99 percent of the infants delivered under spinal anesthesia had scores of 5–10, while only 58 percent of those delivered under general anesthesia had comparable Apgar scores. It is interesting to note, however, that the higher Apgar scores at the time of birth of the infants delivered under conduction anesthesia, indicative of better physical condition, was not reflected in decreased infant mortality rates. Neonatal death rates in each of the four groups studied (elective cesarean sections, premature vaginal deliveries, full-term vaginal deliveries, and breech deliveries) were unaffected by the type of anesthesia (Apgar, et al., 1957). This may imply that the data in this study were weighted by preferential use of regional anesthesia in particularly poor-risk patients. Alternatively, the data may imply that prompt, efficient infant resuscitation eliminated differences in physical condition at the time of birth; or both of the above may be correct.

Fetal hypoxia causes fetal acidosis. The acid-base balance of neonates at the time of delivery is therefore determined by the adequacy of placental blood flow and fetal oxygenation immediately prior to delivery. Marx, et al. (1969) found that umbilical arterial pH, pCO_2, and base deficit were no different in infants delivered by cesarean section under general anesthesia than they were in infants delivered under spinal anesthesia, provided that delivery was not accompanied by maternal hypotension. When spinal anesthesia was complicated by arterial hypotension, umbilical arterial base deficit increased significantly, though pH and carbon dioxide tension were unaffected. Marx, et al. found the prevention of maternal hypotension during spinal anesthesia by prophylactic intravenous fluids or ephedrine to be more effective in maintaining normal neonatal acid-base balance than post facto treatment of hypotension. Both Shnider, et al. (1968; 1970) as well as Eng, et al. (1971, 1973) confirmed the relationship between maternal blood pressure and fetal acid-base balance in experimental animals and emphasized the importance of the type of vasopressor used to treat maternal hypotension. Methoxamine restored maternal blood pressure, but further decreased placental blood flow and so worsened fetal acidosis. Ephedrine restored maternal blood pressure while increasing placental blood flow and partially, if not completely, corrected fetal acidosis.

The preservation of placental blood flow during spinal anesthesia, provided hypotension is avoided, has been demonstrated by Jouppila, et al. (1984). Jouppila, et al. studied nine patients (aged 23–39 yr) undergoing elective cesarean section under spinal anesthesia with isobaric 0.5 percent bupivacaine. The placental blood flow measured by intravenous xenon-133 technique was unchanged by the anesthesia: 101.0 ± 17.7 ml·min^{-1}·dl^{-1} before, and 102.1 ± 8.5 ml·min^{-1}·dl^{-1} after, induction of spinal anesthesia. It should be noted, however, that all patients received Ringer's lactate solution, 1500–2000 ml intravenously prior to initiation of anesthesia, and ephedrine infusion was used to treat hypotension. Interestingly, one of the patients studied had PIH, and her placental blood flow increased markedly (41 to 120 ml·min^{-1}·dl^{-1}) following induction of spinal anesthesia. In contrast, one diabetic patient had a significant decrease (174 to 49 ml·min^{-1}·dl^{-1}) following induction of spinal anesthesia. Nevertheless, all newborns had normal Apgar scores and acid-base status at birth, despite a significant decrease in maternal mean blood pressure from 102 ± 4.6 mmHg to 81 ± 4.9 mmHg during spinal anesthesia. Similar findings of preserved transplacental (fetal aortic and umbilical) blood flows during spinal anesthesia with bupivacaine for cesarean section were reported by Lindblad, et al. (1988). These authors, using real-time ultrasonography and a pulsed Doppler technique to measure fetal blood flow, found that following intravenous fluid preloading with 2000 ml lactated Ringer's solution and prophylaxis with intravenous ephedrine infusion, spinal anesthesia had no effect on fetal aortic or umbilical vein blood flows.

The relationship between maternal hypotension and fetal acidosis is especially evident in diabetic mothers. Datta and Brown (1977) studied 30 mothers and their infants following cesarean section under spinal anesthesia; 15 of the 30 mothers were diabetic. They also studied 30 mothers and their infants following delivery by cesarean section under general anesthesia (thiopental and nitrous oxide-oxygen with infusion of succinylcholine); 15 of the 30 mothers were diabetic. All mothers had a normal acid-base status at the time of delivery. Following general anesthesia, the acid-base status of infants born of diabetic mothers was the same as that of infants born of nondiabetic mothers. Umbilical arterial pH was 7.20, and base deficit was 5.67 $mEq \cdot L^{-1}$ for infants of diabetic mothers delivered under spinal anesthesia. Both values were significantly lower than corresponding values for infants of diabetic mothers who underwent general anesthesia (7.29 and 1.01 $mEq \cdot L^{-1}$). This difference was due largely to maternal hypotension that occurred during spinal anesthesia and resulted in metabolic acidosis in infants. The presence of placental abnormalities, even in mothers with well-controlled diabetes, heightens the susceptibility of placental blood flow to the adverse effects of spinal hypotension (Jouppila, et al., 1984; Datta, et al., 1982). Particular attention must be paid to the diabetic patient, in particular regarding intravenous fluid administration. It has been shown that the incidence of fetal acidosis is increased in diabetic mothers who are rendered hyperglycemic by the administration of dextrose-containing solutions (Datta and Brown, 1977; Datta, et al., 1982). Similarly, Morton, et al., (1985) found that, in women with ketonuria who were receiving 5 percent or 10 percent dextrose solutions during labor, the venous base deficit increased significantly, indicating that the buffering capacity of the blood had been exceeded. Zimmer, et al. (1986) and most recently, Philipson, et al. (1987) also reported that 1000–1500 ml of dextrose-containing solutions infused intravenously prior to cesarean section resulted in significant maternal hyperglycemia, as well as fetal hyperglycemia and metabolic acidosis. Philipson, et al. also reported development of neonatal hypoglycemia following the period of fetal hyperglycemia.

The above findings, however, have been challenged by several recent reports. Loong, et al. (1987) compared two groups of patients receiving intrapartum infusions of 5 percent dextrose or Hartmann's solution to a control group not receiving intravenous hydration, and found that the infusion of dextrose had no adverse effects on fetal blood glucose. Evans, et al., (1986) likewise found that saline plus dextrose infusion prior to epidural anesthesia had no effect on the blood glucose of infants at 12 and 24 hr of age. Grylack, et al. (1984) concluded that administration of a balanced electrolyte solution without excess glucose minimized the incidence of fetal hyperglycemia or neonatal hypoglycemia. In light of the lack of consistency of results regarding effects of exogenous dextrose administration in the above studies, it would seem prudent that intravenous fluids administered for prophylaxis or treatment of hypotension during spinal anesthesia (or other anesthetic techniques) should not contain excessive amounts of dextrose (Wright and Shnider, 1987).

Neonatal neurobehavioral tests have reportedly shown better results following delivery under spinal anesthesia than following delivery under epidural anesthesia. Scanlon, *et al.* (1974) studied 28 infants born of mothers given epidural anesthesia and 13 infants delivered with either low spinal or local infiltration anesthesia. Muscle strength and tone were weaker following epidural anesthesia than following spinal or local infiltration anesthesia. Scores from tests evaluating habituation to repetitive stimuli were the same following epidural, spinal, or local infiltration anesthesia. Unfortunately, in this study, results from patients given spinal anesthesia were combined with those from patients given local infiltration anesthesia. It is thus impossible to determine whether spinal anesthesia differed from local infiltration anesthesia in terms of neonatal responses. Furthermore, no patients were studied who delivered without anesthesia, making it impossible to determine whether neonatal neurobehavioral tests might be different following regional anesthesia than following no anesthesia. The difference noted by Scanlon, *et al.* in neurobehavioral test scores of neonates delivered with epidural and those of neonates delivered with spinal and infiltration anesthesia is, as suggested by the authors, probably related to differences in blood levels of local anesthetics in infants delivered with different types of regional anesthesia.

Stanley, *et al.* (1974), however, found that infants delivered under regional anesthesia had significantly greater irritability and much less motor maturity than those delivered of mothers given systemic analgesics and sedatives (meperidine, promethazine, hydroxyzine). The authors failed to distinguish between the different types of regional anesthesia; 42 mothers had spinal anesthesia, 4 had pudendal nerve blocks, 1 had a paracervical block, 2 had both epidural and spinal anesthesia, and 1 had both spinal anesthesia and pudendal nerve block. The type of regional anesthesia may influence neonatal neurobehavior. Thus, these data do not necessarily prove that spinal anesthesia, or any other specific type of regional anesthesia, is associated with neonatal neurobehavioral activity different from that associated with parenteral medication. Much less do these data prove that spinal, or any other specific type of regional anesthesia, is necessarily worse than parenteral medication for delivery insofar as neonatal behavior is concerned. In fact, Hodgkinson, *et al.* (1978) found spinal anesthesia to be superior to general anesthesia in terms of neonatal neurobehavior. They studied 150 patients having elective cesarean sections: 50 were delivered with spinal anesthesia, 50 with thiopental-nitrous oxide-oxygen anesthesia, and 50 with ketamine-nitrous oxide-oxygen anesthesia. In the first and second days of life, spinal anesthesia was associated with higher neonatal scores for response to pinprick, tone, rooting, sucking, Moro response, alertness, and habituation. Similar results indicating that infants born by cesarean section are affected less by spinal anesthesia than infants born under general anesthesia, have been reported by Marx, *et al.* (1969, 1984), and Abboud, *et al.* (1985). The advantages of spinal anesthesia over general anesthesia, however, only were apparent immediately postpartum, as by 24 hr after birth, differences in infant behavior were no longer present (Abboud, *et al.*, 1985). Recently, Bader, *et al.*, (1990) reported that fetal blood gas values were affected significantly only when uterine incision-to-delivery time interval was prolonged, regardless of the anesthetic technique. These results are similar to those of Datta, *et al.* (1981). Also irrespective of its effect on neonatal behavior, the type of anesthesia used for delivery apparently has no discernible effects on neonatal feeding patterns. Abouleish, *et al.* (1978) found that 5 days postpartum, the weights of neonates were statistically the same following delivery under spinal anesthesia (57 babies), epidural anesthesia (118 babies), general anesthesia (34 babies), or without anesthesia (32 babies).

Role of Spinal Anesthesia in Obstetrics

Spinal anesthesia has now been in use in obstetrics for over 90 yr (Kreis, 1900), during which time it has been both condemned (Greenill, 1952; Crawford, 1988) and praised (Macer, 1956; Lull and Ullery, 1949; de Carle, 1954; Phillips, *et al.*, 1959; Poppers, 1978; Marx, *et al.*, 1984; Carrie, 1988). Past clinical experience, together with a substantial body of experimental data, support neither extreme. Although spinal anesthesia is not the alpha and omega of obstetric anesthesia, it should not be condemned. Obstetric spinal anesthesia has both advantages and disadvantages (Kestin, 1991; Spielman and Corke, 1985). The same is true for any other type of obstetrical anesthesia. This is not surprising. All anesthetics have their risks, obstetric as well as surgical, spinal as well as epidural, inhalation as well as intravenous.

One of the more conspicuous potential advantages of spinal anesthesia for pain relief during childbirth is that it avoids pharmacologic depression of the neonate which may be associated with general anesthesia or other forms of regional anesthesia (Chapter 10). This is of particular importance with premature infants but may be of theoretical advantage with full-term infants. There are no data from prospective studies proving that death rates for full-term infants delivered with well-managed spinal anesthesia are any different from those for infants delivered under equally skillfully administered general anesthesia. In the absence of prematurity, obstetric complications, or excessive narcotic usage, neonatal death rates are similar with both spinal and general anesthesia. This is as true today as it has been in the past, for vaginal delivery as well as for elective cesarean sections (Lund, 1955; McNeill, 1956; Points, 1956; Apgar, 1957). The same applies to comparisons between spinal and epidural anesthesia. Although spinal anesthesia has the possible advantage of producing lower fetal levels of local anesthetics (pp. 372374), its association with a decreased incidence of either neonatal deaths or abnormal neonatal development have yet to be proven, reported alterations in neonatal neurobehavioral activity ascribed to epidural anesthesia notwithstanding. The only large-scale, retrospective study (Ong, et al., 1989) has investigated the effects of general and regional anesthesia (3940 infants) on neonatal outcome. The authors defined neonatal outcome parameters as 1- and 5-min Apgar scores, need for oxygen therapy, and neonatal deaths (i.e., death within the first 30 days postpartum). This study, however, did not differentiate between epidural and spinal techniques (only 1% of regional techniques included spinal anesthesia). Nevertheless, the authors found that the frequency of low Apgar scores (1- and 5-min) was significantly higher in the general anesthesia than in the regional anesthesia groups, even when controlled for the possible bias introduced by the surgical indication for performing cesarean section (Table 8.3). The neonates delivered by nonelective cesarean section under general anesthesia also had more frequent requirements for intubation and artificial ventilation. Although not statistically significant, the percentage of neonatal deaths was higher in the general than in the regional anesthesia group. The authors concluded that "with appropriate neonatal care, the choice of anesthetic technique does not appear to affect neonatal survival in the short term."

Table 8.3.
Neonatal Outcomes After Cesarean Sections by Anesthetic Technique

Indication for Cesarean Section	Anesthetic Technique	Infants with 1-min Apgar Scores 0–4 (%)	Infants with 5-min Apgar Scores 0–4 (%)	Neonates Requiring Oxygen by Mask (%)	Neonates Requiring Tracheal Intubation and Ventilation (%)	Neonatal Deaths (%)
Elective	Regional	2.0	0.2	10.1	1.7	0.5
	General	6.5*	0.4	16.3†	0.8	1.2
Fetal distress	Regional	18.5	2.8	19.7	19.0	3.3
	General	43.5†	8.3†	18.0	42.5‡	6.5
Failure to progress	Regional	9.1	0.5	14.5	10.4	0.7
	General	23.0‡	3.4†	24.0‡	19.6‡	1.4

* $P \leq 0.05$.
† $P \leq 0.01$.
‡ $P \leq 0.001$.

The main advantage of spinal anesthesia for the mother is that along with other forms of regional anesthesia, it substantially reduces the danger of maternal vomiting and aspiration. This complication is one of the major, if not the foremost cause of preventable maternal anesthetic death. Spinal anesthesia is also highly effective in the presence of abnormal fetal positions or presentations, and for multiple births (Levinson and Shnider, 1987). According to reports, the vast majority of maternal deaths associated with spinal anesthesia have been due to one of three factors: the use of spinal anesthesia in cases of hemorrhagic shock, excessive dosage of the spinal anesthetic agent, or inappropriate management of an inadvertently high spinal. Most of these deaths, therefore, can be considered preventable. The low amount of spinal anesthetic agents commonly accepted as the maximal safe doses for obstetric cases should never be exceeded. Additionally, there are few, if any, indications for performing spinal anesthesia in the presence of shock, be it obstetric, surgical, or traumatic in origin. And there is no justification whatsoever for placing a patient with an inadvertently high level of anesthesia into reverse Trendelenburg position, merely to prevent the further cephalad ascent of the anesthetic. This almost certainly results in disaster, namely, cardiac arrest. Maternal death from spinal anesthesia can be prevented by fully understanding the pharmacologic and physiologic principles behind the method. For spinal anesthesia to be safe in obstetrics, it must be given only by those experienced in the technique. While inexperienced anesthetists should probably not administer spinal anesthetics to any patient, they should most certainly never do so to pregnant women.

Perhaps the greatest disadvantage of spinal anesthesia for the mother is that it provides slightly less satisfactory pain control during labor than epidural anesthesia (Chapter 10). Continuous epidural anesthesia is safer and more controllable than either continuous spinal anesthesia or the single injection of local anesthetic with a duration of action sufficient to relieve pain during what may constitute a prolonged labor. Continuous epidural anesthesia also has an advantage in that the height and intensity of anesthesia can be rapidly increased, should an obstetric complication arise that demands immediate cesarean section. On the other hand, if an emergency cesarean section becomes necessary in patient in whom continuous epidural anesthesia has not been established for labor, operative anesthesia can be achieved more rapidly with spinal than with epidural anesthesia.

REFERENCES

ABBOUD, T. K., NAGAPPALA, S., MURAKAWA, K., DAVID, S., HAROUTUNIAN, S., ZAKARIAN, M., YANAGI, T., SHEIKH-OL-ESLAM, A.: Comparison of the effects of general and regional anesthesia for cesarean section on neonatal neurologic and adaptive capacity scores. Anesth. Analg. *64*: 996, 1985.

ABOULEISH, E., VAN DER DONCK, A., MEEUWIS, H., AND TAYLOR, F.: Effect of anaesthesia for delivery on the weight of infants during the first five days of life. Br. J. Anaesth. *50*: 569, 1978.

AHLTORP, G.: Uber Ruckenlagebeschwerden bei Graviden. Acta Obstet. Gynecol. Scand. *15*: 295, 1935.

APGAR, V.: Comparison of results to infant following maternal regional or general anesthesia for delivery. N. Y. St. J. Med. *57*: 2955, 1957.

APGAR, V., HOLADAY, D. A., JAMES, S., PRINCE, C. E., WEISBROT, I. M., AND WEISS, I.: Comparison of regional and general anesthesia in obstetrics with special reference to transmission of cyclopropane across the placenta. J. A. M. A. 165: 2155, 1957.

ASSALI, N. S., KAPLAN, S. A., FOMON, S. J., DOUGLASS, R. A., AND ANDTADA, Y.: The effects of high spinal anesthesia on the renal hemodynamics and the excretion of electrolytes during osmotic diuresis in the hydropenic normal pregnant woman. J. Clin. Invest. *30*: 916, 1951.

ASSALI, N. S., AND PRYSTOWSKY, H.: Studies on autonomic blockade. I. Comparison between the effects of tetraethylammonium chloride (TEAC) and highly selective spinal anesthesia on the blood pressure of normal and toxemic pregnancy. J. Clin. Invest. *29*: 1354, 1950 a.

ASSALI, N. S., AND PRYSTOWSKY, H.: Studies on autonomic blockade. II. Observations on the nature of blood pressure fall with high selective spinal anesthesia in pregnant women. J. Clin. Invest. *29*: 1367, 1950 b.

ASSALI, N. S., AND ROSENKRANTZ, J. G.: Studies on autonomic blockade. V. Inhibition of water diuresis in pregnant women by high spinal anesthesia. Surg. Gynecol. Obstet. *93*: 468, 1951.

AXELSSON, K., AND WIDMAN, B.: Blood concentration of lidocaine after spinal anaesthesia using lidocaine and lidocaine with adrenaline. Acta. Anaesthesiol. Scand. *25*: 240, 1981.

BADER, A. M., DATTA, S., ARTHUR, G. R., BENVENUTI, E., COURTNEY, M., AND HAUCH, M.: Maternal and fetal catecholamines and uterine incision-to-delivery interval during elective cesarean. Obstet. Gynecol. *75*: 600, 1990.

BARCLAY, D. L., RENEGAR, O. J., AND NELSON, JR., E. W.: The influence of inferior vena cava compression on the level of spinal anesthesia. Am. J. Obstet. Gynecol. *101*: 792, 1968.

BONICA, J. J.: Peripheral mechanisms and pathways of parturition pain. Br. J. Anaesth. *51*: 3S, 1979.

BOSOMWORTH, P., SIKORA, F., AND WELCH, C. M.: Fetal ECG and obstetrical blood loss with halothane. Anesthesiology *23*: 140, 1960.

BRETT, C. M.: Cardiovascular physiology in pediatrics, in Gregory, G. A., *Pediatric Anesthesia*. Second Edition. New York: Churchill Livingstone, 1989.

BRIGDEN, W., HOWARTH, S., AND SHARPEY-SCHAFER, E. P.: Postural changes in the peripheral blood-flow of normal subjects with observations on vaso-vagal fainting reactions as a result of tilting, the lordotic posture, pregnancy, and spinal anesthesia. Clin. Sci. *9*: 79, 1950.

BURM, A. G., VAN KLEEF, J. W., GLADINES, M. P., SPIERDIJK, J., BREIMER, D. D.: Plasma concentrations of lidocaine and bupivacaine after subarachnoid administration. Anesthesiology *59*: 191, 1983.

BUTTERWORTH, J. F., IV, WALKER, F. O., AND LYSAK, S. Z.: Pregnancy increases median nerve susceptibility to lidocaine. Anesthesiology 72: 962, 1990.

CAMPBELL, D. M., AND MAC GILLIVRAY, I.: Comparison of maternal response in first and second pregnancies in relation to baby weight. J. Obstet. Gynaecol. Br. Commonw. *79*: 684, 1972.

CARITIS, S. N., ABOULEISH, E., EDELSTONE, D. I., AND MUELLER-HEUBACH, E.: Fetal acid-base state following spinal or epidural anesthesia for cesarean section. Obstet. Gynecol. *56:* 610, 1980.

CARRIE, L. E. S.: Debate on use of spinal anesthesia in obstetrics: spinal anesthesia has definite indications in obstetrics. Acta Anaesth. Belg. *39:* 177, 1988.

CHEEK, T. G., AND GUTSCHE, B. B.: Maternal physiologic alterations during pregnancy, in Shnider, S. M., Levinson, G., *Anesthesia for Obstetrics.* Second Edition. Baltimore: Williams & Wilkins, 1987.

CLARK, R. B., THOMPSON, D. S., AND THOMPSON, C. H.: Prevention of spinal hypotension with cesarean section. Anesthesiology *45:* 670, 1976.

CLELAND, J. P. G.: Paravertebral anesthesia in obstetrics: experimental and clinical basis. Surg. Gynecol. Obstet. *57:* 51, 1933.

CORKE, B. C., DATTA, S., OSTHEIMER, G. W., WEISS, J. B., AND ALPER, M. H.: Spinal anaesthesia for Caesarean section—the influence of hypotension on neonatal outcome. Anaesthesia *37:* 658, 1982.

CRAWFORD, J. S.: There is only a limited place for spinals in obstetrics. Acta Anaesth. Belg. *39:* 181, 1988.

CRAWFORD, M. E., AND MURPHY, J. T.: Spinal abruption. Obstet. Gynecol. *15:* 97, 1960.

DATTA, S., AND BROWN, W. U., JR.: Acid-base status in diabetic mothers and the infant following general or spinal anesthesia for cesarean section. Anesthesiology *47:* 272, 1977.

DATTA, S., KITZMILLER, J. L., NAULTY, J. S., OSTHEIMER, G. W., AND WEISS, J. B.: Acid-base status of diabetic mothers and the infant following spinal anesthesia for Cesarean section. Anesth. Analg. *61:* 662, 1982.

DATTA, S., OSTHEIMER, G. W., WEISS, J. B., BROWN, W. U., JR., AND ALPER, M. H.: Neonatal effect of prolonged anesthetic induction for cesarean section. Obstet. Gynecol. *58:* 331, 1981.

DATTA, S., HURLEY, R. J., NAULTY, J. S., STERN, P., LAMBERT, D. H., CONCEPCION, M., TULCHINSKY, D., WEISS, J. B., AND OSTHEIMER, G. W.: Plasma and cerebrospinal fluid progesterone concentrations in pregnant and nonpregnant women. Anesth. Analg. *65:* 950, 1986.

DATTA, S., LAMBERT, D. H., GREGUS, J., GISSEN, A. J., AND COVINO, B. G.: Differential sensitivities of mammalian nerve fibers during pregnancy. Anesth. Analg. *62:* 1070, 1983.

DATTA, S., OSTHEIMER, G. W., ALPER, M. H., AND WEISS, J. B.: Maternal and fetal lidocaine concentration following subarachnoid block for cesarean section. Anesthesiology *53:* S303, 1980.

DE CARLE, D. W.: Spinal anesthesia in cesarean section: critical analysis of about 1200 cases with no maternal mortality. J. A. M. A. *154:* 545, 1954.

DE JONG, R. H.: Arterial carbon dioxide and oxygen tensions during spinal block. J. A. M. A. *191:* 698, 1965.

DEVORE, J. S., AND EISLER, E. A.: Effects of anesthesia on uterine activity and labor, in Shnider, S. M., Levinson, G., *Anesthesia for Obstetrics.* Second Edition. Baltimore: Williams & Wilkins, 1987.

DUBELMAN, A. M., AND FORBES, A. R.: Does cough increase the spread of subarachnoid anesthesia? Anesth. Analg. *58:* 306, 1979.

DUMITRU, A. P., GARCIA, E. R., BURKHART, S. E., AND POTIER, J. K.: Convulsive seizure following spinal anesthesia for cesarean section. Anesth. Analg. *41:* 422, 1962.

EASTERLING, T. R., BENEDETTI, T. J., SCHMUCKER, B. C., AND MILLARD, S. P.: Maternal hemodynamics in normal and preeclamptic pregnancies: a longitudinal study. Obstet. Gynecol. *76:* 1061, 1990.

EBNER, H., BARCOHANA, J., AND BARTOSHUK, A. K.: Influence of postspinal hypotension on the fetal electrocardiogram. Am. J. Obstet. Gynecol. *80:* 569, 1960.

ECKSTEIN, K. L., AND MARX, G. F.: Aortocaval compression and uterine displacement. Anesthesiology *40:* 92, 1974.

ENG, M., BERGES, P. U., PARER, J. T., BONICA, J. J., AND UELAND, K.: Spinal anesthesia and ephedrine in pregnant monkeys. Am. J. Obstet. Gynecol. *115:* 1095, 1973.

ENG, M., BERGES, P. U., UELAND, K., BONICA, J. J., AND PARER, J. T.: The effects of methoxamine and ephedrine in normotensive pregnant primates. Anesthesiology *35:* 354, 1971.

EVANS, S. E., CRAWFORD, J. S., STEVENS, I. D., DURBIN, G. M., AND DAYA, H.: Fluid therapy for induced labour under epidural analgesia: biochemical consequences for mother and infant. Br. J. Obstet. Gynaecol. *93:* 329, 1986.

FITZGERALD, D. J., ROCKI, W., MURRAY, R., MAYO, G., AND FITZGERALD, G. A.: Thromboxane A_2 synthesis in pregnancy-induced hypertension. Lancet II: 751, 1990.

FLANAGAN, H. L., DATTA, S., LAMBERT, D. H., GISSEN, A. J., AND COVINO, B. G.: Effect of pregnancy on bupivacaine-induced conduction blockade in the isolated rabbit vagus nerve. Anesth. Analg. *66:* 123, 1987.

FLEXNER, L. B., COURIE, D. B., HELLMAN, L. M., WILDE, W. S., AND VOSBURGH, G. J.: The permeability of the human placenta to sodium in normal and abnormal pregnancies and the supply of sodium to the human fetus as determined with radioactive sodium. Am. J. Obstet. Gynecol. *55:* 469, 1948.

FRANKEN, H.: Warum ist die Lumbalanasthesie beim Kiserschnitt besonders gefahrlich. Zentslbl. Gynak. *58:* 2191, 1934.

GIASI, R. M., D'AGOSTINO, E., AND COVINO, B. G.: Absorption of lidocaine following subarachnoid and epidural administration. Anesth. Analg. *58:* 360, 1979.

GREENE, N. M.: Distribution of local anesthetic solutions within the subarachnoid space. Anesth. Analg. *64:* 715, 1985.

GREENHILL, J. P.: *Analgesia and Anesthesia in Obstetrics.* Springfield, Illinois: Charles C. Thomas, 1952.

GREISS, F. C., JR.: Pressure-flow relationship in the gravid uterine vascular bed. Am. J. Obstet. Gynecol. *96:* 41, 1966.

GREISS, F. C., JR., AND CRANDELL, D. L.: Therapy for hypotension induced by spinal anesthesia during pregnancy: observations on gravid ewes. J. A. M. A. *191:* 793, 1965.

GRYLACK, L. J., CHU, S. S., AND SCANLON, J. W.: Use of intravenous fluids before cesarean section. Effects on perinatal glucose, insulin, and sodium homeostasis. Obstet. Gynecol. *63:* 654, 1984.

GUTSCHE, B. B.: Prophylactic ephedrine preceding spinal anesthesia for cesarean section. Anesthesiology *45:* 462, 1976.

GUTSCHE, B. B., AND CHEEK, T. G.: Anesthetic considerations in preeclampsia-eclampsia, in Snider S. M., Levinson, G., *Anesthesia for Obstetrics.* Second Edition. Baltimore: Williams & Wilkins, 1987.

HASELHORST, G., AND STROMBERGER, K.: Ueber den Gasgehalt des Nabelschnurblutes vor und nach der Geburt des Kindes und uber den Gasaustausch in der Plazenta. II. Mitteilung. Ztschr. Geburtsh. u. Gynak. *102:* 16, 1932.

HENDERSON, H., MOSHER, R., AND BITTRICH, N. M.: Oxygen studies of the cord blood of cesarean born infants. Am. J. Obstet. Gynecol. *73:* 664, 1957.

HINGSON, R. A.: New horizons in therapeutic nerve block in the treatment of vascular and renal emergencies with continuous caudal and continuous spinal analgesia and anesthesia. South. Surgeon *13:* 580, 1947.

HODGKINSON, R., BHATT, M., KIM, S. S., GREWAL, G., AND MARX, G. F.: Neonatal neurobehavioral tests following cesarean section under general and spinal anesthesia. Am. J. Obstet. Gynecol. *132:* 670, 1978.

HOLMES, F.: Incidence of supine hypotensive syndrome in late pregnancy. J. Obstet. Gynecol. Br. Commonw. *67:* 254, 1960.

HON, E. H., REID, B. L., AND HEHRE, F. W.: The electronic evaluation of fetal heart rate. II. Changes with maternal hypotension. Am. J. Obstet. Gynecol. *79:* 209, 1960.

HOPKINS, E. L., HENDRICKS, C. M., AND CIBILS, L. A.: Cerebrospinal fluid pressure in labor. Am. J. Obstet. Gynecol. *93:* 907, 1965.

JOHNSON, T., AND CLAYTON, C. G.: Studies in placental action during prolonged and dysfunctional labours using radioactive sodium. J. Obstet. Gynecol. Br. Emp. 62: 513, 1955.

JOHNSON, W. L., WINTER, W. W., ENG, M., BONICA, J. J., AND HUNTER, C. A.: Effect of pudendal, spinal and peridural block anesthesia on the second stage of labor. Am. J. Obstet. Gynecol. 113: 166, 1972.

JOUPPILA, P., JOUPPILA, R., BARINOFF, T., AND KOIVULA, A.: Placental blood flow during caesarean section performed under subarachnoid blockade. Br. J. Anaesth 56: 1379, 1984.

KANG, Y. G., ABOULEISH, E., AND CARITIS, S.: Prophylactic intravenous ephedrine infusion during spinal anesthesia for cesarean section. Anesth. Analg. 61: 839, 1982.

KAPLAN, S. A., AND ASSALI, N. S.: Effects of apresoline, veratrum alkaloids, high spinal anesthesia, and Arfonad on renal hemodynamics of pregnant patients with toxemia and essential hypertension. Surg. Gynecol. Obstet. 97: 501, 1953.

KENNEDY, R. L., FRIEDMAN, D. L., KATCHKA, D. M., SELMANTS, S., AND SMITH, R. N.: Hypotension during obstetrical anesthesia. Anesthesiology 20: 153, 1959.

KESTIN, I. G.: Spinal anaesthesia in obstetrics. Br. J. Anaesth. 66: 596, 1991.

KREIS, O.: Ueber Medullarnarkose bei Gebarenden. Zentalbl Gynak, p. 724, July 14, 1900.

KUHNERT, B. R., PHILIPSON, E. H., PIMENTAL, R., KUHNERT, P. M., ZUSPAN, K. J., AND SYRACUSE, C. D.: Lidocaine disposition in mother, fetus, and neonate after spinal anesthesia. Anesth. Analg. 65: 139, 1986.

LECHNER, R. B., AND CHADWICK, H. S.: Anesthetic care of the patient with preeclampsia, in Reisner, L. S., Obstetric Anesthesia. Anesthesiology Clinics of North America. Vol. 8, No. 1. Philadelphia: W. B. Saunders Co., 1990.

LEVINSON, G., AND SHNIDER, S. M.: Anesthesia for abnormal positions and presentations and multiple births, in: Shnider, S. M., and Levinson, G., Anesthesia for Obstetrics. Second Edition, Baltimore: Williams & Wilkins, 1987.

LINDBLAD, A., BERNOW, J., AND MARSAL, K.: Fetal blood flow during intrathecal anaesthesia for elective caesarean section. Br. J. Anaesth 61: 376, 1988.

LOONG, E. P., LAO, T. T., AND CHIN, R. K.: Effects of intrapartum intravenous infusion of 5% dextrose or Hartmann's solution on maternal and cord blood glucose. Acta. Obstet. Gynecol. Scand. 66: 241, 1987.

LUCAS, W. E., KIRSCHBAUM, T. H., AND ASSALI, N. S.: Effects of autonomic blockade with spinal anesthesia on uterine and fetal hemodynamics and oxygen consumption in sheep. Biol. Neonat. 10: 166, 1966.

LULL, C. B., AND HINGSON, R. A.: Control of Pain in Childbirth; Anesthesia, Analgesia, Amnesia. Philadelphia: J. B. Lippincott Co., 1948.

LULL, C. B., AND ULLERY, J. C.: Continuous spinal anesthesia in cesarean section. Am. J. Obstet. Gynecol. 57: 1199, 1949.

LUND, P. C.: The role of conduction anesthesia in the management of eclampsia. Anesthesiology 12: 693, 1951.

LUND, P. C.: The role of the anesthesiologist in the management of eclampsia. Anesth. Analg. 31: 378, 1952.

LUND, P. C.: Influence of anesthesia on infant mortality rate in cesarean sections. J. A. M. A. 159: 1586, 1955.

McELRATH, P. J., WARE, H. H., JR., WINN, W. C., AND SCHELIN, E. C.: Continuous spinal anesthesia in the treatment of severe pre-eclampsia and eclampsia. Am. J. Obstet. Gynecol. 58: 1084, 1949.

McLENNAN, C. E.: Antecubital and femoral venous pressure in normal and toxemic pregnancy. Am. J. Obstet. Gynecol. 45: 568, 1943.

McNEILL, D. B.: Perinatal mortality associated with cesarean section. Am. J. Obstet. Gynecol. 71: 304, 1956.

MACER, G. A.: Spinal anesthesia in more than thirty-four thousand vaginal deliveries. West. J. Surg. 64: 625, 1956.

MARX, G. F., LUYKX, W. M., AND COHEN, S.: Fetal-neonatal status following caesarean section for fetal distress. Br. J. Anaesth. 56: 1009, 1984.

MARX, G. F., COSMI, E. V., WOLLMAN, S. B.: Biochemical status and clinical condition of mother and infant at cesarean section. Anesth. Analg. 48: 986, 1969.

MARX, G. F., OKA, Y., AND ORKIN, L. R.: Cerebrospinal fluid pressures during labor. Am. J. Obstet. Gynecol. 84: 213, 1962.

MARX, G. F., AND ORKIN, L. R.: Cerebrospinal fluid proteins and spinal anesthesia in obstetrics. Anesthesiology 26: 340, 1965.

MARX, G. F., ZEMAITIS, M. T., AND ORKIN, L. R.: Cerebrospinal fluid pressures during labor and obstetrical anesthesia. Anesthesiology 22: 348, 1961.

MATHRU, M., RAO, T. L. K., KARTHA, R. K., AND SHANMUGHAM, M.: Intravenous albumin administration for prevention of spinal hypotension during Cesarean section. Anesth. Analg. 59: 655, 1980.

MESSMER, K. F. W.: The use of plasma substitutes with special attention to their side effects. World J. Surg. 11: 69, 1987.

MOIR, D. D.: Local anaesthetic techniques in obstetrics. Br. J. Anaesth. 58: 747, 1986.

MORAN, D. H., PERILLO, M., LAPORTA, R. F., BADER, A. M., AND DATTA, S.: Phenylephrine in the prevention of hypotension following spinal anesthesia for cesarean delivery. J. Clin. Anesth. 3: 301, 1991.

MORTON, K. E., JACKSON, M. C., GILLMER, M. D.: A comparison of the effects of four intravenous solutions for the treatment of ketonuria during labour. Br. J. Obstet. Gynaecol. 92: 473, 1985.

MOYA, F., AND SMITH, B.: Spinal anesthesia for cesarean section. J. A. M. A. 179: 609, 1962.

MUNOZ, E.: Costs of alternative colloid solutions (dextran, starch, albumin). Intensive Care World 4: 12, 1987.

MYLKS, G. W., JONES, K., AND DOUGLAS-MURRAY, G. M.: Acute fulminating eclampsia—management in conjunction with prolonged epidural sympathetic block. Can. Med. Assoc. J. 82: 422, 1960.

NORRIS, M. C.: Hypotension during spinal anesthesia for cesarean section: does it affect neonatal outcome? Regional Anesth. 12: 191, 1987.

ONG, B. Y., COHEN, M. M., AND PALAHNIUK, R. J.: Anesthesia for cesarean section—effects on neonates. Anesth. Analg. 68: 270, 1989.

OSKI, F. A., AND DELIVORIA-PAPADOUPOULOS, M.: The red cell, 2,3-diphosphoglycerate, and tissue oxygen release. J. Pediatr. 77: 941, 1970.

PHILLIPS, K. G.: The relative effects of obstetrical anesthesia and analgesia upon the promptness of neonatal respiration. Am. J. Obstet. Gynecol. 77: 113, 1959.

PHILLIPS, O. C., NELSON, A. T., LYONS, W. B., GRAFF, T. D., HARRIS, L. C., AND FRAZIER, T. M.: Spinal anesthesia for vaginal delivery: a review of 2016 cases using Xylocaine. Obstet. Gynecol. 13: 437, 1959.

PHILIPSON, E. H., KALHAN, S. C., RIHA, M. M., AND PIMENTEL, R.: Effects of maternal glucose infusion on fetal acid-base status in human pregnancy. Am. J. Obstet. Gynecol. 157: 866, 1987.

POINTS, T. C.: Premature and term infant mortality as affected by types of anesthesia and delivery. Am. J. Obstet. Gynecol. 71: 1210, 1956.

POPPERS, P. J.: Die Spinalanaesthesie in der Geburtshilfe. Reg. Anaesth. 1: 47, 1978.

PRITCHARD, J. A.: Changes in the blood volume during pregnancy and delivery. Anesthesiology 26: 393, 1965.

PROWSE, C. M., AND GAENSLER, E. A.: Respiratory and acid-base changes during pregnancy. Anesthesiology 26: 378, 1965.

QUILLIGAN, E. J., KATIGBAK, E., NOWACEK, C., AND CZARNECKI, N.: Correlation of fetal heart rate patterns and blood gas values. I. Normal heart rate values. Am. J. Obstet. Gynecol. 90: 1343, 1964.

RALSTON, D. H., AND SHNIDER, S. M.: The fetal and neonatal effects of regional anesthesia in obstetrics. Anesthesiology 48: 34, 1978.

RALSTON, D. H., SHNIDER, S. M., AND DE LORIMIER, A. A.: Effect of equipotent ephedrine, metaraminol, mephentermine, and methoxamine on uterine blood flow in the pregnant ewe. Anesthesiology 40: 354, 1974.

ROGERS, S. F., FLOWERS, C. E., JR., AND ALEXANDER, J. A.: Aggressive toxemia management (pre-eclampsia and eclampsia). Obstet. Gynecol. 33: 724, 1969.

ROLBIN, S. H., LEVINSON, G., SHNIDER, S. M., BIEHL, D. R., AND WRIGHT, R. G.: Dopamine treatment of spinal hypotension decreases uterine blood flow in the pregnant ewe. Anesthesiology 51: 36, 1979.

ROMAN, D. A., AND ADRIANI, J.: Spinal anesthesia for cesarean section. New Orleans Med. Surg. J. 101: 19, 1948.

RUNGE, H.: Ueber den Venedruck in Schwangerschaft, Oeburt, und Wochenbett. Arch. Gynak. 122: 142, 1924.

RUSSELL, I. F.: Spinal anaesthesia for Caesarean section. Br. J. Anaesth. 55: 309, 1983.

RUSSELL, I. F.: Posture and isobaric subarachnoid anaesthesia. Anaesthesia 39: 865, 1984.

RUSSELL, I. F.: Effect of posture during the induction of subarachnoid analgesia for Caesarean section: right v. left lateral. Br. J. Anaesth. 59: 342, 1987.

SCANLON, J. W., BROWN, W. U., JR., WEISS, J. B., AND ALPER, M. H.: Neurobehavioral responses of newborn infants after maternal anesthesia. Anesthesiology 40: 121, 1974.

SHIELDS, L. V., AND TAYLOR, E. S.: Serial oxygen saturation studies of newborn infants following obstetrical complications, difficult deliveries, and cesarean section. Am. J. Obstet. Gynecol. 73: 1011, 1957.

SHNIDER, S. M.: Vasopressors in obstetrics. Regional Anesth. 8: 74, 1983.

SHNIDER, S. M., DE LORIMIER, A. A., ASLING, J. H., AND MORISHIMA, H. O.: Vasopressors in obstetrics. II. Fetal hazards of methoxamine during obstetric spinal anesthesia. Am. J. Obstet. Gynecol. 106: 680, 1970.

SHNIDER, S. M., DE LORIMIER, A. A., HOLL, J. W., CHAPLER, F. K., AND MORISHIMA, H. O.: Vasopressors in obstetrics. I. Correction of fetal acidosis with ephedrine during spinal hypotension. Am. J. Obstet. Gynecol. 102: 911, 1968.

SMITH, B. E., CAVANAGH, D., AND MOYA, F.: Anesthesia for vaginal delivery of the patient with toxemia of pregnancy. Anesthesiology 45: 853, 1966.

SMITH, B. E., MOYA, F., AND SHNIDER, S. M.: The effects of anesthesia on liver function during labor. Anesth. Analg. 41: 24, 1962.

SPIELMAN, F. J., AND CORKE, B. C.: Advantages and disadvantages of regional anesthesia for cesarean section. J. Reprod. Med. 30: 832, 1985.

STANLEY, K., SOULE, A. B., III, COPANS, S. A., AND DUCHOWNY, M. S.: Local regional anesthesia during childbirth: effect on newborn behavior. Science 186: 634, 1974.

STENGER, V., ANDERSON, T., DE PADNA, C., EITZMAN, D., GESSNER, I., AND PRYSTOWSKY, H.: Spinal anesthesia for cesarean section. Physiological and biochemical observations. Am. J. Obstet. Gynecol. 90: 51, 1964.

TAYLOR, E. S., GOVAN, C. D., AND SCOTT, W. C.: Oxygen saturation of the blood of the newborn as affected by maternal anesthetic agents. Am. J. Obstet. Gynecol. 61: 840, 1951 a.

TAYLOR, E. S., SCOTT, W. C., AND GOVAN, C. D.: Studies of blood oxygen saturation and causes of death in premature infants. Am. J. Obstet. Gynecol. 62: 764, 1951 b.

TRONICK, E., WISE, S., ALS, H., ADAMSON, L., SCANLON, J., AND BRAZELTON, T. B.: Regional obstetric anesthesia and newborn behavior: effect over the first ten days of life. Pediatrics 58: 94, 1976.

TUOHY, E. B.: The adaptations of continuous spinal anesthesia. Anesth. Analg. 31: 372, 1952.

TURNER, H. B., AND HOUCK, C. R.: Renal hemodynamics in the toxemias of pregnancy;

alterations of kidney function by regional nerve block. Am. J. Obstet. Gynecol. *60:* 117, 1950.

UELAND, K., GILLS, R. E., AND HANSEN, J. M.: Maternal cardiovascular dynamics. I. Cesarean section under subarachnoid block anesthesia. Am. J. Obstet. Gynecol. *100:* 42, 1968.

VASIKA, A., HUTCHINSON, H. T., ENG, M., AND ALLEN, C. R.: Spinal and epidural anesthesia, fetal and uterine response to acute hypo- and hypertension. Am. J. Obstet. Gynecol. *90:* 800, 1964.

VASIKA, A., AND KRETCHMER, H.: Effect of conduction and inhalation anesthesia on uterine contractions. Am. J. Obstet. Gynecol. *82:* 600, 1961.

WENNBERG, E., FRID, I., HALJAMAE, H., WENNERGREN, M., AND KJELLMER, I.: Comparison of Ringer's acetate with 3% dextran 70 for volume loading before extradural caesarean section. Br. J. Anaesth. *65:* 654, 1990.

WHITACRE, F. E., HINGSON, R. A., AND TURNER, H. D.: The treatment of eclampsia by means of regional nerve block. South. Med. J. *41:* 920, 1948.

WOLLMAN, S. B., AND MARX, G. F.: Acute hydration for prevention of hypotension of spinal anesthesia in parturients. Anesthesiology *29:* 374, 1968.

WRIGHT, J. P.: Anesthetic considerations in preeclampsia-eclampsia. Anesth. Analg. *62:* 590, 1983.

WRIGHT, R. G., AND SHNIDER, S. M.: Hypotension and regional anesthesia in obstetrics, in Schnider, S. M. and Levinson, G., *Anesthesia for Obstetrics*. Second Edition. Baltimore: Williams & Wilkins, 1987.

ZIMMER, E. Z., GOLDSTEIN, I., FELDMAN, E., AND GLIK, A.: Maternal and newborn levels of glucose, sodium and osmolality after preloading with three intravenous solutions during elective cesarean sections. Eur. J. Obstet. Gynecol. Reprod. Biol. *23:* 61, 1986.

CHAPTER 9

Gastrointestinal Tract

The effect of spinal anesthesia on the gastrointestinal tract is related to the extent of subarachnoid preganglionic sympathetic block. The reader is referred to Tables 1.7 and 1.8, p. 24 and 25, for an outline of the sympathetic innervation of intraperitoneal organs.

The motor innervation of the esophagus is mainly (White, *et al.*, 1952), if not entirely (Ingram, 1947), parasympathetic in origin. Therefore, spinal anesthesia has no significant effect on normal esophageal motility or tone. Despite this, spinal anesthesia has been reported as being of therapeutic value in the treatment of cardiospasm (Telford and Simmons, 1939). However, in view of the complex pathogenesis of cardiospasm and in view of what is known of the motor innervation of esophageal musculature, it is doubtful whether spinal anesthesia is of any value as a reliable diagnostic or therapeutic technic in cases of lower esophageal obstructions.

Sympathetic nerves to the stomach serve to inhibit peristalsis and gastric secretion, to contract the pylorus, and to produce constriction in gastric vessels. Spinal anesthesia high enough to produce sympathetic block of the fifth thoracic segmental level would, therefore, be expected to be associated with increased peristalsis, increased secretion, and relaxation of the pylorus. Few studies have been reported, however, on gastric changes during spinal anesthesia. Those published indicate that there is complete gastric inhibition (Curtis and Barron, 1936). However, the inhibition may have been due to factors other than spinal anesthesia (e.g., narcotics), as suggested by the fact that inhibition persisted for 24 hr after anesthesia.

Sympathetic denervation produced by spinal anesthesia causes contraction of the bowel, including jejunum, ileum, and colon, due to the unopposed action of the parasympathetic nervous system. It is associated with an increase in propulsive force of peristalsis, but not usually with an increase in frequency of peristaltic waves (Burstein, 1939; Golden and Mann, 1943; Sarnoff, *et al.*, 1948). Spinal anesthesia is also associated with an increase in intraluminal pressure within the intestinal tract, the degree of elevation ranging from 15 percent to 100 percent (Eckenhoff and Cannard, 1960).

Contraction of the intestine caused by spinal anesthesia, especially when accompanied by relaxation of the abdominal wall, provides operating conditions that are nearly ideal for intra-abdominal surgery—a long-recognized attraction of this technique. Contraction of the intestine during spinal anesthesia has, however, also led to the suggestion on the part of some anesthetists (and fewer surgeons) that the incidence of postoperative disruption of intestinal anastomoses is increased by spinal anesthesia. Indeed, it has been stated (Treissman, 1980) that this danger is so great that "surgery of the colon should be considered a relative contraindication for epidural anesthesia," a conclusion that, if correct, should also apply to spinal anesthesia, since it has the same effect on the intestine as epidural anesthesia. Objective clinical data fail to support such a conclusion, however. In the only objective retrospective study of this problem based on statistically valid numbers of patients, Aitkenhead, et al. (1978 b) found that the incidence of anastomotic breakdown following large bowel surgery was 7.0 percent (3 in 43 patients) when spinal anesthesia was used, 8.0 percent (2 in 25 patients) when epidural anesthesia was used, and 23.1 percent (6 in 26 patients) when general anesthesia was used. The differences were not statistically significant. A subsequent prospective study by the same group (Worsley, et al., 1988) confirmed these findings: colonic anastomotic dehiscence occurred in 17.0 percent of 47 patients having large bowel surgery under spinal anesthesia with light general anesthesia, and in 17.6 percent of 51 patients having general anesthesia (thiopental induction and nitrous oxide-halothane-morphine maintenance of anesthesia), a difference that was not statistically significant. Objective data to date fail to confirm the hypothetical advantages of spinal anesthesia for surgery involving intestinal anastomoses. The question deserves further study, however, if for no other reason that, while not statistically significant, the difference in frequency of postoperative anastomotic dehiscence was so great between spinal anesthesia (7.4 percent) and general anesthesia (23 percent) in the paper by Aitkenhead, et al. (1978 b).

The studies of Aitkenhead, et al. (1988 b) and of Worsley, et al. (1988) also fail to support the contention that the incidence of anastomotic breakdown associated with neostigmine is increased because of the increased intestinal tone caused by neostigmine (Bell and Lewis, 1968; Bell, 1970). In both studies neostigmine was always given at the end of general anesthesia to reverse intraoperatively administered neuromuscular relaxants, but was never used with spinal anesthesia; yet, the incidence of anastomotic disruption was similar after both spinal and general anesthesia. The same was true for morphine: the frequency of anastomotic breakdown was the same with and without intraoperatively administered morphine.

Contraction of the bowel produced by the sympathetic denervation associated with spinal anesthesia has led to the early suggestion that not only can the incidence of postoperative ileus be decreased by spinal anesthesia but so, too, spinal anesthesia can be used in management of postoperative ileus (Ochsner, *et al.*, 1930). Indeed, Shaw and Wolcott (1963) found, after a variety of operations, that return of normal intestinal activity, as measured by the presence of flatus within 48 hr and the occurrence of bowel movements within 72 hr, was significantly more rapid after spinal than after general anesthesia. Aitkenhead, *et al.* (1978 b), on the other hand, found no statistically significant difference in the frequency of paralytic or mechanical ileus following colon surgery that could be related to the type of anesthesia. Ileus occurred within the first 3 postoperative days in 19.2 percent of 26 patients undergoing general anesthesia, and, in 23.1 percent, it occurred more than 3 days postoperatively. Corresponding values for spinal anesthesia were 11.6 and 11.6 percent (of 43 patients), and 12 percent and 4 percent (of 25 patients) for epidural anesthesia. The site and type of operation, narcotics, age, obesity, and the presence of concurrent diseases are such major factors in determining the rate at which intestinal function returns postoperatively that the type of anesthesia probably plays little, if any, role of clinical significance.

A hypothetical, and not yet quantitated, advantage of spinal anesthesia in patients having colectomies for carcinoma centers about the observation that for some yet unexplained reason, patients having this type of surgery survive longer if they are not given blood transfusions intraoperatively (Burrows and Tartter, 1982; Foster, *et al.*, 1985; Blumberg, *et al.*, 1985). In the patients studied by Aitkenhead, *et al.*, none of 43 patients given spinal anesthesia (mean intraoperative blood loss 27 ± 4 ml) required an intraoperative transfusion; 8 of the 26 patients given general anesthesia (mean intraoperative blood loss 430 ± 109 ml) required intraoperative transfusion. The difference in frequency of the need for intraoperative transfusion was statistically significant. Worsley, *et al.* (1988), however, reported that 10.6 percent of 47 patients given spinal anesthesia for surgery requiring large bowel anastomoses (mean intraoperative blood loss 105 ± 205 ml) needed intraoperative transfusion, and 21.6% of 51 patients having general anesthesia (mean intraoperative blood loss 288 ± 288 ml) needed intraoperative transfusion; this difference was not statistically significant (although this difference may be clinically relevant). In these two studies, the frequency of transfusion was related to the degree of intraoperative decrease in mean arterial pressure below preoperative levels. No data were given on the frequency of recurrence of carcinoma in the two groups. The relationship, if any, between type of anesthesia, intraoperative transfusion and postoperative recurrence of cancer following colonic anastomoses for cancer deserves further study.

The increase in propulsive activity of the bowel caused by spinal anesthesia has led to its therapeutic application in cases of intestinal obstruction following paralytic ileus, and as a diagnostic measure in cases of megacolon (Mayer 1921, 1922; Wagner, 1922; Asteriades, 1925; Markowitz and Campbell, 1927; Scott and Morton, 1930; Ochsner, et al., 1930; Stabins, et al., 1935; Härtel, 1936; Sarnoff, et al., 1948; Tuohy, 1952). With regard to paralytic ileus, it should be emphasized that the beneficial effects of spinal anesthesia may be offset by the simultaneous administration of morphine or atropine. Such drugs effectively prevent the contraction of the bowel that normally occurs after spinal anesthesia (Domenech, 1929; Helm and Ingelfinger, 1944). Spinal anesthesia is not as effective in the treatment of paralytic ileus as decompression of the bowel by gastric or intestinal intubation; it can give only temporary relief in ileus and always carries the risk of perforation of previously weakened areas in the bowel wall when organic obstruction is superimposed on paralytic obstruction.

Spinal anesthesia has also been suggested as a diagnostic and therapeutic measure in so-called "spastic" intestinal obstruction, that is, obstruction caused by neurogenic imbalance resulting in abnormally strong contraction of one or more segments of bowel. Parasympathetic activity increases the tone of intestinal smooth muscle, and activity of the sympathetic nervous system decreases it. It is, therefore, difficult to understand how sympathetic hyperactivity would result in neurogenic spastic intestinal obstruction or how sympathetic denervation by spinal anesthesia would be expected to relieve neurogenic spastic disorders involving jejunum or ileum. It might, however, in some cases relieve neurogenic spasm of the colon. Here, the relief, if any, would be due to subarachnoid block of the parasympathetic fibers from the second, third, and fourth sacral segments, rather than to preganglionic sympathetic block.

The changes in the gastrointestinal tract just discussed are not attended by changes in splanchnic vascular resistance or total splanchnic blood flow during spinal anesthesia (Mueller, et al., 1952; Sancetta, et al., 1952; Sivarajan, et al., 1975). Regional blood flow and vascular resistance within the splanchnic bed, however, may change during spinal anesthesia and thereby produce areas of relative hyper- or hypoperfusion, even in the absence of changes in total flow to the splanchnic circulation (Chapter 2). Thus, Aitkenhead, et al. (1978 a) reported in an abstract that (in dogs) spinal anesthesia was associated with a 22 percent increase in colonic blood flow and a 45 percent decrease in colonic vascular resistance. In the more detailed report of the same study (Aitkenhead, et al., 1980), colon blood flow was found to increase 22.3 percent over baseline levels during spinal anesthesia, concurrent with decreases in both colonic vascular resistance (43.9 percent) and total peripheral vascular resistance (31.5 percent), and a parallel decrease in mean arterial blood pressure (31.4 percent). The increase in colon blood flow during spinal anesthesia occurred during both hyper- and hypocapnia. In this study, a statistically significant 17.3 percent decrease in colon oxygen consumption was observed, which was associated with statistically significant increases in the differences between both arteriovenous oxygen content and tension. This suggests that, during spinal anesthesia, the decrease in oxygen consumption reflected decreases in oxygen demand, that is, work, not decreases in availability or delivery of oxygen to the colon. Bohlen and Gore (1977) suggested that the increase in intestinal blood flow associated with sympathetic denervation is related not to increased pressure of the arterioles induced by vasodilation, but instead to a decrease in venular back pressure which increases the effective perfusion pressure across the capillary bed. This assumption is consistent with the data reported by Aitkenhead, *et al.* (1980). Bohlen and Gore found that the increase in intestinal blood flow that occurs following denervation involves intestinal smooth muscle. Whether it also involves intestinal mucosa, submucosa, and adventitia is undetermined.

The influence of spinal anesthesia on absorption of fluids and other substances across the mucosal wall of the gastrointestinal tract has been little studied. The only report dealing with this subject is that by Howard and David (1954). They found, in a limited number of patients, that following oral ingestion of water labeled with deuterium oxide, venous blood levels of deuterium oxide reached higher levels more rapidly during spinal anesthesia than they did in the same patients when not under spinal anesthesia. The results could be explained either on the basis of alterations in permeability of the mucosa to water or to changes in blood flow to the intestines. The blood levels of deuterium oxide also remained elevated for longer periods of time during spinal anesthesia, but this was probably the result of decreased urinary output.

Nausea and vomiting frequently accompany spinal anesthesia and are most likely to happen when the level of sensory anesthesia extends to above the tenth thoracic segment (Crocker and Vandam, 1959). Sometimes such disturbances are caused by traction on the vagi during intra-abdominal manipulations; sometimes they are caused by psychogenic factors. Nausea and vomiting may occur, however, even before surgery has been started. In such circumstances spinal anesthesia is clearly to blame and for two main reasons. One is cerebral hypoxia, the other increased gastric motility.

If arterial blood pressure decreases to the extent that cerebral blood flow is decreased, central hypoxia will occur and will be followed by nausea and vomiting. Observations on this phenomenon have been made by Kety, *et al.* (1950), who found during differential spinal anesthesia in humans that when the blood pressure fell low enough to cause a reduction in cerebral blood flow, nausea and vomiting occurred. The significant factor is not hypotension *per se* but rather the reduction in cerebral blood flow that may be associated with it. During clinical spinal anesthesia, the same degree of hypotension is not always accompanied by nausea and vomiting. This occurs because, in some patients, cerebral blood flow remains relatively unchanged during hypotension.

On the other hand, there are patients who experience nausea and vomiting even when not hypotensive. There are other patients in whom nausea and vomiting persist after elevation of low blood pressure to normal and, presumably, restoration of cerebral blood flow to normal. In these patients, nausea and vomiting are probably the result of increased gastric peristalsis following preganglionic sympathetic denervation of the stomach. This type of nausea and vomiting is usually transitory in nature. Apparently, the changes in gastric physiology produced by the high spinal blockade that cause nausea and vomiting may spontaneously regress with time. The fact that rapidly obtained high levels of sensory anesthesia are more frequently accompanied by nausea and vomiting than are equally high levels achieved more gradually (Sancetta, et al., 1952), is probably due to the fact that in the former cases the changes in gastric motility, and especially the increased peristalsis, are brought about more rapidly.

The nausea and vomiting that accompany spinal anesthesia are not caused by anoxia. Measurements of arterial oxygen content during such nausea and vomiting show normal oxygenation (Latterell and Lundy, 1949), and the successful treatment of the condition once it has become established during anesthesia may be accomplished without changing arterial oxygen tension (de Jong, 1965).

The various factors involved in vomiting during spinal anesthesia have been evaluated by Ratra, et al. (1972) in a study that is especially useful because of careful patient selection to control many of the etiologic factors involved in vomiting during spinal anesthesia. All of the 133 patients studied were females, all were aged 35–40 yr, all had either perineal operations or abdominal hysterectomies, and all had, of course, spinal anesthesia. Nausea, a subjective sensation notoriously difficult to quantitate, was not evaluated, only retching and emesis were. When oxygen was administered during anesthesia to unpremedicated patients, the incidence of vomiting was significantly less (16.6 percent) than it was when oxygen was not administered to similarly unpremedicated patients having the same operation (64.7 percent). Premedication with chlorpromazine significantly decreased the incidence of vomiting (30.7 percent). Premedication with meperidine (90.0 percent of the patients had vomiting) or atropine (54.0 percent had vomiting) had no statistically significant effect. Hypotension was associated with a significant increase in the incidence of vomiting: 70.6 percent of patients in whom systolic blood pressure decreased below 80 mmHg vomited; 37.7 percent of patients in whom systolic pressure was maintained above 80 mmHg by intravenous fluids or vasopressors had vomiting.

That the data derived from the all-female population of patients studied by Ratra *et al.* may be applicable to males is suggested by data in Crocker and Vandam's (1959) study, which showed that the incidence of intraoperative nausea and vomiting was unrelated to gender. The clinical impression that the incidence of nausea and vomiting is increased during spinal anesthesia for cesarean section in term parturients has never been subjected to a prospective, statistically valid study in which the frequency of intraoperative nausea and vomiting was measured, not only during spinal anesthesia for cesarean section, but also simultaneously in patients (both male and female) of similar ages who had similar anesthetic management, including equal sensory levels of spinal anesthesia for lower abdominal surgery. Also, an age-related increase in the frequency of nausea and vomiting in both males and females during spinal anesthesia has been reported in geriatric patients by Chunt, *et al.*, 1987.

The correlation of hypotension with nausea and vomiting so widely observed during spinal, and so well quantitated by Ratra, *et al.*, by Crocker and Vandam, and others may, however, represent just that: a correlation, not proof positive, that a cause-and-effect relation exists. Hypotension is not the single, sole cause of nausea and vomiting during spinal anesthesia, and nausea and vomiting can occur in the absence of hypotension during spinal anesthesia. Conversely, hypotension can occur without development of nausea and vomiting. Indeed, Spelina, *et al.* (1984) found in their study of 77 patients that mean arterial blood pressure did not differ significantly in patients with and without intraoperative nausea and vomiting. Confusion arises about this conclusion, however, because these authors also state that mean arterial blood pressure was significantly lower in patients who developed nausea and vomiting than in those patients who did not. In their study of nausea and vomiting during spinal anesthesia for cesarean section, Santos and Datta (1984) also reported that nausea and vomiting occurred at a time when blood pressure was unchanged from baseline levels.

As far as prevention of nausea and vomiting during spinal anesthesia is concerned, there are no data to prove that any particular preoperative medication decreases to any statistically significant degree the incidence of this intraoperative complication. Even promising antiemetics such as metoclopramide, a centrally acting dopamine receptor antagonist, or domperidone, a peripherally acting dopamine blocker (Spelina, *et al.*, 1984) have not decreased the incidence significantly. It remains to be determined whether the new, selective 5-hydroxytryptamine subtype 3-receptor antagonist ondansetron will be as effective in preventing nausea and vomiting associated with spinal anesthesia as it was in preventing postoperative nausea and vomiting following general anesthesia (Leeser and Lip, 1991; Bodner and White, 1991). However, Santos and Datta

(1984) found that, at least in term parturients having cesarean sections under spinal anesthesia, the incidence of nausea and vomiting could be significantly decreased by intravenous droperidol given immediately after delivery of the infant and clamping of the umbilical cord. The frequency of nausea and vomiting was also decreased by prompt correction of hypotension during spinal anesthesia. Datta, et al. (1982) found that none of 20 patients given enough intravenous ephedrine to restore blood pressure immediately to preoperative levels developed nausea and vomiting during spinal anesthesia for cesarean section. In this setting, promptness was of the essence: 66 percent of patients given repeated small intravenous doses of ephedrine after arterial pressure had already decreased more than 30 mmHg below baseline or below 100 mmHg developed nausea and vomiting, despite restoration of blood pressure to preoperative baseline levels.

Treatment of intraoperative nausea and vomiting, once established, is most effective if based on prompt restoration of blood pressure using vasopressors and methods described in pp. 163–176, and prompt administration of 100 percent oxygen, together with reassurance of the patient. Overtreatment should be avoided; in most instances vomiting during spinal anesthesia lasts only relatively briefly. Intravenous atropine, though ineffective in prevention of intraoperative nausea and vomiting when administered preoperatively, has been said to be effective in treatment of this problem (Ward, et al., 1966; Graves, et al., 1966). The above-mentioned methods of treatment are, however, more reliable than atropine and intravenous antiemetics, which carry the potential for unwanted side effects.

Postoperative nausea and vomiting are related to a number of factors, particularly the site and type of operation, as well as the type, frequency, and amount of postoperative medications given for management of pain. There is no compelling evidence as to the existence of a relationship between type of anesthesia, be it spinal , epidural, nerve block or general anesthesia, and either frequency or severity of postoperative vomiting. Reports of decreased incidence of nausea and vomiting following spinal anesthesia are most frequently related to differences in types and sites of operations performed (Dent, et al., 1955; Bonica, et al., 1958). Of particular interest is the fact that the incidence of vomiting after regional plus general anesthesia was greater than the sum of the incidences of vomiting after spinal anesthesia alone and after general anesthesia alone (Bonica, 1958).

Pancreatic exocrine function has been studied only little during spinal anesthesia. It is unlikely, however, to be affected significantly. While sympathetic fibers to the pancreas innervate pancreatic blood vessels, their stimulation results in vasodilation and an increase in blood flow (Richins, 1953). Thus, spinal anesthesia might be associated with a slight decrease in pancreatic blood flow, but under normal conditions this would probably be of little or no physiologic consequence. The release of digestive enzymes by the pancreas is controlled primarily by the blood level of secretin. Although exocrine glands of the pancreas do have dual innervation from sympathetic and parasympathetic nerves (Kuntz and Richins, 1947; Lowenstein, 1960), their output is normally regulated more by secretin than by neural stimuli. Since secretin output is not under sympathetic control, pancreatic denervation by high spinal anesthesia would have little effect on the output of digestive enzymes by the pancreas (Crider and Thomas, 1944).

Sympathetic denervation produced by spinal anesthesia or by other methods has been advocated in the treatment of hemorrhagic pancreatitis (Ott and Warren, 1950; Berk and Krumperman, 1952; Dale, 1952; Thistlethwaite, et al., 1953; Berk, 1953; Walker and Pembleton, 1953). The rationale of such therapy is that the pain of pancreatitis can be more readily controlled with sympathetic block than with analgesics and that the sphincter of Oddi is relaxed by sympathetic denervation, thereby allowing biliary secretions to pass into the duodenum instead of refluxing up the pancreatic duct. In addition, sympathetic block increases blood flow to the pancreas, and so decreases pancreatic necrosis. Sympathetic blockade can control the pain of pancreatitis. Sympathetic denervation also relaxes the sphincter of Oddi (White, et al., 1952). This may be a considerable advantage in certain cases. It is questionable, however, whether sympathetic block increases pancreatic blood flow and so reduces necrosis. Experimental evidence indicates that sympathetic denervation would have the opposite effect (Richins, 1953). The clinical value of sympathetic blockade during acute pancreatitis remains to be proven. Even though the pain of pancreatitis may be relieved in this way, and that is certainly an advantage, there is still no evidence, as determined by controlled studies, to prove that outcome, both morbidity and mortality, is improved by sympathetic blockade.

REFERENCES

AITKENHEAD, A. R., GILMORE, D. G., HOTHERSALL, A. P., AND LEDINGHAM, I. McA: The effects of subarachnoid spinal block of colonic blood flow in the dog. Br. J. Anaesth. 50: 77, 1978 a.

AITKENHEAD, A. R., WISHART, H. Y., AND PEEBLES-BROWN, D. A.: High spinal nerve block for large bowel anastomosis. Br. J. Anaesth. 50: 177, 1978 b.

AITKENHEAD, A. R., GILMOUR, D. G., HOTHERSALL, A. P., AND LEDINGHAM, I. McA.: Effects of subarachnoid spinal nerve block and arterial PCO_2 on colon blood flow in the dog. Br. J. Anaesth. 52: 1071, 1980.

ASTERIADES, T.: Sur le traitement de l'iléus spasmodique post-opératoire aigu par la simple rachianesthésie. Presse Méd. 33: 1480, 1925.

BELL, C. M. A.: Neostigmine and anastomosis dehiscence. Proc. R. Soc. Med. 63: 752, 1970.

BELL, C. M. A., AND LEWIS, C. B.: Effect of neostigmine on integrity of ileo-rectal anastomoses. Br. Med. J. 3: 587, 1968.

BERK, J. E.: Management of acute pancreatitis. J. A. M. A. 152: 1, 1953.

BERK, J. E., AND KRUMPERMAN, L. W.: The use of fractional epidural block in the management of acute pancreatitis. Am. J. Med. Sci. 224: 507, 1952.

BLUMBERG, N., AGARWAL, M. M., AND CHUENG, C.: Relationship between recurrence of cancer of the colon and blood transfusion. Br. Med. J. 290: 1037, 1985.

BODNER, M., AND WHITE, P. F.: Antiemetic efficacy of ondansetron after outpatient laparoscopy. Anesth. Analg. 73: 250, 1991.

BOHLEN, H. G., AND GORE, R. W.: Comparison of microvascular pressures and diameters in the innervated and denervated rat intestine. Microvasc. Res. 14: 251, 1977.

BONICA, J. J., CREPPS, W., MONK, B., AND BENNETT, B.: Postanesthetic nausea, retching and vomiting: evaluation of cyclizine (Marezine) suppositories for treatment. Anesthesiology 19: 532, 1958.

BURROWS, L., AND TARTTER, P.: Effect of blood transfusion on colon malignancy recurrence rate. Lancet 2: 662, 1982.

BURSTEIN, C. L.: Effect of spinal anesthesia on intestinal activity. Proc. Soc. Exp. Biol. Med. 42: 291, 1939.

CHUNG, F., MEIER, R., LAUTENSCHLAGER, E., CARMICHAEL, F. J., AND CHUNG, A.: General or spinal anesthesia: which is better in the elderly? Anesthesiology 67: 422, 1987.

CRIDER, J. O., AND THOMAS, J. E.: Secretion of pancreatic juice after cutting the extrinsic nerves. Am. J. Physiol. 141: 730, 1944.

CROCKER, J. S., AND VANDAM, L. D.: Concerning nausea and vomiting during spinal anesthesia. Anesthesiology 20: 587, 1959.

CURTIS, G. M., AND BARRON, L. E.: Influence of laparotomy on the gastric motor mechanism. J. Clin. Invest. 15: 462, 1936.

DALE, W. A.: Splanchnic block in the treatment of acute pancreatitis. Surgery 32: 606, 1952.

DATTA, S., ALPER, M. H., OSTHEIMER, G. W., AND WEISS, J. B.: Method of ephedrine administration and nausea and hypotension during spinal anesthesia for cesarean section. Anesthesiology 56: 68, 1982.

DE JONG, R. J.: Arterial carbon dioxide and oxygen tensions during spinal block. J. A. M. A. 191: 698, 1965.

DENT, S., RAMACHANDRA, V., AND STEPHEN, C. R.: Postoperative vomiting: incidence, analysis and therapeutic measures in 3000 patients. Anesthesiology 16: 564, 1955.

DOMENECH, F.: Action de l'anesthésie, rachidienne sur la motilité intestinale. Presse Méd. 37: 66, 1929.

ECKENHOFF, J. E., AND CANNARD, T. H.: Influence of anesthetic agents and adjuvants upon intestinal tone. Anesthesiology 21: 96, 1960.

FOSTER, R. S., COSTANZA, M. C., FOSTER, J. C., WANNER, M. C., AND FOSTER, C. B.: Adverse relationship between blood transfusion and survial after colectomy for colon cancer. Cancer 55: 1195, 1985.

GOLDEN, R. F., AND MANN, F. C.: The effects of drugs in anesthesiology on the tone and motility of the small intestine: an experimental study. Anesthesiology 4: 577, 1943.

GRAVES, C. L., UNDERWOOD, P. S., KLEIN, R. L., AND KIM, Y. I.: Intravenous fluid administration as therapy for hypotension secondary to spinal anesthesia. Anesth. Analg. 47: 548, 1966.

HÄRTEL, F.: Zur Vehandlung der postoperativen Darmatonie. Arch. Klin. Chir. 186: 445, 1936.

HELM, J. D., JR., AND INGELFINGER, F. J.: Effect of spinal anesthesia on the motility of the small intestine. Surg. Gynecol. Obstet. 79: 553, 1944.

HOWARD, J. M., AND DAVIS, J. H.: Studies on the absorption and equilibration of water (deuterium oxide) from the gastrointestinal tract following abdominal surgery under spinal anesthesia. Surgery 36: 1127, 1954.

INGRAM, W. R.: The visceral functions of the nervous system. Annu. Rev. Physiol. 9: 163, 1947.

KETY, S. S., KING, B. D., HORVATH, S. M., JEFFERS, W. A., AND HAFKENSCHIEL, J. H.: The effects of an acute reduction in blood pressure by means of differential spinal sympathetic block on the cerebral circulation of hypertensive patients. J. Clin. Invest. 29: 402, 1950.

KUNTZ, A., AND RICHINS, C. A.: Effects of direct and reflex nerve stimulation on exocrine pancreatic function. J. Neurophysiol. 12: 29, 1947.

LATTERELL, K. E., AND LUNDY, J. S.: Oxygen and carbon dioxide content of arterial blood before and during spinal analgesia. Anesthesiology 10: 677, 1949.

LESSER, J., AND LIP, H.: Prevention of postoperative nausea and vomiting using ondansetron, a new, selective 5-HT₃ receptor anatagonist. Anesth. Analg. 72: 751, 1991.

LOWENSTEIN, W. R.: Neural control of mucous gland cells of the pancreatic duct. Am. J. Dig. Dis. 5: 126, 1960.

MARKOWITZ, J., AND CAMPBELL, W. R.: The relief of experimental ileus by spinal anesthesia. Am. J. Physiol. 81: 101, 1927.

MAYER, A.: Ueber die wirkung der Lumbalanästhesie auf die glatte Muskulatur. Dtsch. Med. Wochenschr. 47: 1454, 1921.

MAYER, A.: Ueber spastischen Ileus and Ileusbehandlung mit Lumbalanästhesie. Zentralbl. Chir. 49: 1882, 1922.

MUELLER, R. P., LYNN, R. B., AND SANCETTA, S. M.: Studies of hemodynamic changes in humans following induction of low and high spinal anesthesia. II. The changes in splanchnic blood flow, oxygen extraction and consumption, and splanchnic vascular resistance in humans not undergoing surgery. Circulation 6: 894, 1952.

OCHSNER, A., GAGE, I. M., AND CUTTING, H. A.: Comparative value of splanchnic and spinal analgesia in treatment of experimental ileus. Arch. Surg. 20: 802, 1930.

OTT, R. B., AND WARREN, K. W.: Continuous epidural analgesia in acute pancreatitis. Lahey Clin. Bull. 6: 204, 1950.

RATRA, C. K., BADOLA, R. P., AND BHARGAVA, K. P.: A study of factors concerned in emesis during spinal anaesthesia. Br. J. Anaesth. 44: 1208, 1972.

RICHINS, C. A.: The innervation of the pancreas. J. Comp. Neurol. 83: 223, 1945.

RICHINS, C. A.: Effects of sympathetic nerve stimulation on blood flow and secretion in the pancreas. Am. J. Physiol. 173: 467, 1953.

SANCETTA, S. M., LYNN, R. B., SIMEONE, F. A., AND SCOTT, R. W.: Studies of hemodynamic changes in humans following induction of low and high spinal anesthesia. I. General consideration of the problem. The changes in cardiac output, brachial arterial pressure, peripheral and pulmonary oxygen contents and peripheral blood flows induced by spinal anesthesia in humans not undergoing surgery. Circulation 6: 559, 1952.

SANTOS, A., AND DATTA, S.: Prophylactic use of droperidol for control of nausea and vomiting during spinal anesthesia for cesarean section. Anesth. Analg. 63: 85, 1984.

SARNOFF, S. J., ARROWOOD, J. G., AND CHAPMAN, W. P.: Differential spinal block. IV. The investigation of intestinal dyskinesia, colonic atony, and visceral afferent fibers. Surg. Gynecol. Obstet. 86: 571, 1948.

SCOTT, W. J. M., AND MORTON, J. J.: Sympathetic inhibition of the large intestine in Hirschsprung's disease. J. Clin. Invest. 9: 247, 1930.

SHAW, W., AND WOLCOTT, M. W.: A triple-blind study for the clinical evaluation of dextropantothenyl alcohol and dextropantothenyl alcohol plus choline chloride. Surg. Gynecol. Obstet. 116: 489, 1963.

SIVARAJAN, M., AMORY, D. W., LINDBLOOM, L. E., AND SCHWETTMAN, R. S.: Systemic and regional blood-flow changes during spinal anesthesia in Rhesus monkeys. Anesthesiology 43: 78, 1975.

SPELINA, K. R., GERBER, H. R., AND PAGELS, I. L.: Nausea and vomiting during spinal anaesthesia. Anaesthesia 39: 132, 1984.

STABINS, S. J., MORTON, J. J., AND SCOTT, W. J. M.: Spinal anesthesia in the treatment of megacolon and obstinate constipation. Am. J. Surg. 27: 107, 1935.

TELFORD, E. D., AND SIMMONS, H. T.: Treatment of gastrointestinal achalasia by spinal anaesthesia. Br. Med. J. 2: 1224, 1939.

THISTLETHWAITE, J. R., EDISON, T. G., GRUENWALD, C., AND HARRISON, I.: Experiences with epidural analgesia for sympathetic block. Surgery 33: 818, 1953.

TREISSMAN, D. A.: Disruption of colonic anastomosis associated with epidural anesthesia. Regional Anesth. 5: 22, 1980.

TUOHY, E. B.: The adaptations of continuous spinal anesthesia. Anesth. Analg. 31: 372, 1952.

WAGNER, G. A.: Zur Behandlung des Ileus mit Lumbalanästhesie. Zentralbl. Gynäk 46: 1225, 1922.

WALKER, I., AND PEMBLETON, P. E.: Continuous epidural block in the treatment of pancreatitis. Anesthesiology 14: 33, 1953.

WARD, R. J., KENNEDY, W. F., JR., BONICA, J. J., MARTIN, W. E., TOLAS, A. G., AND AKAMATSU, T.: Experimental evaluation of atropine and vasopressors for the treatment of hypotension of high subarachnoid anesthesia. Anesth. Analg. 45: 621, 1966.

WHITE, J. C., SMITHWICK, R. H., AND SIMEONE, F. A.: The Autonomic Nervous System. Third Edition. New York: The Macmillan Company, 1952.

WORSLEY, M. H., WISHART, H. Y., PEBBLES-BROWN, D. A., AND AITKENHEAD, A. R.: High spinal nerve block for large bowel anastomosis: a prospective study. Br. J. Anaesth. 60: 836, 1988.

CHAPTER 10

Epidural Anesthesia

The physiologic changes induced by spinal anesthesia and epidural anesthesia are similar in many respects. Both techniques produce sympathetic denervation, and both involve blockade of somatic sensory and motor fibers. Important differences exist, however. It is appropriate to consider briefly the nature of, and reasons for, these differences and their clinical significance. In view of the material in the preceding chapters, as well as Bromage's review (1978) of the physiology and pharmacology of epidural anesthesia, it is necessary only to compare the physiological responses to the two types of anesthesia, rather than considering the physiology of epidural anesthesia *per se*.

The difference between the physiologic responses to spinal and epidural anesthesia may be explained by one of the five factors listed in Table 10.1. But before dealing with these five factors, we must first underscore the difficulty of comparing the systemic changes produced by two such different techniques as spinal and epidural anesthesia. There are no controlled, prospective, double-blind studies comparing the two techniques, whether in patients or in volunteers. Furthermore, studies that do exist generally employed different local anesthetics, both with and without additives such as epinephrine or sodium bicarbonate; this resulted in varying levels of motor and sensory denervation, and the volunteers or patients studied were given varying amounts of intravascular fluids. Perhaps even more important, there is a lack of uniformity in reporting of results: "sensory" denervation does not always distinguish between light touch or pinprick modalities. The two are not synonymous. Perhaps the best example of this lack of uniformity (or agreement) pertains to the definition of "level of sympathetic denervation." For over 30 years, the level of temperature discrimination block has been used as a clinical correlate of the level of sympathetic denervation during spinal anesthesia, and there are no data to support the contention that this correlation is invalid during epidural anesthesia. Many reports, however, have used liquid crystal contact thermography (Hardy, 1988), muscle sympathetic activity (Lundin, *et al.*, 1989), regional skin temperatures (Peters, *et al.*, 1989), strain gauge plethysmography, and Doppler ultrasound (Perhoniemi and Linko, 1987) to assess the level of sympathetic blockade; most of these studies reported different results. This lack of uniformity adds to the difficulty of comparing data among studies. And

---

Table 10.1.
Factors Determining the Differences in Physiologic Responses to Spinal and Epidural Anesthesia

---

- Extent of sensory-to-sympathetic zone of differential blockade
- Extent of sensory-to-motor zone of differential blockade
- Intensity of denervation within the sensory-to-sympathetic zone of differential blockade
- Systemic effects of local anesthetic and epinephrine absorption from the epidural space
- Cerebrospinal fluid pressure achieved following local anesthetic injection

---

lastly, it must be noted that segmental level of anesthesia (dermatomes) are ordinal data, and as such, they should be analyzed statistically and reported as medians, not means $\pm$ SD. With the above-mentioned caveats, the following discussion serves as an attempt to explain the differences in systemic effects induced by spinal and epidural anesthesia.

Extent of Sensory-to-Sympathetic Zone of Differential Blockade

During spinal anesthesia the level of sympathetic denervation exceeds the level of somatic sensory anesthesia by two or more spinal segments (pp. 33–38). The corresponding zone of differential blockade during epidural anesthesia, however, has been the focus of some debate. Some investigators have reported that the levels of both sympathetic denervation and sensory blockade are the same (Bromage, 1967; Wugmeister and Hehre, 1967). Wugmeister and Hehre (1967), using loss of temperature discrimination as an indication of the extent of sympathetic denervation (p. 33), were unable to detect any significant difference during epidural anesthesia between the level made anesthetic to pinprick and the level made anesthetic to cold, a difference readily apparent during spinal anesthesia (Greene, 1958). However, it is not clear in their study (Wugmeister and Hehre, 1967) whether "touching the skin with a needle point at 1-cm intervals" measured loss of pinprick sensation, or loss of light touch sensibility. Even more importantly, however, this study employed two different concentrations of lidocaine (1.2 percent and 2.0 percent), and some of their patients received a mixture of local anesthetic with 1:200,000 epinephrine, while some received plain lidocaine. It is not stated in their report how many of the 45 patients (aged 19–75 yr) were given the different local anesthetic solutions, and the data were pooled and expressed as means. The authors concluded that "a large zone of differential blockade does not exist" during epidural anesthesia.

The findings of Bigler, *et al.* (1986) were different: they found that during bupivacaine epidural anesthesia, the "segmental spread of loss of temperature discrimination was invariably larger" (one to two segments both cephalad and caudad) than the spread of pinprick anesthesia. Similarly, Peters, *et al.* (1989) found in dogs that the level of sympathetic denervation (assessed by regional skin temperatures) produced by upper thoracic epidural anesthesia "induced a decrease in sympathetic tone distal to the area of analgesia." Recently, Brull and Greene (1991) also evaluated the zone of differential sensory blockade during epidural anesthesia with 2 percent lidocaine plus epinephrine (1:200,000) and sodium bicarbonate, 0.1 mmol·L^{-1} per ml of solution. The authors performed assessments of the levels of denervation to light touch, sharp (pinprick), and cold temperature discrimination in 22 patients (aged 22–76 yr), and the results were reported as both means and medians (Fig. 10.1). In this study, the zone of differential sensory blockade between pinprick and cold temperature discrimination reached statistical significance (mean of 1.3 ± 0.6 dermatomes) 5 min after epidural injection of local anesthetic,

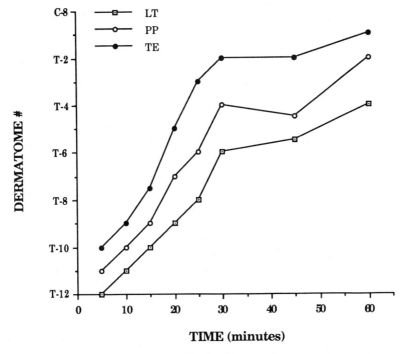

Figure 10.1. Thoracic (T) or cervical (C) dermatomal levels of light touch (LT), pinprick (PP) and cold temperature (TE) denervation as a function of time (min) during epidural anesthesia with lidocaine. (Redrawn with permission from Brull and Greene, Br. J. Anaesth. *66:* 651, 1991.)

Table 10.2.
Mean (SD) Width (dermatomes) of Light Touch to Pinprick (LT-PP) and Pinprick to Temperature (PP-TE) Zones of Differential Anesthesia as a Function of Time[a]

Time (min)	LT-PP		PP-TE	
	N[b]	Width	N	Width
5	8	1.0 (0.5)	12	1.3 (0.6)
10	13	1.8 (2.0)	22	1.1 (0.9)
15	18	1.5 (0.7)	22	1.1 (1.2)
20	20	1.8 (0.9)	22	1.4 (0.8)
25	19	2.3 (1.3)	21	1.6 (1.4)
30	21	2.3 (1.6)	21	1.6 (1.3)
45	10	2.6 (1.6)	10	1.3 (1.0)
60	5	2.8 (3.1)	5	1.2 (1.6)

[a] From Brull and Greene, Br. J. Anaesth. 66: 651, 1991.
[b] N = number of observations at each time interval.

and this significance was maintained during the entire 60-min study. Similar results were obtained for the zone of differential sensory blockade between light touch and pinprick sensation (Table 10.2). The zones of differential sensory blockade in their study did not appear to be influenced by age when patients were grouped according to the median age of 35 yr. The results of this study appear to contradict those of Wugmeister and Hehre (1967). However, the findings in these two studies are not necessarily at odds with each other, and some of the differences can be explained based on the mechanisms of differential blockade so elegantly proposed by Fink (1989) and concurrently supported by work of Raymond and Strichartz (Raymond and Strichartz, 1989; Raymond, et al., 1989). In his article, Fink (1989) proposes two mechanisms, derived from *in vitro* study of myelinated axons, that can explain the mechanism by which zones of differential blockade develop during spinal and epidural anesthesia. The first principle, which applies to epidural anesthesia, proposes that neuronal conduction can still occur by saltatory means, as long as a maximum of two consecutive nodes are blocked. During epidural blockade, the segmental nerve extending extradurally in the intervertebral foramen is exposed to the local anesthetic injected epidurally for only a few millimeters. Therefore, the large (and long-internode) fibers such as motor nerves will not have enough length (i.e., less than three nodes) exposed to the local anesthetic for conduction to be blocked. In contrast, the smaller (and shorter internode) fibers will have three or more nodes exposed to local anesthetic blockade. The second principle proposed by Fink applies to differential blockade that occurs during spinal anesthesia (Fink, 1989) (Chapter 1).

Thus, taking into account the above-mentioned principle, it is not known how many of the 45 patients in the study by Wugmeister and Hehre received the weak 1.2 percent lidocaine solution, which, according to Fink (1989), may not be strong enough to produce significant differential sensory blockade. Also unknown are the possible effects, if any, of adding epinephrine to some, but not all, local anesthetic solutions (Wugmeister and Hehre, 1967), or of adding sodium bicarbonate to the local anesthetic solution (Brull and Greene, 1991). As shown by Sharrock (1978), Park, *et al.* (1982), and Grundy, *et al.* (1978), age also may significantly influence the segmental dose requirement of local anesthetic. The results of Wugmeister and Hehre and those of Brull and Greene must therefore be viewed in this context; the preponderance of data nevertheless indicate that epidural anesthesia is associated with a zone of differential blockade which is very similar in its extent to the zone which develops during clinical spinal anesthesia. Any differences can be explained on methodologic grounds (pp. 27–37).

Extent of Sensory-to-Motor Zone of Differential Blockade

Epidural anesthesia is associated with a small (one to two dermatomes) but statistically significant zone of differential blockade involving sympathetic and sensory fibers (Chapter 1), and is accompanied by a zone of differential anesthesia involving sensory and somatic motor nerves. However, the difference between the sensory and motor levels of anesthesia are considerably larger during epidural anesthesia than during spinal anesthesia. Freund, *et al.* (1967) evaluated this point in 18 subjects who served as their own controls during spinal and epidural anesthesia. At a time when the sensory levels of denervation averaged $T_{2.3}$ during spinal anesthesia, the level of somatic motor paralysis averaged $T_{5.1}$, a difference of 2.8 spinal segments. During epidural anesthesia, on the other hand, when the sensory level of anesthesia averaged $T_{3.6}$, the level of motor paralysis averaged $T_{8.2}$, a difference of 4.6 spinal segments. One result of this difference is the contrast in ventilatory responses to the two types of anesthesia. Since epidural and spinal anesthesia affect pulmonary function according to the degree of respiratory muscle paralysis, epidural anesthesia alters respiratory function less than does spinal anesthesia in the presence of equal sensory levels of anesthesia. This was demonstrated in the study by Freund, *et al.* (1967). Spinal anesthesia reduced inspiratory capacity from average control values of 3.20 to 2.93 L, and reduced expiratory reserve volume from 0.74 to 0.38 L. Significantly fewer changes were produced by epidural anesthesia: inspiratory capacity decreased from 3.22 to 3.12 L, expiratory reserve volume decreased from 0.75 to 0.59 L. The differences between spinal and epidural anesthesia are most evident, however, in pulmonary function studies such as maximum inspiratory capacity, which depend on the subject's ability to force ventilate. Conversely, there are no differences in ventilatory response during quiet respiration under resting conditions of clinical anesthesia. Arterial gas tensions are not altered significantly by either spinal or epidural anesthesia (de Jong, 1965; Bonica, et al., 1966). Differences in blood gas tensions observed during spontaneous, quiet breathing under equal levels of spinal and epidural anesthesia (Ward, et al., 1965), usually result from other factors (p. 221), rather than from different degrees of motor paralysis. Other effects of epidural anesthesia on the respiratory system have also been described. Segmental sensory (and necessarily, also sympathetic) denervation, such as produced by thoracic epidural block, has been shown to improve diaphragmatic function following upper abdominal surgery (Mankikian, et al., 1988). Other benefits include decreased incidence of postoperative atelectasis and decreased convalescence time (Pflug, et al., 1974), and improved postoperative lung function (Spence and Smith, 1971). Similarly, the sympathetic blockade produced by epidural anesthesia has been shown to attenuate the normal cardiovascular responses to severe hypoxemia (Peters, et al., 1990). In dogs without sympathetic blockade, hypoxemia induced an increase in blood pressure and heart rate by 37 mmHg and 50 beats/min, respectively. In contrast, in the presence of sympathetic blockade, the same degree of hypoxemia induced no change in blood pressure, and heart rate increased by only 15 beats/min. Regardless of presence of sympathectomy, hypoxemia induced hypocarbia, indicating preservation of normal ventilatory response.

Despite the demonstration that during epidural anesthesia the level of temperature sensibility denervation extends further cephalad from the site of local anesthetic injection than do the levels of pinprick, light touch, and motor denervation (similar to the sequence of denervation observed during spinal anesthesia), differences in physiologic responses induced by spinal and epidural anesthesia remain. The minor differences in the extent of zones of differential blockade during spinal anesthesia (two levels or more) and epidural anesthesia (one to two levels) only partially explain the observation that, as sensory anesthesia wears off postoperatively, the rate of regression of sympathetic and motor paralysis is different following spinal than following epidural anesthesia (Daos and Virtue, 1963). The reasons for these differences may be one or a combination of the remaining factors discussed below.

Intensity of Denervation Within the Sensory-to-Sympathetic Zone of Differential Blockade

There may be less profound (but equal extent of) sympathetic denervation with epidural than with spinal anesthesia. Bromage (1978) for instance, stated that epidural blockade does not usually result in complete block of sympathetic fibers, but merely in a reduction in neural traffic. Further, both spinal (Chapter 6) and epidural anesthesia can alter the stress response, depending on the site of surgery and level of blockade (Kehlet, 1984; Bigler, et al., 1986; Peters, et al., 1990; Roizen, et al., 1981; Pflug and Halter, 1981; Stevens, et al., 1991). However, when used as an adjunct to general anesthesia, epidural anesthesia with sensory blockade extending to mid-thoracic levels (i.e., below T_4) does not completely block the increases in plasma catecholamines during upper abdominal surgery. This finding has been attributed to unblocked nociceptive and autonomic afferents (Rutberg, et al., 1984; Kehlet, et al., 1980). Similarly, Stevens, et al. (1990) suggested that high epidural block with 2 percent lidocaine attenuated but did not completely block efferent sympathetic transmission in dogs. Recently, maintenance of blood pressure at normal levels and maintenance of baseline concentrations of catecholamines in humans have been attributed to the fact that "sympathectomy produced by even high levels of epidural anesthesia is not complete compared to that produced by a spinal anesthetic of the same extent" (Stevens, et al., 1991). Another study that supports the theory that sensory (and, therefore, sympathetic) denervation may be less profound during epidural than during spinal anesthesia (Arendt-Nielsen et al., 1990) has demonstrated that pain caused by one needle was blocked during bupivacaine epidural anesthesia at a time when stimulation by 10 needles (spatial summation) or by laser (temporal summation) caused pain. Similar studies comparing the ability of spinal anesthesia to block spatial or temporal summation, however, have not been reported. A similarly incomplete blockade of somatosensory evoked potentials during bupivacaine epidural anesthesia was reported by Lund, et al. (1987). Lundin, et al. (1989) made direct intraneural recordings of muscle sympathetic activity (MSA) in the peroneal nerve during mepivacaine epidural anesthesia in humans. They found that "the sympathetic fibers to the lower extremities were completely blocked when sensory anesthesia was present up to or above the T_{10} level," supporting the theory that sympathetic denervation beyond (i.e., cephalad to) the level of sensory denervation is incomplete. Other studies reporting the inability of epidural anesthesia to provide adequate analgesia from tourniquet pain likewise support the possibility of incomplete blockade (Valli and Rosenberg, 1985; Lee, *et al.*, 1990; Brown, *et al.*, 1990; Rucci, *et al.*, 1987). Finally, Hardy (1988) reported that bupivacaine epidural anesthesia resulted in a zone of differential blockade in which cold temperature discrimination was noted three to four segments cephalad to the corresponding "sympathetic" level as assessed by liquid crystal contact thermography.

In contrast to the above-mentioned studies, Perhoniemi and Linko (1987) concluded that "epidural anaesthesia with bupivacaine causes a more intensive sympathetic block than does spinal anaesthesia." The authors based their conclusions on the fact that the increase in skin temperature was more pronounced, and the arterial blood flow was significantly higher, following epidural than following spinal anesthesia. It must be noted, however, that spinal anesthesia blocked an average of 12.7 ± 0.7 spinal segments, while the extent of blockade during epidural anesthesia was relatively larger (14.4 ± 0.7 segments). The difference in extent of anesthesia between spinal and epidural may therefore explain the changes in temperature and blood flow reported in this study. However, it is not only epidural anesthesia that is sometimes inadequate in providing anesthesia or analgesia. Incomplete relief from tourniquet pain has been reported during spinal anesthesia, as well (Bonnet, *et al.*, 1989; Concepcion, 1989; Brun-Buisson, *et al.*, 1988; Stewart, *et al.*, 1988; Concepcion, *et al.*, 1988).

Systemic Effects of Local Anesthetic and Epinephrine Absorption from the Epidural Space

Since most physiologic responses to spinal and epidural anesthesia result from sympathetic denervation, particularly with regard to the cardiovascular system, the "physiologic trespass" associated with epidural anesthesia, if indeed less than that associated with spinal anesthesia of equal sensory extent, must be due to factors other than the relatively minor differences in the extent of pinprick-to-temperature zone of differential blockade. Differences between cardiovascular responses to spinal and to epidural anesthesia, however, have been reported.

Ward, *et al.* (1965) studied the cardiovascular responses of 14 subjects (volunteers and patients, aged 21–42 yr) who served as their own controls during both lumbar epidural anesthesia (with 2 percent lidocaine) and spinal anesthesia (with 5 percent hyperbaric lidocaine). The level of

Table 10.3.
**Cardiovascular Responses (% Change from Control) to Equal Sensory Levels of
Spinal and Epidural Anesthesia**[a]

Parameter	Spinal	Epidural Without Epinephrine	Epidural With Epinephrine
Mean arterial pressure	− 21.3	− 8.9	− 22.0
Pulse rate	+ 3.7	+ 6.7	+ 15.8
Cardiac output	− 17.7	− 5.4	+ 30.2
Stroke volume	− 25.4	− 10.2	+ 30.2
Total peripheral vascular resistance	− 5.0	− 2.9	− 39.6

[a] Reproduced with permission from Ward, *et al.*, J. A. M. A. *191*: 99, 1965.

sensory (pinprick) anesthesia was the same (T_5) for both anesthetics. In these subjects, spinal anesthesia induced a 21.3 percent decrease in mean arterial blood pressure, a 17.7 percent decrease in cardiac output, a 25.4 percent decrease in stroke volume, and a 5.0 percent decrease in total peripheral resistance. Significantly less alteration of cardiovascular function was observed when equal levels of sensory anesthesia were obtained with epidural anesthesia (Table 10.3). Mean arterial blood pressure averaged 8.9 percent, cardiac output 5.4 percent, stroke volume 10.2 percent, and total peripheral resistance 2.9 percent below preanesthetic control values. Bonica, *et al.* (1966) studied 37 subjects and found that with equal sensory levels of anesthesia there was no significant difference in mean arterial blood pressure following either spinal anesthesia or lumbar epidural anesthesia (2 percent lidocaine without epinephrine); however, spinal anesthesia produced a significant decrease in cardiac output (8 percent) and total peripheral resistance (15 percent), while epidural anesthesia produced no change in either. Comparable data have also been reported by Ward, *et al.* (1966). Since the zones of differential sensory blockade that develop during spinal anesthesia are not as different from those that develop during epidural anesthesia as once thought, other factors must explain the different hemodynamic responses induced by the two techniques. Local anesthetics (75 mg lidocaine) can be detected in peripheral blood during both spinal (0.32 ± 0.07 mg·ml^{-1}) and epidural (0.41 ± 0.07 mg·ml^{-1}) anesthesia (Giasi, *et al.*, 1979). However, the total dose of local anesthetic injected during spinal anesthesia is so insignificant that resulting blood levels of anesthetic are below those associated with systemic pharmacologic responses. On the other hand, the amount of local anesthetic employed during epidural anesthesia may result in pharmacologically active levels of local anesthetic in peripheral blood. Following their absorption into the blood, local anesthetics can affect the hemodynamic parameters in several ways (Blair, 1975):

- Direct action on cardiac muscle or vascular smooth muscle
- Direct action on the autonomic nervous system
- Direct action on the central nervous system
- Indirectly via evoked reflexes

The different levels of local anesthetics in the blood associated with spinal and epidural anesthesia are not the result of differences in the percentage of injected drug absorbed into the vascular system. Blood levels of local anesthetic are similar when the same amounts of anesthetic are injected intrathecally or epidurally (Giasi, et al., 1979). Instead, the reason for the difference in blood levels is due to the fact that a given level of epidural anesthesia requires a much greater amount (i.e., total dose) of local anesthetic to produce an equal level of anesthesia injected epidurally than when injected into the subarachnoid space (Greene, 1979). Because blood levels are primarily a function of the total amount of local anesthetic injected, blood levels of local anesthetic are greater during epidural anesthesia than during equal levels of spinal anesthesia. In light of recent reports of neurologic complications (extreme agitation) following the use of continuous epidural anesthesia even with dilute (0.125–0.25 percent) bupivacaine (Dunne and Kox, 1991), it is therefore prudent to maintain a high index of suspicion for local anesthetic toxicity and even monitor plasma concentrations if toxicity is suspected.

Blood levels of local anesthetics during epidural anesthesia frequently are great enough to have significant systemic effects (Tuvemo and Willdeck-Lund, 1982; Albright, 1979; Dunne and Kox, 1991; Lofgren and Hahn, 1991; Kerkkamp and Gielen, 1991). The drug-induced systemic changes that may be associated with epidural anesthesia are additive to changes resulting from the sympathetic and motor denervations produced by the anesthetic technique itself. In the presence of equal sensory levels of anesthesia, the combined effects of drug and of denervation during epidural anesthesia often exceed the effects of denervation alone produced during spinal anesthesia. In some clinical series that did not employ epinephrine during epidural anesthesia, the incidence of hypotension has been shown to be greater with epidural than with spinal anesthesia (Defalque, 1962). In this study, the difference may have been due to drug-induced peripheral vasodilation following absorption of the local anesthetic (lidocaine given in a dose of 5.5 mg·kg^{-1}) from the epidural space, or to the different local anesthetics that were used in spinal (pontocaine) and epidural (1.5 percent lidocaine) anesthesia.

The role of drug-induced changes during epidural anesthesia is best evaluated by comparing the cardiovascular responses to both spinal and epidural anesthesia. Such comparisons should be made between two groups of subjects, each having the same proven level of sympathetic denervation, produced by different amounts of the same drug (without epinephrine). Unfortunately, no such studies have been reported. Some investigations have compared patient populations with equal sensory levels of anesthesia, but have not documented drug plasma levels during spinal and epidural anesthesia (Ward, et al., 1966). Others have compared spinal anesthesia with epidural anesthesia that had epinephrine added to the local anesthetic solution (Moore, et al., 1968). Epinephrine has a pronounced effect in such a situation, and illustrates well the degree to which drugs used to produce epidural anesthesia may themselves alter the response to anesthesia. This has been demonstrated by investigators from the University of Washington (Ward, et al., 1965; Bonica et al., 1966; Ward, et al., 1966) who compared the cardiovascular effects of spinal anesthesia, epidural anesthesia without epinephrine, and epidural anesthesia with 1:200,000 epinephrine in 14 subjects with equivalent levels of sensory denervation (T_5). During epidural anesthesia with epinephrine, mean arterial blood pressure decreased 22.0 percent below control values, while during spinal and epidural anesthesia without epinephrine mean arterial pressure averaged 21.3 and 8.9 percent, respectively, below control levels (Table 10.3). With epidural anesthesia, pulse rate increased more when the local anesthetic contained epinephrine than when epinephrine was absent, and stroke volume increased with epinephrine but decreased without it. Stroke volume also decreased significantly during spinal anesthesia. Most significant was the fact that cardiac output increased 30.2 percent and total peripheral resistance decreased 39.6 percent during epidural anesthesia with epinephrine, while without it, cardiac output and peripheral resistance decreased 5.4 percent and 2.9 percent, respectively. During spinal anesthesia cardiac output decreased 17.7 percent and peripheral resistance decreased 5.0 percent. As the authors suggest, the difference in response between epidural anesthesia with epinephrine and epidural anesthesia without epinephrine is most likely related to the vascular absorption of epinephrine which takes place in the former. The effects of epinephrine absorption from the epidural space into the blood also have been documented recently by Salevsky, et al. (1990). The authors found that patients receiving epidural bupivacaine (12 ml) plus epinephrine (5 $\mu g \cdot ml^{-1}$) experienced a significantly greater decrease in mean blood pressure and systemic vascular resistance (beta-adrenergic effects), and a significantly greater increase in cardiac output than patients receiving the same dose of plain epidural bupivacaine (79.3 percent vs. 94.6 percent, 61.6 percent vs. 91.6 percent, and 130.8 percent vs. 105.0 percent, respectively). These differences were no longer evident 45 min after epidural injection (Tables 10.4 and 10.5).

Epinephrine absorption from the epidural space into the blood occurs in amounts sufficient to improve fibrinolytic function (Modig, 1988; Mannucci, et al., 1975), to produce beta-adrenergic stimulation (increased

Table 10.4.
Hemodynamic Data[a]

	HR (beats/min)	MBP (mmHg)	CO ($L \cdot min^{-1}$)	SVR ($dynes \cdot sec \cdot cm^{-5} \cdot 10^{-3}$)	PWP (mmHg)
Control					
B	71.8 ± 9.5	106.3 ± 18.9	4.62 ± 1.58	2.13 ± 1.61	15.0 ± 6.2
B + E	76.3 ± 15.3	104.2 ± 18.2	4.50 ± 1.50	1.82 ± 0.41	13.6 ± 5.5
15 min					
B	68.9 ± 8.7	99.6 ± 19.2	4.64 ± 1.32	1.80 ± 0.85	13.1 ± 5.4
B + E	78.3 ± 15.3	83.1 ± 22.0	5.81 ± 2.07	1.11 ± 0.31	11.3 ± 3.8
45 min					
B	62.7 ± 7.8	92.2 ± 17.1	4.58 ± 1.01	1.58 ± 0.54	12.9 ± 3.2
B + E	71.2 ± 11.8	86.0 ± 21.5	5.25 ± 1.68	1.30 ± 0.47	13.1 ± 4.4

Abbreviations: B, bupivacaine 0.75 percent; B + E, bupivacaine 0.75 percent plus epinephrine 5 $\mu g \cdot mL^{-1}$. CO, cardiac output; HR, heart rate; MBP, mean arterial blood pressure; PWP, pulmonary capillary wedge pressure; SVR, systemic vascular resistance.
[a] From Salevsky, *et al.*, Can. J. Anaesth. *37:* 160, 1990.
[b] Mean ± SD.

Table 10.5.
Hemodynamic Data as Percentage of Control[a,b]

	HR	MBP	CO	SVR	PWP
15 min					
B	96.3 ± 7.3	94.5 ± 15.8[c]	105.0 ± 20.8[c]	91.6 ± 19.2[c]	99.8 ± 29.2
B + E	104.0 ± 17.4	79.3 ± 11.6[c]	130.8 ± 23.0[c]	61.6 ± 9.0[c]	79.4 ± 20.5
45 min					
B	87.7 ± 7.6	87.5 ± 13.7	107.8 ± 35.5	84.9 ± 19.9	101.3 ± 23.9
B + E	94.7 ± 12.9	82.4 ± 14.1	118.1 ± 22.1	71.3 ± 16.4	92.2 ± 25.4

Abbreviations: As in Table 10.4.
[a] From Salevsky, *et al.*, Can. J. Anaesth. *37:* 160, 1990.
[b] Mean ± SD.
[c] $P < 0.05$ between groups.

cardiac output, increased stroke volume, increased pulse rate, peripheral vasodilation), but not enough to produce alpha-adrenergic stimulation (vasoconstriction). Epinephrine absorption into plasma following administration of 10 ml of 2 percent lidocaine (1:200,000 epinephrine) was effective in lowering the plasma level of lidocaine following bolus administration, but not during continuous epidural infusion at a rate of 10 $ml \cdot hr^{-1}$ (Takasaki and Kajitani, 1990) (Fig. 10.2). The hemodynamic effects of intravenous epinephrine infusion (i.e., preservation of cardiac output) during hypotensive epidural anesthesia in man have recently been reported (Sharrock, *et al.*, 1990, 1991).

The difference in cardiovascular responses between patients undergoing spinal anesthesia and patients undergoing epidural anesthesia without epinephrine may be due to one or a combination of three factors: (a) the difference may be due to a reflex initiated by an increase in cerebrospinal fluid pressure produced by epidural anesthesia (p. 371); (b) the extent of sympathetic denervation may be relatively less during epidural than during spinal anesthesia even though sensory levels are the same (pp. 358–361); (c) subconvulsive concentrations of local anesthetics may have positive inotropic and chronotropic effects. These latter effects have been observed in patients given intravenous lidocaine for treatment of arrhythmias, and when enough local anesthetics have been infused intravenously to produce blood levels equal to those obtained during epidural anesthesia (Jorfeldt, et al., 1968).

Few studies in humans have measured plasma levels of local anesthetics following their injection epidurally. Therefore, most data on their systemic effects must be derived from studies in which local anesthetics have been injected directly intravenously. It is reasonable to expect that, except for the hemodynamic changes induced by the sympathetic denervation of epidural anesthesia, the remaining systemic effects would be similar at equivalent plasma concentrations, regardless of whether local anesthetics were first injected epidurally or directly intravenously. Thus, several groups of investigators have reported on the cardiovascular side effects of different local anesthetics given intravenously. Buffington (1989) injected lidocaine and bupivacaine into the left coronary artery of

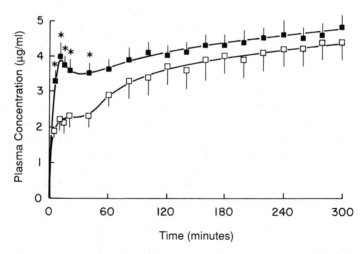

Figure 10.2. Mean plasma concentrations of lidocaine during epidural anesthesia induced by continuous infusion of plain (solid squares) and epinephrine-containing (open squares) 2% lidocaine. Means ± SEM. *Denotes significant differences ($P <$ 0.05). (Redrawn with permission from Takasaki and Kajitani, Can. J. Anaesth. 37: 166, 1990.)

dogs and found that both agents depressed contractility and coronary blood flow. In a series of investigations, Johns, *et al.* (Johns, *et al.*, 1985; Johns, *et al.*, 1986; Johns, 1989) studied the effects of local anesthetics on rat muscle arteries and arterioles. These investigators found that at low plasma concentration, lidocaine was a vasoconstrictor, while at higher plasma concentrations, such as those occurring during epidural anesthesia, lidocaine produced vasodilation. In contrast, bupivacaine produced vasoconstriction, even at plasma levels that were "at the upper limits of those expected to occur during regional anesthesia" (Johns, *et al.*, 1986; Norén, *et al.*, 1991). Some vasoconstriction (exerted by inhibition of the endothelium-dependent relaxant factor) (pp. 103–104) was reported with etidocaine and 2-chloroprocaine (Johns, 1989), and with intravenous bupivacaine infusion in humans (Hasselstrom, *et al.*, 1984).

Injection of the local anesthetic agent into the epidural space may also affect ventilation (Chapter 3). With equal levels of sensory anesthesia, Ward, *et al.* (1965) noted that arterial carbon dioxide tension increased slightly during epidural anesthesia and decreased slightly during spinal anesthesia. Since both epidural and spinal anesthesia are associated with similar interference with respiratory muscles, the changes in carbon dioxide tension (PCO_2) observed were different from those expected if the effects of the anesthetic techniques on respiration were solely the result of somatic motor paralysis. The subjects studied by Ward, *et al.*, appeared to be less apprehensive during epidural anesthesia than during spinal anesthesia. This was probably the result of sedation produced by lidocaine after its absorption from the epidural space. Consequently, subjects sedated by lidocaine were less likely to hyperventilate and thereby lower their levels of arterial PCO_2. Similarly, blood levels of local anesthetics equal to those observed during clinical epidural anesthesia have been shown to depress the ventilatory response to carbon dioxide during general anesthesia (Himes, *et al.*, 1979).

Though in awake humans carbon dioxide-ventilatory response curves have not been reported with blood levels of local anesthetics similar to those known to accompany epidural anesthesia, it is possible that local anesthetics in systemic blood during epidural anesthesia may effect, however subtly, central respiratory control mechanisms. It seems unlikely that blood levels of local anesthetics capable of depressing the ventilatory response to carbon dioxide in the presence of general anesthetics (Himes, *et al.*, 1979) would have no affect whatsoever in the absence of general anesthesia. That the intravenous infusion of local anesthetics in amounts adequate to produce subconvulsive plasma levels of anesthetics has no effect on resting arterial PCO_2 (Jorfeldt, *et al.*, 1968) does not preclude such a possibility.

The systemic effects of local anesthetics used for epidural anesthesia are of particular concern in obstetrics. Ralston and Shnider (1978) have summarized the numerous reports claiming that local anesthetics appearing in the systemic blood of parturients given epidural anesthesia appear in the fetus as well. Ralston and Shnider also summarized a considerable body of information indicating that local anesthetics in the circulating blood of neonates may be associated with both neonatal depression and reduced Apgar scores and with alterations in neurobehavioral activity which may persist for several days after delivery. The specific effects of local anesthetics absorbed from the epidural space into the blood are discussed below (pp. 372–374). For the purposes of the present discussion, it is sufficient to emphasize that absorption of local anesthetics from the epidural space does take place, and it does so in amounts sufficient to have some effects on both mother and fetus. Debate exists as to whether these effects, direct or indirect, are significant (pp. 372–374).

Cerebrospinal Fluid Pressure Following Local Anesthetic Injection

Injection of a large volume of local anesthetic solution into the lumbar epidural space produces an increase in cerebrospinal fluid pressure (Buchholz and Lesse, 1951; Usubiaga, et al., 1967; Bromage, 1967). The increase in intracranial pressure, though often marked, is transient and does not last more than 3–10 min. It may, however, produce dizziness, nausea, and frontal headache (Usubiaga, et al., 1967). It may also contribute to cardiovascular (Ward, et al., 1965) and respiratory changes following induction of epidural anesthesia. Similar increases in cerebrospinal fluid pressure do not occur with spinal anesthesia, and physiologic changes produced through this mechanism during epidural anesthesia are absent during spinal anesthesia. In addition to the above-mentioned side effects of epidural injection of large volumes of local anesthetic, other local tissue responses have been noted. Most recently, Loughnan, et al. (1990), demonstrated that epidural administration of 10 ml of either lidocaine 2 percent or normal saline significantly increased the latency of somatosensory evoked potentials for at least 50 min following epidural injection. Finally, an epidural dose of 20 ml of bupivacaine plus a continuous infusion (8 ml·hr^{-1}) have been associated with an increase in epidural blood flow (Mogensen, et al., 1988), although when given intravenously, bupivacaine induces vasoconstriction (p. 370).

Thoracic Epidural Anesthesia

Plasma concentration of local anesthetic is a function of dose injected (p. 366). Furthermore, similar peak plasma concentrations are achieved regardless of whether the local anesthetic was injected in the subarachnoid or in the epidural space (Giasi, *et al.*, 1979). Because much smaller total doses of local anesthetic are used, segmental thoracic epidural anesthesia is a technique that may allow delineation of cardiovascular responses to sympathetic denervation relatively separately from the additive (and confounding) systemic effects of local anesthetic absorption. Spinal anesthesia with an equivalent segmental level of denervation would also result in low plasma levels of spinal anesthetic, but the physiologic trespass (i.e., total sympathetic blockade) would certainly exceed that of epidural anesthesia involving only the upper thoracic dermatomes. The following discussion therefore focuses on the cardiovascular effects of limited, thoracic segmental epidural anesthesia.

Segmental epidural anesthesia, and in particular, thoracic epidural anesthesia, has received a great deal of attention, especially with regard to its cardiovascular effects in patients with coronary artery disease. Klassen, *et al.* (1980) studied the effects of epidurally induced sympathectomy in dogs and found an 18 percent increase in the endocardial-to-epicardial ratio under control conditions, and a 76 percent increase in the ratio following myocardial infarction. These beneficial effects on the myocardial perfusion and oxygen demand were independent of systemic factors. Similar beneficial effects of thoracic epidural anesthesia (TEA) have been reported by Hotvedt, *et al.* (1984), and by Reiz, *et al.* (1980), who found that TEA decreased myocardial oxygen demand. Other reported benefits of TEA include relief of chest pain, decrease in pulmonary artery and pulmonary capillary wedge pressures, and improvement in the myocardial oxygen supply-to-demand ratio (Blomberg, *et al.*, 1989), protection against malignant ventricular arrhythmias following myocardial infarction (Blomberg and Ricksten, 1988), increase in luminal diameter (vasodilation) of stenotic coronary arteries and improvement in ischemic chest pain (Blomberg, *et al.*, 1990), and improved ischemia-induced left ventricular wall motion and improvement of ST segment depression on the electrocardiogram (Kock, *et al.*, 1990; Tsuchida, *et al.*, 1991).

Epidural Anesthesia in Obstetrics

Although many benefits have been reported for both spinal anesthesia (Chapter 8) and epidural anesthesia, the latter also involves a different and specific set of consequences and side effects for both mother and fetus. Initial reports indicated that lidocaine and mepivacaine epidural anesthesia caused some depression of motor performance in the neonate (Scanlon, *et al.*, 1974; Tronick, *et al.*, 1976). Subsequent studies, however, failed to substantiate these findings (Abboud, *et al.*, 1983, 1984, 1986;

Cole, *et al.*, 1984; Corke, 1986). Furthermore, mepivacaine is rarely, if ever, used in obstetric anesthesia, as its elimination half-life in the neonate is 8.5–9.4 hr, depending on the concurrent use of epinephrine (Brown, *et al.*, 1975). The literature also contains conflicting reports with regard to the effects of chloroprocaine and bupivacaine on the neonate (Kileff, *et al.*, 1984; Kuhnert, *et al.*, 1988), although these effects are so transient and minimal as to lack clinical significance (Corke, 1986; Tronick, *et al.*, 1976). In general, therefore, it is unlikely that the direct effects of local anesthetics absorbed from the maternal epidural space into the fetal blood is significant (Chapter 8).

Possible effects of blood levels of local anesthetics associated with epidural anesthesia on the progression of labor, however, have not been clearly defined. Vasicka and Kretchmer (1961) found that spinal anesthesia to T_{2-6} had no effect on the frequency, intensity or tonus of uterine contractions. Epidural anesthesia to T_6, however, produced an immediate but transient decrease in the intensity of contractions. This may have been related to maternal blood levels of local anesthetic associated with epidural anesthesia. There are no data, however, to prove that the duration of labor and the frequency with which mid-forceps have to be used to accomplish delivery are any different with spinal anesthesia than with epidural anesthesia. Data exist, however, on the effects of continuous epidural anesthesia on second stage of labor and method of delivery. Phillips and Thomas (1983) found that when compared to a group of parturients in whom epidural anesthesia was allowed to wear off for the second stage of labor, the group that continued to receive epidural anesthesia experienced less pain, labor was not prolonged, the forceps delivery rate was lower, and there were fewer fetal malrotations. A lack of effects of 0.75 percent lidocaine infused epidurally on the duration of second stage of labor was also reported by Chestnut, *et al.* (1987 a).

Somewhat different results were obtained by Chestnut, *et al.* (1987 b) who reported better analgesia, similar incidence of fetal malrotation, and similar rates of cesarean section (13 percent) between two groups of nulliparous parturients, only one of which was given a continuous epidural infusion of 0.125 percent bupivacaine. Duration of second stage and frequency of instrumental delivery were, in contrast, statistically higher in the group of patients receiving epidural anesthesia. Most recently, Chestnut, *et al.* (1988) again reported a prolongation of the second stage of labor when patients received either 0.125 percent bupivacaine or 0.062 percent bupivacaine plus fentanyl 2 µg/ml.

Although the vast majority of studies appear to demonstrate that epidural anesthesia may have no effects on uterine activity during the first stage of labor (Jouppila, *et al.*, 1979; Abboud, *et al.*, 1984; Phillips, *et al.*, 1977), while increasing the duration of the second stage (Chestnut, *et al.*, 1987 b; Chestnut, *et al.*, 1988; Abboud, *et al.*, 1984; Bates, *et al.*, 1985), fetal well-being at delivery is the best indicator of the safety of this technique. It has been shown that the acid-base status of the neonate is either normal or even improved following delivery under epidural anesthesia (Chestnut, *et al.*, 1987 b, 1988; Abboud, *et al.*, 1984; Thorp, *et al.*, 1989; Noble, *et al.*, 1991). Similarly, Apgar scores are not affected negatively (Chestnut, *et al.*, 1987 b, 1988; Thorp, *et al.*, 1989). Therefore, the increased duration of the second stage of labor that may be associated with epidural anesthesia is not detrimental to fetal well-being, as long as fetal heart rate and acid-base status remain normal.

Possible inhibition of uterine contractility (beta-adrenergic effect) caused by increased blood levels of epinephrine as used during obstetric epidural anesthesia has not been shown to be a problem in clinical practice (Eisenach, *et al.*, 1987). It has been reported, however, that the addition of epinephrine to local anesthetic infusions during labor increased the incidence of profound motor block (Lysak, *et al.*, 1988), intensified the quality of the epidural bupivacaine and fentanyl analgesia (Youngstrom, *et al.*, 1984), and decreased uptake of local anesthetic from site of injection (Abboud, *et al.*, 1984).

The effects of epidural anesthesia on the rate of cesarean section are controversial. Chestnut, *et al.* (1987 b), found the rate of cesarean section to be 13 percent, regardless of whether or not epidural anesthesia was used. This report is in contrast to the experience on rate of cesarean section reported by Thorp, *et al.* (1989). In their series of 711 consecutive nulliparous females at term, the incidence of cesarean section for dystocia was significantly greater in the epidural group (10.3 percent) than in the control group (3.8 percent). In this study, however, selection bias may have been introduced as patients were not randomized before the onset of labor.

In passing, it should also be mentioned that although it has been claimed that maternal arterial hypotension is more frequent and more severe following spinal anesthesia than following epidural anesthesia (e.g., Stenger, *et al.*, 1965), such reports are based on studies that have used inadequate controls and inappropriate statistical methods (pp. 361–364).

REFERENCES

ABBOUD, T. K., DAVID, S., NAGAPPALA, S., COSTANDI, J., YANAGI, T., HAROUTUNIAN, S., AND YEH, S-U.: Maternal, fetal, and neonatal effects of lidocaine with and without epinephrine for epidural anesthesia in obstetrics. Anesth. Analg. 63: 973, 1984.

ABBOUD, T. K., KERN, S., AND JACOBS, J.: The neonatal neurobehavioral effects of mepivacaine for epidural anesthesia during labor. Reg. Anaesth. 11: 143, 1986.

ABBOUD, T. K., SARKIS, F., BLIKIAN, A., VARAKIAN, L., EARL, S., AND HENRIKSEN, E.: Lack of adverse neonatal neurobehavioral effects of lidocaine. Anesth. Analg. 62: 473, 1983.

ABBOUD, T. K., AFRASIABI, A., SARKIS, F., DAFTARIAN, F., NAGAPPALA, S., NOUEIHED, R., KUHNERT, B. R., AND MILLER, F.: Continuous infusion epidural analgesia in parturients receiving bupivacaine, chloroprocaine, or lidocaine—maternal, fetal, and neonatal effects. Anesth. Analg. 63: 421, 1984.

ALBRIGHT, G. A.: Cardiac arrest following regional anesthesia with etidocaine or bupivacaine (Editorial). Anesthesiology 51: 285, 1979.

ARENDT-NIELSEN, L., OBERG, B., AND BJERRING, P.: Quantitative assessment of extradural bupivacaine analgesia. Br. J. Anaesth. 65: 633, 1990.

BATES, R. G., DUNCAN, A., AND EDMONDS, D. K.: Uterine activity in the second stage of labour and the effect of epidural analgesia. Br. J. Obstet. Gynecol. 92: 1246, 1985.

BIGLER, D., HJORTSO, N. C., AND KEHLET, H.: Variation in spread of analgesia and loss of temperature discrimination during intermittent postoperative epidural bupivacaine administration. Acta Anaesthesiol. Scand. 30: 289, 1986.

BLAIR, M. R.: Cardiovascular pharmacology of local anaesthetics. Br. J. Anaesth. 47: 247, 1975.

BLOMBERG, S., EMANUELSSON, H., KVIST, H., LAMM, C., PONTÉN, J., WAAGSTEIN, F., AND RICKSTEN, S-E.: Effects of thoracic epidural anesthesia on coronary arteries and arterioles in patients with coronary artery disease. Anesthesiology 73: 840, 1990.

BLOMBERG, S., EMANUELSSON, H., AND RICKSTEN, S-E.: Thoracic epidural anesthesia and central hemodynamics in patients with unstable angina pectoris. Anesth. Analg. 69: 558, 1989.

BLOMBERG, S., AND RICKSTEN, S-E.: Thoracic epidural anaesthesia decreases the incidence of ventricular arrhythmias during acute myocardial ischaemia in the anaesthetized rat. Acta Anaesthesiol. Scand. 32: 173, 1988.

BONICA, J. J., KENNEDY, W. F., JR., WARD, R. J., AND TOLAS, A. G.: A comparison of the effects of high subarachnoid and epidural anaesthesia. Acta Anaesthesiol. Scand. (Suppl.) 23: 429, 1966.

BONNET, F., DIALLO, A., SAADA, M., BELON, M., GUILBAUD, M., AND BOICO, O.: Prevention of tourniquet pain by spinal isobaric bupivacaine with clonidine. Br. J. Anaesth. 63: 93, 1989.

BROMAGE, P. R.: Physiology and pharmacology of epidural anesthesia. Anesthesiology 28: 592, 1967.

BROMAGE, P. R.: Epidural Analgesia. Philadelphia: W. B. Saunders Co., 1978.

BROWN, D. L., CARPENTER, R. L., AND THOMPSON, G. E.: Comparison of 0.5% ropivacaine and 0.5% bupivacaine for epidural anesthesia in patients undergoing lower-extremity surgery. Anesthesiology 72: 633, 1990.

BROWN, W. U., JR., BELL, G. C., LURIE, A. O., WEISS, J. B., SCANLON, J. W., AND ALPER, M. H.: Newborn blood levels of lidocaine and mepivacaine in the first postnatal day following maternal epidural anesthesia. Anesthesiology 42: 698, 1975.

BRULL, S. J., AND GREENE, N. M.: Zones of differential sensory block during extradural anaesthesia. Br. J. Anaesth. 66: 651, 1991.

BRUN-BUISSON, V., BONNET, F., BOICO, O., AND SAADA, M.: Failure of spinal anesthesia: evaluation of the practice at a university hospital. Ann. Fr. Anesth. Reanim. 7: 383, 1988.

BUCHHOLZ, H. W., AND LESSE, K. T.: Druckverhaltnisse im Periduralraum und im Liquorraum bei periduralen Injektionen. Chirurg (Berlin) 22: 11, 1951.

BUFFINGTON, C. W.: The magnitude and duration of direct myocardial depression following intracoronary local anesthetics: a comparison of lidocaine and bupivacaine. Anesthesiology 70: 280, 1989.

CHESTNUT, D. H., BATES, J. N., AND CHOI, W. W.: Continuous infusion epidural analgesia with lidocaine: efficacy and influence during the second stage of labor. Obstet. Gynecol. 69: 323, 1987 a.

CHESTNUT, D. H., VANDEWALKER, G. E., OWEN, C. L., BATES, J. N., AND CHOI, W. W.: The influence of continuous epidural bupivacaine analgesia on the second stage of labor and method of delivery in nulliparous women. Anesthesiology 66: 774, 1987 b.

CHESTNUT, D. H., OWEN, C. L., BATES, J. N., OSTMAN, L. G., CHOI, W. W., AND GEIGER, M. W.: Continuous infusion epidural analgesia during labor: a randomized, double-blind comparison of 0.0625% bupivacaine/0.0002% fentanyl versus 0.125% bupivacaine. Anesthesiology 68: 754, 1988.

COLE, C. P., McMORLAND, G. H., AND AXELSON, J. E.: Comparison of neonatal neurobehavioral responses after lidocaine-HCl and lidocaine hydrocarbonate epidural anaesthesia for caesarean section. Can. Anaesth. Soc. J., 31: S68, 1984.

CONCEPCION, M. A.: Spinal anesthetic agents. Int. Anesthesiol. Clin. 27: 21, 1989.

CONCEPCION, M. A., LAMBERT, D. H., WELCH, K. A., AND COVINO, B. G.: Tourniquet pain during spinal anesthesia: a comparison of plain solutions of tetracaine and bupivacaine. Anesth. Analg. 67: 828, 1988.

CORKE, B. C.: Neonatal neurobehavior II: Current clinical status. Clin. Anaesth. 4: 219, 1986.

DAOS, F. G., AND VIRTUE, R. W.: Sympathetic block persistence after spinal or epidural anesthesia. J. A. M. A. 183: 285, 1963.

DEFALQUE, R. J.: Compared effects of spinal and extradural anesthesia upon the blood pressure. Anesthesiology 23: 627, 1962.

DE JONG, R. H.: Arterial carbon dioxide and oxygen tensions during spinal block. J. A. M. A. 191: 698, 1965.

DUNNE, N. M., AND KOX, W. J.: Neurological complications following the use of continuous extradural analgesia with bupivacaine. Br. J. Anaesth. 66: 617, 1991.

EISENACH, J. C., GRICE, S. C., AND DEWAN, D. M.: Epinephrine enhances analgesia produced by epidural bupivacaine during labor. Anesth. Analg. 66: 447, 1987.

FINK, B. R.: Mechanisms of differential axial blockade in epidural and subarachnoid anesthesia. Anesthesiology 70: 851, 1989.

FREUND, F. G., BONICA, J. J., WARD, R. J., AKAMATSU, T. J., AND KENNEDY, W. F., JR.: Ventilatory reserve and level of motor block during high spinal and epidural anesthesia. Anesthesiology 28: 834, 1967.

GIASI, R. M., D'AGOSTINO, E., AND COVINO, B. G.: Absorption of lidocaine following subarachnoid and epidural administration. Anesth. Analg. 58: 360, 1979.

GREENE, N. M.: The area of differential block during spinal anesthesia with hyperbaric tetracaine. Anesthesiology 19: 45, 1958.

GREENE, N. M.: Blood levels of local anesthetics during spinal anesthesia. Anesth. Analg. 58: 357, 1979.

GRUNDY, E. M., RAMAMURTHY, S., PATEL, K. P., MANI, M., AND WINNIE, A. P.: Extradual analgesia revisited: a statistical study. Br. J. Anaesth. 50: 805, 1978.

HARDY, P. A. J.: Differential cold and sympathetic blockade during obstetric epidural analgesia: a pilot study. Regional Anesth. 4: 162, 1988.

HASSELSTRØM, L. J., MOGENSEN, T., KEHLET, H., AND CHRISTENSEN, N. J.: Effects of intravenous bupivacaine on cardiovascular function and plasma catecholamine levels in humans. Anesth. Analg. 63: 1053, 1984.

HIMES, R. S., JR., MUNSON, E. S., AND EMBRO, W. J.: Enflurane requirement and ventilatory response to carbon dioxide during lidocaine infusion in dogs. Anesthesiology 51: 131, 1979.

HOTVEDT, R., PLATOU, E. S., AND REFSUM, H.: Effects of thoracic epidural analgesia on cardiovascular function and plasma concentration of free fatty acids and catecholamines in the dog. Acta Anaesthesiol. Scand. 28: 132, 1984.

JOHNS, R. A.: Local anesthetics inhibit endothelium-dependent vasodilation. Anesthesiology 70: 805, 1989.

JOHNS, R. A., DIFAZIO, C. A., AND LONGNECKER, D. E.: Lidocaine constricts or dilates rat arterioles in a dose-dependent manner. Anesthesiology 62: 141, 1985.

JOHNS, R. A., SEYDE, W. C., DIFAZIO, C. A., AND LONGNECKER, D. E.: Dose-dependent effects of bupivacaine on rat muscle arterioles. Anesthesiology 65: 186, 1986.

JORFELDT, L., LOFSTROM, B., PERNOW, B., PERSSON, B., WAHREN, J., AND WIDMAN, B.: The effects of local anaesthetics on the central circulation and respiration in man and dog. Acta Anaesthesiol. Scand. 12: 153, 1968.

JOUPPILA, R., JOUPPILA, P., KARINEN, J. M., ET AL.: Segmental epidural analgesia in labour: related to the progress of labour, fetal malposition and intrumental delivery. Acta Obstet. Gynecol. Scand. 58: 135, 1979.

KEHLET, H.: The stress response to anaesthesia and surgery: release mechanisms and modifying factors. Clin. Anaesthesiol. 2: 315, 1984.

KEHLET, H., BRANDT, M. R., AND REM, J.: Role of neurogenic stimuli in mediating the endocrine-metabolic response to surgery. J. Parent. Ent. Nutr. 4: 152, 1980.

KERKKAMP, H. E. M., AND GIELEN, M. J. M.: Cardiovascular effects of epidural local anaesthetics: comparison of 0.75% bupivacaine and 0.75% ropivacaine, both with adrenaline. Anaesthesia 46: 361, 1991.

KILEFF, M. E., JAMES, F. M., III, DEWAN, D. M., AND FLOYD, H. M.: Neonatal neurobehavioral responses after epidural anesthesia for cesarean section using lidocaine and bupivacaine. Anesth. Analg. 63: 413, 1984.

KLASSEN, G. A., BRAMWELL, R. W., BROMAGE, P. R., AND ZBOROWSKA-SLUIS, D. T.: Effect of acute sympathectomy by epidural anesthesia on the canine coronary circulation. Anesthesiology 52: 8, 1980.

KOCK, M., BLOMBERG, S., EMANUELSSON, H., LOMSKY, M., STROMBLAD, S-O., AND RICKSTEN, S-E.: Thoracic epidural anesthesia improves global and regional left ventricular function during stress-induced myocardial ischemia in patients with coronary artery disease. Anesth. Analg. 71: 625, 1990.

KUHNERT, B. R., KENNARD, M. J., AND LINN, P. L.: Neonatal neurobehavior after epidural anesthesia for cesarean section: a comparison of bupivacaine and chloroprocaine. Anesth. Analg. 67: 64, 1988.

LEE, Y., TUNG, M. C., WHO, L. H., LAI, K. B., WONG, K. L., WU, K. H., WEI, T. T., AND PAN, P. M.: The effect of epidural anesthesia on tourniquet pain: a comparison of 2% lidocaine and 0.5% bupivacaine. Ma. Tsui. Hsueh. Tsa. Chi. 28: 459, 1990.

LOFGREN, A., AND HAHN, R. G.: Serum potassium levels after induction of epidural anaesthesia using mepivacaine with and without adrenaline. Acta Anaesthesiol. Scand. 35: 170, 1991.

LOUGHNAN, B. A., MURDOCH, L. J., HETREED, M. A., HOWARD, L. A., AND HALL, G. M.: Effects of 2% lignocaine on somatosensory evoked potentials recorded in the extradural space. Br. J. Anaesth. 65: 643, 1990.

LUND, C., SELMAR, P., HANSEN, O. B., HJORTSO, N-C., AND KEHLET, H.: Effect of epidural bupivacaine on somatosensory evoked potentials after dermatomal stimulation. Anesth. Analg. 6: 34, 1987.

LUNDIN, S., WALLIN, B. G., AND ELAM, M.: Intraneural recording of muscle sympathetic activity during epidural anesthesia in humans. Anesth. Analg. 69: 788, 1989.

LYSAK, S. Z., EISENACH, J. C., AND DOBSON, C. E.: Patient controlled epidural analgesia (PCEA) during labor: a comparison of three solutions with continuous epidural infusion (CEI) control. Anesthesiology 69: A690, 1988.

MANKIKIAN, B., CANTINEAU, J. P., BERTRAND, M., KIEFFER, E., SARTENE, R., AND VIARS, P.: Improvement of diaphragmatic function by a thoracic extradural block after upper abdominal surgery. Anesthesiology 68: 379, 1988.

MANNUCCI, P. M., ABERG, M., NILSSON, I. M., AND ROBERTSON, B.: Mechanism of plasminogen activator and factor VIII increase after vasoactive drugs. Br. J. Haematol. 30: 81, 1975.

MODIG, J.: Influence of regional anesthesia, local anesthetics, and sympathicomimetics on the pathophysiology of deep vein thrombosis. Acta Chir. Scand. (Suppl.) 550: 119, 1989.

MOGENSEN, T., HOJGAARD, L., SCOTT, N. B., HENRIKSEN, J. H., AND KEHLET, H.: Epidural blood flow and regression of sensory analgesia during continuous postoperative epidural infusion of bupivacaine. Anesth. Analg. 67: 809, 1988.

MOORE, D. C., BRIDENBAUGH, L. D., BAGDI, P. A., BRIDENBAUGH, P. O., AND STANDER, H.: The present status of spinal (subarachnoid) and epidural (peridural) block. Anesth. Analg. 47: 40, 1968.

NOBLE, H. A., ENEVER, G. R., AND THOMAS, T. A.: Epidural bupivacaine dilution for labour. A comparison of three concentrations infused with a fixed dose of fentanyl. Anaesthesia 46: 549, 1991.

NORÉN, H., LINDBLOM, B., AND KÄLLFELT, B.: Effects of bupivacaine and calcium antagonists on the rat uterine artery. Acta Anaesthesiol. Scand 35: 77, 1991.

PARK, W. Y., HAGINS, F. M., RIVAT, E. L., AND MACNAMARA, T. E.: Age and epidural dose response in adult men. Anesthesiology 56: 318, 1982.

PERHONIEMI, V., AND LINKO, K.: Effect of spinal versus epidural anaesthesia with 0.5% bupivacaine on lower limb blood flow. Acta Anaesthesiol. Scand. 31: 117, 1987.

PETERS, J., KOUSOULIS, L., AND ARNDT, J. O.: Effects of segmental thoracic extradural analgesia on sympathetic block in conscious dogs. Br. J. Anaesth. 63: 470, 1989.

PETERS, J., KUTKUHN, B., MEDERT, H. A., SCHLAGHECKE, R., SCHUTTLER, J., AND ARNDT, J. O.: Sympathetic blockade by epidural anesthesia attenuates the cardiovascular response to severe hypoxemia. Anesthesiology 72: 134, 1990.

PFLUG, A. E., AND HALTER, J. B.: Effect of spinal anesthesia on adrenergic tone and the neuroendocrine responses to surgical stress in humans. Anesthesiology 55: 120, 1981.

PFLUG, A. E., MURPHY, T. M., BUTLER, S. H., AND TUCKER, G. T.: The effects of postoperative peridural analgesia on pulmonary therapy and pulmonary complications. Anesthesiology 41: 8, 1974.

PHILLIPS, J. C., HOCHBERG, C. J., PETRAKIS, J. K., AND VAN WINKLE, J. D.: Epidural analgesia and its effects on the "normal" progress of labor. Am. J. Obstet. Gynecol. 129: 316, 1977.

PHILLIPS, K. C., AND THOMAS, T. A.: Second stage of labour with or without extradural analgesia. Anaesthesia 38: 972, 1983.

RALSTON, D. H., AND SHNIDER, S. M.: The fetal and neonatal effects of regional anesthesia in obstetrics. Anesthesiology 48: 34, 1978.

RAYMOND, S. A., STEFFENSEN, S. C., GUGINO, L. D., AND STRICHARTZ, G. R.: The role of length of nerve exposed to local anesthetics in impulse blocking action. Anesth. Analg. 68: 563, 1989.

RAYMOND, S. A., AND STRICHARTZ, G. R.: The long and short of differential block (Editorial). Anesthesiology 70: 725, 1989.

REIZ, S., NATH, S., AND RAIS, O.: Effects of thoracic epidural block and prenalterol on coronary vascular resistance and myocardial metabolism in patients with coronary artery disease. Acta Anaesthesiol. Scand. 24: 11, 1980.

ROIZEN, M. F., HORRIGAN, R. W., AND FRAZER, B. M.: Anesthetic doses blocking adrenergic (stress) and cardiovascular responses to incision—MAC BAR. Anesthesiology 54: 390, 1981.

RUCCI, F. S., TRAFFICANTE, F. G., AND PIPPA, P.: Fentanyl and bupivacaine mixture for extradural blockade in orthopaedic surgery: effects on haemodynamic responses and pain related to the use of thigh tourniquet. Eur. J. Anaesthesiol. 4: 167, 1987.

RUTBERG, H., HAKANSON, E., ANDERBERG, B., JORFELDT, L., MARTENSSON, J., AND SCHILDT, B.: Effects of the extradural administration of morphine, or bupivacaine, on the endocrine response to upper abdominal surgery. Br. J. Anaesth. 56: 233, 1984.

SALEVSKY, F. C., WHALLEY, D. G., KALANT, D., AND CRAWHALL, J. Epidural epinephrine and the systemic circulation during peripheral vascular surgery. Can. J. Anaesth. 37: 160, 1990.

SCANLON, J. W., BROWN, W. U., JR., WEISS, J. B., AND ALPER, M. H.: Neurobehavioral responses of newborn infants after maternal epidural anesthesia. Anesthesiology *40:* 121, 1974.

SHARROCK, N. E.: Epidural anesthetic dose responses in patients 20 to 80 years old. Anesthesiology *49:* 425, 1978.

SHARROCK, N. E., MINEO, R., AND URQUHART, B.: Haemodynamic effects and outcome analysis of hypotensive extradural anaesthesia in controlled hypertensive patients undergoing total hip arthroplasty. Br. J. Anaesth. *67:* 17, 1991.

SHARROCK, N. E., MINEO, R., AND URQUHART, B.: Hemodynamic response to low-dose epinephrine infusion during hypotensive epidural anesthesia for total hip replacement. Regional Anesth. *15:* 295, 1990.

SPENCE, A. A., AND SMITH, G.: Postoperative analgesia and lung function: a comparison of morphine with extradural block. Br. J. Anaesth. *43:* 144, 1971.

STENGER, V., ANDERSEN, T., EITZMAN, D., AND PRYSTOWSKY, H.: Extradural anesthesia for cesarean section: physiologic and biochemical observations. Obstet. Gynecol. *25:* 802, 1965.

STEVENS, R. A., ARTUSO, J. D., KAO, T.-C., BRAY, J. G., SPITZER, L., AND LOUWSMA, D. L.: Changes in human plasma catecholamine concentrations during epidural anesthesia depend on the level of block. Anesthesiology *74:* 1029, 1991.

STEVENS, R. A., LINEBERRY, P. J., ARCARIO, T. J., BACON, G. S., AND CRESS, L. W.: Epidural anaesthesia attenuates the catecholamine response to hypoventilation. Can. J. Anaesth. *37:* 867, 1990.

STEWART, A., LAMBERT, D. H., CONCEPCION, M. A., DATTA, S., FLANAGAN, H., MIGLIOZZI, R., AND COVINO, B. G.: Decreased incidence of tourniquet pain during spinal anesthesia with bupivacaine: a possible explanation. Anesth. Analg. *67:* 833, 1988.

TAKASAKI, M., AND KAJITANI, H.: Plasma lidocaine concentrations during continuous epidural infusion of lidocaine with and without epinephrine. Can. J. Anaesth. *37:* 166, 1990.

THORP, J. A., PARISI, V. M., BOYLAN, P. C., AND JOHNSTON, D. A.: The effect of continuous epidural analgesia on cesarean section for dystocia in nulliparous women. Am. J. Obstet. Gyn. *161:* 670, 1989.

TRONICK, E., WISE, S., ALS, H., ADAMSON, L., SCANLON, J., AND BRAZELTON, T. B.: Regional obstetric anesthesia and newborn behavior: effect over the first ten days of life. Pediatrics *58:* 94, 1976.

TSUCHIDA, H., OMOTE, T., MIYAMOTO, M., NAMIKI, A., ICHIHARA, K., AND ABIKO, Y.: Effects of thoracic epidural anaesthesia on myocardial pH and metabolism during ischaemia. Acta Anaesthesiol. Scand. *35:* 508, 1991.

TUVEMO, T., AND WILLDECK-LUND, G.: Smooth muscle effects of lidocaine, prilocaine, bupivacaine and etidocaine on the human umbilical artery. Acta Anaesthesiol. Scand. *26:* 104, 1982.

USUBIAGA, J. E., USUBIAGA, L. E., BREA, L. M., AND GOYENA, R.: Effect of saline injections on epidural and subarachnoid space pressures and relation to postspinal anesthesia headache. Anesth. Analg. *46:* 293, 1967.

VALLI, H., AND ROSENBERG, P. H.: Effects of three anaesthesia methods on haemodynamic responses connected with the use of thigh tourniquet in orthopaedic patients. Acta Anaesthesiol. Scand. *29:* 142, 1985.

VASICKA, A., AND KRETCHMER, H.: Effect of conduction and inhalation anesthesia on uterine contractions. Am. J. Obstet. Gynecol. *82:* 600, 1961.

WARD, R. J., BONICA, J. J., FREUND, F. G., AKAMATSU, T., DANZIGER, F., AND ENGLESSON, S.: Epidural and subarachnoid anesthesia: cardiovascular and respiratory effects. J. A. M. A. *191:* 99, 1965.

WARD, R. J., DANZIGER, F., AKAMATSU, T., FREUND, F., AND BONICA, J. J.: Cardiovascular response of oxygen therapy for hypotension of regional anesthesia. Anesth. Analg. *45:* 140, 1966.

WUGMEISTER, M., AND HEHRE, F. W.: The absence of differential blockade in peridural anaesthesia. Br. J. Anaesth. *39:* 953, 1967.

YOUNGSTROM, P., EASTWOOD, D., PATEL, H., ET AL.: Epidural fentanyl and bupivacaine in labor: double-blind study. Anesthesiology *62:* A414, 1984.

INDEX

Acid-base balance, 297–306, 326, 330–332
Acidosis, see *Acid-base balance*
Acquired immunodeficiency syndrome (AIDS), 292
Adrenal
  cortex, 149–150, 282–285, 287–288
  medulla, 285–287
Adrenocorticotropic hormone (ACTH), 284, 288, 291
Afferent nerves, 41–47
Age, 157, 176–177
Alanine aminotransferase, see *Glutamic, pyruvic transaminase*; see *Transferase*
Albumin, 246
Alcohol, 19–20, 251
Aldosterone, 273–275, 282, 285
Alkalosis, see *Acid-base balance*
Alkaline phosphatase, 234–237, 239, 245
Alveolar gas exchange, 203
Amino acid nitrogen, 304
Amylase, 233–237
Anastomotic breakdown, 346
Anemia, 309
Anesthesia
  hypotensive
    spinal, 39–40, 114, 132, 164, 220, 250, 256–257, 259, 287
    epidural, 368
    total spinal, 92, 166, 223
Angiotensin, 285
Angiotensin-coverting enzyme (ACE), 104
Antidiuretic hormone (ADH), 275, 290
Aortic compression, see *Hypotension*
Anuria, 273
Apgar scores, 322, 330–331, 335, 371, 374
Apnea, see *Lungs*
Arrhythmias, see *Heart*
Arteries, 87–94
Arterioles, 87–122
Arterio-venous anastomoses, 88

Artificial ventilation, 223–224
Aspartate aminotransferase (AST), see *Glutamic, oxaloacetic transaminase*; see *Transferase*
Aspiration, gastric contents, 166, 336
Asthma, see *Lungs*
Atelectasis, see *Lungs*
Atropine, 127, 169

Ballistocardiography, 92
Baricity, local anesthetic solutions, 5
Bilirubin, 234–237, 239–240, 244, 249, 251
Blood
  coagulation, 120–122, 175, 225, 321
  fibrinolysis, 367
  hematocrit, 89, 100, 119–120
  hemodilution, 119–120, 173
  hemorrhage, 121–122, 158–160
  hemorrhagic shock, 159–160, 267
  hypercoagulability, 121
  pH, 305
  plasma volume, 119
  pressure, see *Pressure*
  transfusion, 347
  rheology, 265
  velocity of flow, 265
  viscosity, 90, 121, 173–175, 215, 265
  volume, 118–119, 309
Bradycardia, see *Heart, rate*
Brain
  cerebral blood flow, 55–61
  cortical function, 64–71
  glucose consumption, 59, 300
  medullary function, 61–64
  oxygen consumption, 59
Bromsulfalein, 233–237, 238–241, 243, 246–250, 258, 326
Bronchiectasis, see *Lungs*
Bronchitis, see *Lungs*
Bronchospasm, see *Lungs*

oxaloacetic transaminase (SGOT),
235, 245, 251, 257
pyruvic transaminase (SGPT), 235,
245, 251, 257
Gonadotropin, 290
Growth hormone, 289, 300

Hearing, 71
Heart
afterload, 86–87, 142
arrhythmias, 144–145, 372
asystole, 144
athletic heart syndrome, 128
atrial pressure, right, see *Heart,
venous return*
Bezold-Jarisch reflex, 128, 133,
164–165
bradycardia, fetal, 312, 328
cardiac
accelerator fibers, 129
arrest, 221, 223
function, 126–149, 372
output, 86, 118, 124–125, 132–144,
154–155, 165–167, 213–214, 223,
253–254, 270–271, 309–310,
318–319, 323, 365–368, 372
coronary
artery disease, 372
blood flow, 145–149, 370, 372
contractility, 86–87, 130, 144, 370, 372
infarction, myocardial, 372
innervation, 129
ischemia, 147–149, 169, 372
oxygen demand, 169, 372
preload, see *Heart, venous return*
pulmonary capillary wedge pressure
(PWCP), see *Lung, pulmonary*
rate, 86–87, 126–134, 142–143, 169,
213, 362, 365, 367–368
rate-pressure product, 148–149
right ventricular output, 211
sick sinus syndrome, 144
stroke volume, 86, 142–144, 367–368,
372
venous return, 86, 122–126, 129–130,
142, 223, 310, 319, 321
ventricular end-diastolic volume, 122,
131, 133, 136
ventricular wall tension, 87, 372
work, 130, 141–145
Hematocrit, see *Blood*
Hemorrhage, see *Blood*
Hemorrhagic shock, see *Blood*
Hepatic, see *Liver*
Hepatitis, 251
Hippuric acid, 233–237, 238–242, 244,
246, 257
Histamine, 102

Hormones, see *Endocrine function*
Hypercarbia, see *Carbon dioxide*
Hypercoagulability, see *Blood*
Hyperemia, 106–107
Hyperemia, reactive, 102
Hypertension, 57–60, 155–158, 271, 287,
323–324
Hyperthermia, malignant, 304
Hyperthyroidism, 292
Hyperventilation, 152, 220–221, 226,
306, 326, 370
Hypervolemia, 290
Hypocarbia, see *Carbon dioxide*
Hypoglycemia, 303, 332
Hypotension, see also *Pressure*
arterial, 161–163, 255, 257–258,
272–273
etiology, 149–176, 275, 309, 312, 318,
350–352, 366
maternal, 318–324, 328–332, 374
supine, syndrome, 309–310
treatment, 163–176, 274–275, 318–323,
331, 349–352
Hypothalamus, 291, 299
Hypothermia, 299
Hypoventilation, 205–208, 221
Hypovolemia, 266
Hypoxia, see *Oxygen*

Ileus, 346–348
Immunocompetence, 292–293
Inotropy, 369
Indocyanine green, 253
Insulin, 301–303
Intercostals, see *Muscle*
Ischemia
myocardial, see *Heart*
placental, 327
Isoproterenol, 171

Kidney
blood flow, 264, 267–272, 325
chronic renal failure (CRF),
274
cortex, 265
filtration fraction, 263–264, 266
function, 263–276, 324
glomerular
perfusion, 264
filtration, 266, 270, 272–273
plasma flow, 266–267, 270
tubular reabsorption, 263
vascular resistance, 265, 271

Labor
first stage, 313, 373